THE IMPERILED RED CROSS
AND THE PALESTINE—ERETZ-YISRAEL CONFLICT 1945–1952

A PUBLICATION OF THE GRADUATE INSTITUTE OF INTERNATIONAL STUDIES, GENEVA

Also published in this series:

The United States and the Politicization of the World Bank
Bartram S. Brown

Trade Negotiations in the OECD
David J. Blair

World Financial Markets after 1992
Hans Genberg and Alexander K. Swoboda

Succession Between International Organisations
Patrick R. Myers

Ten Years of Turbulence: The Chinese Cultural Revolution
Barbara Barnouin and Yu Changgen

The Islamic Movement in Egypt: Perceptions of International Relations 1967–81
Walid M. Abdelnasser

Namibia and Southern Africa: Regional Dynamics of Decolonization 1945–90
Ronald Dreyer

The International Organization of Hunger
Peter Uvin

Citizenship East and West
Edited by André Liebich and Daniel Warner with Jasna Dragovic

Introduction to the Law of Treaties
Paul Reuter

THE IMPERILED RED CROSS
AND THE PALESTINE—ERETZ-YISRAEL CONFLICT 1945–1952

The Influence of Institutional Concerns on a Humanitarian Operation

Dominique-D. Junod

KEGAN PAUL INTERNATIONAL
London and New York

First published in 1996 by
Kegan Paul International
UK: P.O. Box 256, London WC1B 3SW, England
Tel: (0171) 580 5511 Fax: (0171) 436 0899
E-mail: books@keganpau.demon.co.uk
Internet: http://www.demon.co.uk/keganpaul/
USA: 562 West 113th Street, New York, NY 10025, USA
Tel: (212) 666 1000 Fax: (212) 316 3100

Distributed by

John Wiley & Sons Ltd
Southern Cross Trading Estate
1 Oldlands Way, Bognor Regis
West Sussex, PO22 9SA, England
Tel: (01243) 779 777 Fax: (01243) 820 250

Columbia University Press
562 West 113th Street
New York, NY 10025, USA
Tel: (212) 666 1000 Fax: (212) 316 3100

Copyright © The Graduate Institute of International Studies, Geneva, 1996

Set in 10/12 Palatino by Intype, London

Printed in Great Britain by TJ Press Ltd, Padstow, Cornwall

All rights reserved. No part of this book may be reprinted
or reproduced or utilized in any form or by any electronic,
mechanical or other means, now known or hereafter invented,
including photocopying and recording, or in any information
storage or retrieval system, without permission in writing
from the publishers.

ISBN 0-7103-0519-2

British Library Cataloguing in Publication Data
Junod, Dominique-D.
Imperiled Red Cross and the Palestine/
Eretz-Yisrael Conflict, 1945-52:
Influence of Institutional Concerns on a
Humanitarian Operation
I. Title
361.77

ISBN 0-7103-0519-2

Library of Congress Cataloging-in-Publication Data
Junod, Dominique-D., 1945-
The imperiled Red Cross and the Palestine–Eretz-Yisrael conflict.
1945–1952: the influence of institutional concerns on a
humanitarian operation / Dominique-D. Junod.
340pp.   23 cm. – (A Publication of the Graduate Institute of
International Studies, Geneva)
Includes bibliographical references (p. –) and index.
ISBN 0-7103-0519-2
1. International Committee of the Red Cross—History. 2. Jewish–
Arab relations—1917–1949. 3. Jewish–Arab relations—1949–1967.
4. Israel-Arab conflicts.   I. Title.   II. Series: Publications de
l'Institut universitaire des hautes études internationales, Genève.
HV568.J86   1995
361.7'634'095694—dc20   95-8732
CIP

To my daughter, Caroline Emmanuelle

Notice to the reader: The author takes sole responsibility for this work. Although the International Committee of the Red Cross (ICRC) authorized its publication, the ICRC does not necessarily concur with the content of the book and the opinions expressed therein.

CONTENTS

Preface   xi
Acknowledgements   xiii
Abbreviations   xv
Introduction   1

1 THE RED CROSS IN PERIL AND THE INTERNATIONAL COMMITTEE OF THE RED CROSS (ICRC)   6
  The International Committee of the Red Cross   7
  The International Red Cross in peril   13
  The development of a strategy   32
  ICRC administration and operation between 1945 and 1952   37
  Interpreting an ICRC operation: a challenge for the historian   48

2 ACTING IN MANDATORY PALESTINE: MOTIVES AND STRATEGIES   50
  1945: a distant conflict   50
  1947: the ICRC changes course   65
  Objective: neutral intermediary   70
  The vote on the partition of Palestine: a new deal   89

3 THE ICRC ACHIEVES ITS AIM   91
  The Palestine government's appeal to the ICRC   91
  Evaluation: the first mission   98
  Fitting the operation to a strategy   112
  The ICRC's conditions are met   122
  Deploying forces   132

4 THE RED CROSS IN PALESTINE–ERETZ-YISRAEL: FUNCTION, SIGNIFICANCE, AND USAGE 134

The flag	134
Acceptance of the red cross by the local communities	145
In Jerusalem: the flag in the service of politics	155
Bernadotte in Palestine	179

5 FROM HEROISM TO TRADITIONAL ACTIVITIES: THE EVOLUTION FROM IDEALS TO STRATEGY 187

From ideals to strategy	187
From the heroic period to traditional activities	209
The operation in Palestine: an asset in Stockholm	231

6 FROM STOCKHOLM TO TORONTO: THE RED CROSS RECOVERS ITS BALANCE 236

The ICRC on the eve of the Stockholm Conference	236
The conference of Stockholm	248
The refugees of Palestine and the Red Cross's quest for balance	253
For destitute Arabs: a major enterprise	261
Staying in the Near East while waiting for the USSR in Toronto	267
Epilogue	268

Conclusion	280
Chronology	293
List of the delegates and nurses of the ICRC delegation	317
Bibliography	319
Index	333

ILLUSTRATIONS

Plates

between pages 144 and 145

1. 'All day long, you can see the schools studying on the decks. . . .' Picture Marti.
2. School on the *Runnymede Park*. Picture and caption ICRC.
3. The King David Hotel under the Red Cross flag. Picture ICRC. Caption D.D.J.
4. Jerusalem, May 10, 1948. Picture and caption ICRC.
5. The positioning of the red cross and the red crescent for a joint repatriation convoy. Picture ICRC. Caption D.D.J.
6. President Ruegger attending to the evacuation of the inhabitants of the Jewish Quarter. Picture de Reynier. Caption D.D.J.
7. Evacuation of the inhabitants of the Jewish Quarter of the Old City. Picture de Reynier. Caption D.D.J.
8. Kfar Yona, June 18, 1948. Picture and caption ICRC.
9. The ICRC's delegates prepare an exchange of civilians. Picture ICRC. Caption D.D.J.
10. Moshe Dayan and Abdullah Tel meet for the repatriation of wounded Arab prisoners. Picture Munier. Caption D.D.J.
11. Munier wearing the *keffiyeh* in Petra. Picture Munier. Caption D.D.J.
12. 'Repatriation of Arab POWs. Two wounded.' Picture and caption Munier.
13. 'Transferring some of the Arab old people and wounded from Tel Aviv to Jaffa. Summer 1948.' Picture H. Pinn. Caption ICRC.

14. 'ICRC's activities in the Middle East.' Picture ICRC. Caption D.D.J.

Maps

	page
1. Mandatory Palestine and the UN partition plan, 1947	130
2. ICRC's security zones	160
3. ICRC's security zone no. 1	171
4. Two days with an ICRC delegate in Galilee	189

Figure

General organization of the Committee's departments   43

PREFACE

Dominique-Debora Junod has written an important book, a description and analysis of the activity of the International Committee of the Red Cross in a conflict which still concerns us. This study is based on material in the ICRC archives, to which the author had unrestricted access. She has scrutinized the institution from the viewpoint of an historian and at the same time from the privileged position of someone who actually worked for it. In doing so, Dominique Junod took a major responsibility and must be congratulated for her moderation and her tact.

The study presented to us here follows several channels of investigation. It seeks primarily to piece together the strategy adopted by an institution that stood accused after the Second World War of failings with regard to the victims of Nazi persecution, in particular the Jews. The objective of that strategy was to regain and consolidate its position on the international scene. Ms Junod's approach reveals the links and interactions between the ICRC's activities in favor of the victims of armed conflicts and the creation or reform of relevant legal instruments such as the Geneva Conventions and the Statutes of the International Red Cross. The actions of individual high officials and delegates of the ICRC with regard to the Palestine–Eretz Yisrael conflict and its victims are elucidated and shown to be consistent in terms of the political stakes and the philosophy of the institution. One example is provided by the little known and highly interesting episode of the neutral zones set up in Jerusalem in mid-1948.

The approach adopted in this work sheds fresh light on both recent problems and old but recurring issues such as structural reform of the International Red Cross, conflicts over spheres of competence between humanitarian organizations, whether governmental or not, and recognition in international law of the emblem of the Red Star of David for functions identical to those of the Red Cross, Red Crescent and Red Lion and Sun.

It is clear that Dominique-D. Junod had to look beyond these questions at the thinking and attitudes of the men who served and identified with the ICRC, at their perceptions, their relationship with an ideal anchored in a noble principle, and in some cases at prejudices that unfortunately came into play. All this gives the book a depth which is emphasized by the wealth of information that has gone into it.

The author's way of tackling her task leads us to ponder anew the motives and mechanisms of an institution which, while pursuing laudable aims, has tended to protect itself since the Second World War through a sometimes dogmatic discourse.

Finally, what we are witnessing today in the field of humanitarian diplomacy in general, and sometimes in the behavior of individual ICRC delegates, makes this book, spanning history of international relations and international humanitarian law and institutions, so intensely topical.

Saul Friedländer
UCLA and Tel Aviv University

ACKNOWLEDGEMENTS

This book began as a doctoral thesis written in French and defended at the Graduate Institute of International Studies (GIIS) in Geneva in October, 1993. I would like to express here my deep appreciation to Professor Saul Friedlander (UCLA and Tel Aviv University) for motivating me to write this work; to Professors Miklos Molnar and Philippe Burrin (GIIS) who successively and expertly directed the writing of my thesis; and, finally, to Jean-Claude Favez (former rector of the University of Geneva and professor of modern history) for his valuable encouragement. The usual formulas of acknowledgement are inadequate to convey the extent of my gratitude to each of them.

My very sincere appreciation goes as well to the International Committee of the Red Cross (ICRC) for giving me the run of its archives, and in particular to Jacques Moreillon, former director-general of the ICRC, who in his official capacity accorded me facilities without which I could never have brought this work to term. I am also indebted to Lady Mountbatten, who did me the honor of carrying out research in the archives of her late father for the purposes of this work.

In addition, many thanks to: Geoffrey Best (St. Antony's College, Oxford); Daniel Bourgeois (Swiss Federal Archives, Bern); Anne-Claire Daeniker (Institüt für Zeitgeschichte, Zurich); Yehoshua Freundlich (Israel State Archives, Jerusalem); Floresca and Paul Lalor (St. Antony's College, Oxford); M. Mayorek (Central Zionist Archives, Jerusalem); Mara Meriboute (ICRC Library, Geneva); Michael Meyer (British Red Cross, London); Martin Morger (ICRC Archives, Geneva); Jean and Maurice de Reynier (Rolle, Switzerland); Liliane Rytz, former ICRC delegate; Shmuel Spektor (Yad Vashem, Jerusalem); Klaus Urner (Institüt für Zeitgeschichte, Zurich); and Francine Wilcoks (ICRC Archives, Geneva), for their contributions to my research.

I am also indebted to the following:

– Jean Courvoisier, Michel Doret, Robert Gouy, Arieh Harel (Steinberg), Hillel Kook, Zvi Loker, Netanel Lorch, and Jean Munier for their testimony;
– Marion Droz and Avner and Isabelle Levi for their translations from Hebrew;
– Jonathan Breen for his attentive perusal of my manuscript and his competent and invaluable advice;
– Elinore Ben-Shaul (Jerusalem) and Gilbert Koull (Geneva), for their inestimable assistance in drawing the maps used in this book;
– The ICRC, Peter Peeters (Geneva) and Mario Cherubini (Rome), for their financial contributions;
– Martine Callendrier (ICRC, Geneva), for coming to my aid with her computer expertise.

Last, but not least, I would like to express my warmest thanks to Martha Grenzeback (Tel-Aviv) for her excellent translation of my manuscript.

ABBREVIATIONS

ADPF	Archives du Département Politique fédéral
AHC	Arab Higher Committee
AICRC	Archives of the International Committee of the Red Cross
CICR	Comité international de la Croix-Rouge
CO	Colonial Office
CP	Communiqué de presse
CZA	Central Zionist Archives
EY	Eretz-Yisrael
FO	Foreign Office
HCNL	Hebrew Committee of National Liberation
HDI	Henry Dunant Institute
ICRC	International Committee of the Red Cross
IHD	Institut Henry Dunant
IRC	International Red Cross
ISA	Israel State Archives
IUHEI	Institut Universitaire de Hautes Etudes Internationales
IZG	Institüt für Zeitgeschichte
IZL	Irgun Zva'i Le'umi
JA	Jewish Agency
Lehi	Lohamei Herut Israel
LRCS	League of Red Cross Societies
LSCR	Ligue des Sociétés de la Croix-Rouge
MDA	Magen David Adom
MEA	Ministry of External Affairs
PIC	Prisonniers et Internés Civils
PR	Press release
PRO	Public Record Office

PUF	Presses Universitaires de France
RC	Red Cross
RICR	*Revue internationale de la Croix-Rouge*
UNICEF	United Nations International Children's Emergency Fund
UNO	United Nations Organization
UNRPR	United Nations Relief for Palestine Refugees
UNRWAPR	United Nations Relief and Work Agency for Palestine Refugees
UNSCOP	United Nations Special Commission on Palestine

INTRODUCTION

Purpose of the research and definition of the subject

I did not begin the research and analysis for this work with the idea of writing a book, but rather with the more modest ambition of preparing a monograph on 'the ICRC's action in aid of the victims of the Palestine–Eretz-Yisrael conflict from 1945 to 1952.' This title in itself merits some explanation.

From 1945 to 1947, Jewish extremists fought Great Britain in Mandatory Palestine. After the United Nations resolved, in November 1947, to partition Palestine into an Arab state and a Jewish state, the conflict became one between Arabs and Jews. This conflict, in turn, developed into an Arab-Israeli war, after the British left and the State of Israel declared its independence, on May 14, 1948. This war ended in 1949 with an armistice between Israel and its Arab adversaries.

The British and the Arabs called the territory concerned 'Palestine.' For the Jews it was 'Eretz-Yisrael' (hereafter EY), or, 'the Land of Israel.' The three successive conflicts – Jewish-British, Arab-Jewish, and Arab-Israeli – were all waged over the same territory, called Palestine by one side and Eretz-Yisrael by the other. That is why I speak of the 'Palestine–Eretz-Yisrael' conflict.

For the ICRC, the operation it conducted in the Palestine-EY conflict during the decisive years of 1945–1951 was of great significance. This is indicated by its contemporary publications on the subject, which were relatively more numerous and detailed than those covering ICRC activities in other parts of the world during the same period. These publications also convey the impression that the organization's achievements in this particular sphere were very satisfactory from the humanitarian point of view; yet, although works on the 1948 Arab-Israeli war and its antecedents and direct consequences do mention certain ICRC actions, they do not accord them the same importance that the organization's public documents do. This might indicate that the ICRC's achievements were not commensurate with its efforts. If such was the case – and that remains to be seen – why did the ICRC attribute such great significance to its activities in the Palestine-EY conflict? That question is the basis of this study.

Comparing the content and tone of the ICRC's publications with those of the documents in its archives, I noticed that the contemporary communications revealed a certain tendentiousness, an awareness of the historical moment. In describing its operations, particularly the one it was conducting in Mandatory Palestine, it was actually transmitting messages to public opinion that went beyond the purpose of simply providing information. Did these messages have an ideological or political function?

There was, therefore, reason to wonder about the ICRC's own situation during the period extending from the immediate aftermath of World War II to the beginning of the Cold War – the same years that the ICRC was active in the Near East. The dearth of detailed, unbiased works on the ICRC during the years 1945–1952 seemed to call for a meticulous reconstructive study of the structure, functioning, frame of reference, and values of the International Red Cross in general and of the ICRC in particular.

As it proceeded, this analytical research gradually uncovered the political challenges the ICRC faced between 1945 and 1952, a time when the organization was in great difficulty; for despite the ICRC's substantial humanitarian efforts during World War II (which earned it the Nobel Peace Prize in 1944), when the fighting stopped, the organization was put on trial. It was accused of not having done enough for Soviet prisoners of war, the partisans and resistance members who had fought against the Fascists and the Nazis, and the victims of Hitler's racial persecution – particularly the European Jews, who had been the victims of a systematic massacre without precedent in history.

The criticisms of the ICRC came principally from the Soviet Union and its allies; but they were heard as well from within the International Red Cross, in which the Committee held a central position as the guarantor of the entire movement's unity

INTRODUCTION

and equilibrium. Beleaguered, threatened with extinction – which would have brought about the scission of an International Red Cross torn by the ideological differences of the Cold War – the ICRC devised a strategy to re-establish and reinforce its position. This strategy was partly reflected in its approach to preparing the Geneva Conventions for the protection of war victims, which were to be adopted by a diplomatic conference in 1949. It was also reflected in the organization's reactions to attempts to revise the structure of the International Red Cross and to redefine the roles of its components. The reforms envisioned were the brainchild of Count Folke Bernadotte, who from the end of May, 1948, combined key functions in the International Red Cross with the position of United Nations mediator in Palestine, and they could be expected to result in a paralysis of ICRC activities in the middle term, or even in the extinction of the organization itself.

An intriguing question was whether the ICRC's efforts in the arena of the Palestine-EY conflict might have been influenced by the crucial problems the organization faced at the time, notably the fact that it was fighting for its own survival and for the unity of the International Red Cross. My attempt to answer that question led me to modify my original plan considerably – in fact, to change the focus of my research. Instead of merely writing a history of the ICRC's activities in the Palestine-EY conflict, I decided to trace, in counterpoint, the evolution of the ICRC, its politics, and its strategy during the relevant period, pinpointing wherever possible any interaction between the ICRC's activities in Palestine, on one hand, and its more general challenges between 1945 and 1952, on the other – hence the title of this work.

Sources

For the purposes of this study, I was able to consult all the files in the archives of the International Committee of the Red Cross for the period in question. These archives are incomplete, however, and the documents produced by the ICRC itself are subject to a certain degree of self-censorship. The procès-verbaux are not verbatim. Moreover, the ICRC archives do not contain related documents, concerning the International Red Cross as a whole or the Palestine-EY conflict. For these reasons I drew on the following additional sources:

- the Swiss federal archives, because of the ICRC's special ties with Switzerland;
- the Public Record Office in Great Britain (Kew Gardens), which houses documents on the International Red Cross in general as well as on the ICRC's relations with the British government;
- the Central Zionist Archives and the Israel State Archives, which I considered likely to throw light on items in the ICRC archives, particularly on the reports by ICRC delegates in Palestine during the first Arab-Israeli conflict.

Finally, invaluable material was furnished by private collections, such as the archives of Paul Ruegger, president of the ICRC from the end of 1947 to 1956, which are now located at the Institute of Contemporary History in Zurich, and the archives of Sir Alan Cunningham, the last high commissioner in Palestine, which are housed in the Middle East Library of St. Antony's College at Oxford. I also had access to documents belonging to former ICRC delegates, and took the opportunity to question these individuals personally as well.

Some readers may be surprised to find no primary Arab sources on this list; attempts, from Jerusalem, to contact Arab circles or documents produced no results. This failure can be attributed to the fact that these attempts were made at a time when the Gulf War was brewing, and the atmosphere was not conducive to calm tempers. Although this objective restriction was regrettable, the Arab sources seemed less important for the purposes of this study than the sources mentioned above, in particular the Israeli archives, since the reports from ICRC delegates (particularly those of the head of the ICRC delegation in Palestine, Jacques de Reynier) indicated that their relations with the local Jews were difficult. The problems that both the delegates and the Committee itself encountered in their contacts with the Arab world were less significant than those entailed by their relations with the Jewish and, subsequently, Israeli authorities. Nonetheless, the aspect of the ICRC's relations with the Arab world has not been neglected; the ICRC archives contain extensive documentation on the subject, which proved adequate for this research.

INTRODUCTION

Having chosen to examine the ICRC both as it was and as an entity in process of evolution, influenced by its prospects and perspectives, I relied most heavily on archival sources and direct, contemporary testimony. As a rule, public institutional documents have been used only to underline the significance the ICRC tried to attribute to them in terms of its general objectives.

Finally, it is assumed that the reader is familiar with the context of the ICRC's actions in Mandatory Palestine and in the first Arab-Israeli conflict. To avoid interrupting the flow of the text with parenthetical reminders, I have appended a chronology encompassing some of the stages of the nascent Cold War and of the evolving Palestine-EY conflict. Those diplomatic or strategic circumstances that directly influenced the ICRC's humanitarian policy are briefly described in the course of the book.

Chapter One

THE RED CROSS IN PERIL AND THE INTERNATIONAL COMMITTEE OF THE RED CROSS (ICRC)

The International Committee of the Red Cross

The origin and the heart of the International Red Cross

Our first step must be to look at the ICRC as it was in 1947, and to examine the relation between it and the International Red Cross. The International Red Cross adopted its first statutes at The Hague in 1928. Those statutes, still in force during the period that concerns us, defined the International Red Cross as comprising the International Committee of the Red Cross, the National Red Cross Societies, and the League of Red Cross Societies.[1]

The 1928 Statutes in fact constituted formal confirmation of a structure that had already evolved, the result of an empirical but purposeful process that had determined the relationship between the different components of the movement and the division of humanitarian tasks between them. The Statutes were drafted by two men who helped establish the International Red Cross's spheres of action, its limits, its orientation: Max Huber, an eminent jurist and a member of the ICRC, and Paul Drauldt, vice-chairman of the League of Red Cross Societies. In formulating these Statutes, they considered the Red Cross organizations in the context of their historical evolution, and tried to identify and codify those elements they considered essential in order to

---

[1] Art. 1, p. 305, of 'Statutes of the International Red Cross (adopted by the XIIIth International Red Cross Conference, The Hague, 1928),' pp. 305–309, in ICRC/LRCS, *Handbook of the International Red Cross*, 1st English edition (Geneva: ICRC, 1951).

maintain the equilibrium of the International Red Cross and to remain faithful to its ideals.

The 1928 Statutes of the International Red Cross defined the International Committee as 'an independent institution, governed by its own Statutes and recruited by co-optation from among Swiss citizens.'[2] The ICRC is therefore international in nothing but its name, which is a relic from the end of the nineteenth century. Founded in 1863 to aid soldiers wounded in battle, the ICRC called itself international to show that it excluded no nation from its philanthropic project. From the legal point of view, however, the ICRC is a private association with civil capacity, governed by the section of the Swiss Civil Code beginning with Article 60.[3] Its headquarters are in Geneva.

As a Swiss private body, independent of any government, the ICRC differs from the other components of the IRC. The national Red Cross societies are actually auxiliary branches of the health services of their respective countries, so consequently the League of Red Cross Societies, in which they are federated, is multinational.

The ICRC was the founder of the International Red Cross, its inspiration provided by a citizen of Geneva, Henry Dunant, who had witnessed the horrors of the aftermath of battle. In 1859, business affairs led Dunant to a region not far from Solferino, Italy, where the Austrian army had just fought against the French and Sardinian troops. There he was shocked to see wounded soldiers abandoned to their fate, the sick and dying lying unattended. Outraged, he improvised a rescue operation, using local volunteers, and after returning to Switzerland, he described what he had seen in all its horror, in a little book published in 1862. In this book, *Un Souvenir de Solferino* (A Memory of Solferino),[4] he described at almost indecent length the terrible scenes he had witnessed, wanting to shock his readers, to jolt them into taking steps to prevent such incidents from ever happening again. To that end, he proposed the establishment of voluntary relief societies that would ensure that care was pro-

[2]'Statutes of the International Red Cross,' Art. 7, in ICRC/LRCS, *Handbook*, p. 307.
[3]'Statuts du Comité international de la Croix-Rouge du 10 mars 1921, modifiés le 12 octobre 1928, le 28 août 1930 et le 2 mars 1939,' Art. I, in CICR/LSCR, *Manuel de la Croix-Rouge internationale* (Geneva: CICR/LRCS, 1942), p. 174.
[4]Henry Dunant, *Un Souvenir de Solferino*, 1st ed. (Geneva: Fick, 1862), 115 pp.

vided to wounded military personnel in wartime. In addition, he suggested that it might be possible to 'formulate some international principle, sanctioned by a Convention inviolate in character'[5] that, adopted and ratified by many nations, would give such societies a legal basis for intervention. Dunant exhorted his readers to consider these ideas.

The Committee was set up in Geneva in 1863 to find concrete responses to Dunant's proposals. Following his suggestions to the letter, it encouraged the establishment in several European countries of national aid societies whose main purpose was to assist the military medical services and, in peacetime, to work towards improving the means of assisting military personnel in wartime. With the encouragement of military and medical experts from a number of European countries, it drew up a draft convention to improve the conditions of military personnel wounded in battle, which gave rise to the adoption by a diplomatic conference, on August 22, 1864, of the Geneva Convention for the Amelioration of the Condition of the Wounded in Armies in the Field. This treaty established the principle of immunity for sick and wounded soldiers, who were to be collected and cared for regardless of their nationality.[6] It also proclaimed the neutrality of hospital and ambulance personnel and equipment, to be identified by a distinctive, uniform emblem on armbands or flags: a red cross on a white background.[7]

Neutral, independent intermediary

A philanthropic ideal had been established, national societies had been founded to put it into practice, an international convention had been adopted to give it a basis in law, and the International Red Cross had been created; at this point the International Committee of the Red Cross could have disappeared from the scene. Instead, however, encouraged by the existing national societies, it developed a role closely linked to its nature as a uninational, private Swiss organization located in Switzerland, that perpetually neutral country: that of neutral

---

[5] Henry Dunant, *A Memory of Solferino*, English version reprinted by courtesy of American Red Cross (Geneva: ICRC, 1986), p. 126.
[6] 'Geneva Convention of August 22, 1864, for the Amelioration of the Condition of the Wounded in Armies in the Field,' Art. 6, in ICRC/LRCS, *Handbook*, p. 8.
[7] Ibid., Art. 7., p. 8.

intermediary between the national aid societies in wartime. Its task was to collect information from the national societies of belligerent countries concerning their needs and to pass it to national societies of other countries, whether belligerent or not, that wanted to lend material support. It also transmitted their correspondence.

Its first major initiative of this type was the creation, in July, 1870, of an information and liaison agency in Basle to serve military personnel wounded in the Franco-Prussian War. The Basle agency also transmitted letters from the wounded soldiers to their families. Shortly afterwards, the ICRC set up an aid committee for prisoners of war, an operation it repeated during World War I in conjunction with other humanitarian efforts. Its tasks were to visit prisoners and ensure that they were treated properly by the detaining states.[8]

These activities, among others, exemplify the role of neutral intermediary between combatants that the ICRC gradually took upon itself in the wars that followed. During the conflicts in Hungary in 1919 and Upper Silesia in 1921, the ICRC decisively expanded its field of activities to include internal strife and civil war, in which it tried to act as a neutral intermediary between the parties in conflict. In that capacity it concentrated mostly on visiting prisoners.

Accordingly, the 1928 Statutes of the International Red Cross confirmed that the ICRC would 'continue to be a neutral intermediary whose intervention is recognized as necessary, especially in time of war, civil war or civil strife.'[9] When the conflict ended, the ICRC would 'work for the relief of distress considered to be a result of war.'[10] One way that the ICRC fulfilled this mission was by taking care of the victims of war; another was by fostering the development of international humanitarian law, drawing on its knowledge of the ravages of battle and the practical experience it had gained in wartime.

---

[8]Boissier, Pierre, *From Solferino to Tsushima* (Geneva: Henry Dunant Institute, 1985), pp. 263–265.
[9]'Statutes of the International Red Cross,' Art. 7, in ICRC/LRCS, *Handbook*, p. 307.
[10]Ibid.

Main author of the Law of Geneva

The ICRC had made a considerable contribution to the international humanitarian law applicable at the time of the Palestine-EY conflict. It was largely due to the ICRC's labors that the Geneva Convention was revised in 1906 and again in 1929, and that its principles were extended to other categories of victims in addition to the war-wounded – notably, prisoners of war. In 1929, besides the Geneva Convention of July 27, 1929, for the Amelioration of the Condition of the Wounded and Sick in Armed Forces in the Field, the body of humanitarian law protecting war victims consisted notably[11] in the Convention of July 27, 1929, concluded at Geneva Relative to the Treatment of Prisoners of War, more commonly known as the Prisoners of War Convention. These conventions, primarily the work of the ICRC, were still relevant after World War II and during the Palestine-EY conflict.

It should be noted that from 1906 on the Geneva Convention stated that the distinctive emblem of the red cross on a white background, an inversion of the colors of the Swiss flag, had been chosen as a compliment to Switzerland.[12] The 1929 Geneva Convention recognized two additional emblems equivalent to the red cross: the red crescent, a Moslem symbol, and the red lion and sun espoused by Persia. Both these symbols could be used by the countries already employing them.[13] The 1929 Conventions of humanitarian law were applicable to international wars, but not civil wars or internal strife.

---

[11]Only the conventions relevant to the subject of this book are mentioned here. Besides the ones listed in the text, the 1929 humanitarian law included principally these treaties:
- The Annex to the Hague Convention of 1907, Regulations Concerning the Laws and Customs of War on Land;
- The Hague Convention of October 18, 1907, for the Adaptation to Maritime Warfare of the Principles of the Geneva Convention of July 6, 1906;
- The Geneva Protocol of June 17, 1925, for the Prohibition of the Use in War of Asphyxiating, Poisonous or Other Gases, and of Bacteriological Methods of Warfare.

[12]'Geneva Convention of July 6, 1906, for the Amelioration of the Condition of the Wounded and Sick in Armed Forces in the Field,' Chapter VI, 'The Distinctive Emblem,' Art. 18, p. 22, and 'Geneva Convention of July 27, 1929, for the Amelioration of the Condition of the Wounded and Sick in Armed Forces in the Field,' Chapter VI, 'The Distinctive Emblem,' Art. 19, p. 64, in ICRC/LRCS, *Handbook*.

[13]Ibid.

From practice to tradition

As the main author of the Geneva Conventions, the ICRC naturally was obliged to operate within their limits. Indeed, the 1928 Statutes of the International Red Cross stated that the ICRC would carry out all humanitarian activity, in particular, 'in conformity with international conventions.'[14] However, since the conventions lagged behind the provisions of the 1928 Statutes, which covered civil wars and internal strife, the ICRC decided after World War II that conforming to the international conventions meant acting in their general spirit[15] and promoting that spirit in all types of armed conflict.

The ICRC was not actually bound by the 1929 Convention. The Geneva Convention entrusted the task of collecting and caring for wounded soldiers to the military medical corps. The relief society volunteers who assisted it were subject to the military authority. In fact, the Geneva Convention did not explicitly define any role at all for the ICRC, which had not originally been a component of the system imagined by Dunant. The Prisoners of War Convention, in contrast, granted the ICRC the right to propose to the belligerents the organization in a neutral country of a central information agency for prisoners of war, if it judged this to be necessary.[16] 'This agency shall be charged with the duty of collecting all information regarding prisoners which they may be able to obtain through official or private channels, and the agency shall transmit the information as rapidly as possible to the prisoners' own country or the Power in whose service they have been.'[17]

The ICRC was not expressly given the mandate of monitoring the application of the 1929 Conventions. That work was to be carried out by the 'protecting Powers,'[18] powers which in war-

---

[14]'Statutes of the International Red Cross,' Art. 7, in ICRC/LRCS, *Handbook*, p. 307.

[15]ICRC, procès-verbal, Bureau meeting of April 11, 1946 (AICRC, no file number).

[16]'Geneva Convention of July 27, 1929, Relative to the Treatment of Prisoners of War,' Part VI, 'Bureaux of Relief and Information Concerning Prisoners of War,' Art. 79, in ICRC/LRCS, *Handbook*, p. 91.

[17]Ibid., p. 92. The Prisoners of War Convention also obliged states to set up national information bureaux in their respective countries at the commencement of hostilities. *Cf.* Ibid., Art. 77, p. 90.

[18]Ibid., Part VIII, 'Execution of the Convention,' in ICRC/LRCS, *Handbook*, pp. 92–94.

time were assigned the task of protecting the belligerent country's interests on the adverse party's territory. These arrangements, however, were not to stand in the way of any measures the ICRC might feel obliged to take on behalf of the prisoners of war.[19] All these provisions were derived from the ICRC's practice in previous wars.

The 1928 Statutes of the International Red Cross established a relationship between the existing conventions and the ICRC's activities, which had to conform to those treaties. The relation worked in reverse, as well: The ICRC's initiatives and practices were likely to receive official sanction in the evolving international humanitarian law. As new legal instruments were adopted, the ICRC could cite them as a legal basis for intervention. Consequently, if the ICRC wanted to expand the purview assigned to it by the community of nations, it had an interest in seeing the humanitarian conventions develop as well. The same was true for the powers attributed to it by the Statutes of the International Red Cross, which institutionalized existing practice and could always be revised.

This symbiosis meant that the ICRC gradually developed a traditionally humanitarian role as a neutral intermediary which was consistent with the philosophy behind the Geneva Convention – that is, the principle that a soldier who is no longer fit for armed combat should not be warred against, but treated humanely, since he no longer poses any physical threat. This principle was extended to include prisoners of war in 1929. The ICRC thus sought to act on behalf of different categories of war victims covered, by extension or analogy, by the philosophy of the Geneva Convention. In its own Statutes, too, the organization had given itself the legal means to develop its tradition in this respect. Besides the functions explicitly attributed to it by the Statutes of the International Red Cross and the Prisoners of War Convention, it in fact reserves the right to undertake 'any humanitarian initiative which comes within its traditional role.'[20]

---

[19]Ibid., Part VI, 'Bureaux of Relief and Information Concerning Prisoners of War,' Art. 79, p. 91, and Part VIII, 'Execution of the Convention,' Art. 88, p. 94, in ICRC/LRCS, *Handbook*.

[20]'Statuts du Comité international de la Croix-Rouge,' Art. 5, in CICR/LSCR, *Manuel*, p. 176.

THE RED CROSS IN PERIL AND THE ICRC

The International Red Cross in peril

At this point, it might be helpful to compare the ICRC with the other components of the International Red Cross – the National Societies and their federation, the League of Red Cross Societies – as they were in 1947. The National Societies were still, as they had always been, auxiliary branches of the army medical services. To join the International Red Cross, they had to meet the requirements that had been established at the Conference of National Societies in Karlsruhe in 1887 and set down as formal regulations by the ICRC. Essentially, each national society had to belong to a country where the Geneva Convention was in force, to be the only recognized national society there, and to adopt as its emblem a red cross on a white background.[21] The ICRC was supposed to 'notify the existing National Societies of the establishment of new societies after having verified the bases on which they [were] founded.'[22]

As time passed, circumstances and experience led the National Red Cross Societies – created to aid soldiers wounded in war – to expand their sphere of operations to include national health and social programs, which they directed in peacetime. The 1928 International Red Cross Statutes did not define the tasks of the National Societies within their own countries; that was a matter for each country's internal law. The Statutes established only the duties of the League. Unlike the ICRC, which is a uninational private body empowered to act in wartime and its aftermath, the League of Red Cross Societies is a multinational organization defined by the 1928 Statutes as an 'association of National Red Cross Societies bound together for practical co-operation in peacetime, for mutual assistance, and the pursuit of common activities.'[23] Thus, in defining spheres of operation the 1928 Statutes gave the ICRC the wartime role and the League the peacetime role, while the National Societies could be involved in the activities of both on the international level.

[21]'Reconnaissance des nouvelles Sociétés nationales de la Croix-Rouge, formulées par le Comité international de la Croix-Rouge à la suite de la Conférence de Carlsruhe en 1887,' Art. 1, 2, and 5, in CICR/LSCR, *Manuel*, pp. 255–256. See also *Quatrième conférence internationale des Sociétés de la Croix-Rouge. Compte rendu* (Karlsruhe, 1887), *passim*.

[22]'Reconnaissance des nouvelles Sociétés nationales de la Croix-Rouge,' in CICR/LSCR, *Manuel*, p. 256. [Translation: M.G.]

[23]'Statutes of the International Red Cross,' Art. 8, in ICRC/LRCS, *Handbook*, p. 308.

The rules governing the division of responsibilities between the League and the ICRC were essential to the equilibrium of the Red Cross movement, for they served as points of reference in conflicts of authority. But this was not the only factor that helped maintain harmony in the International Red Cross; another element was a set of principles established by the ICRC to preserve the uniformity of the International Red Cross as it grew and developed. These principles consisted in *impartiality*, which was supposed to characterize IRC actions; the *political, religious*, and *economic independence* of the National Societies; the *universality* of the International Red Cross, which had to be ready to accept any duly established national society; and *equality* between National Societies.

These principles – which can be considered as historical traits of the IRC – were not mentioned in the 1928 IRC Statutes, but only in the ICRC Statutes.[24] This was a shrewd arrangement, since only the ICRC had the power to amend its own Statutes; the principles laid down in them were therefore protected from possible modifications by the other bodies of the International Red Cross. Furthermore, the IRC Statutes confirm that the International Committee of the Red Cross 'shall remain the guardian of the principles of the Red Cross,'[25] making it the implicit guarantor of the unity of the International Red Cross. Thus, in the 1928 Statutes of the International Red Cross, which were still in effect in 1947, the ICRC held a central position in the International Red Cross, largely because it was private, uninational, Swiss, and elected its members by co-optation: These factors made it independent, a prerequisite for the neutrality it needed in order to serve as an effective intermediary and to safeguard the principles that preserved Red Cross unity. Any infringement of these characteristics could be expected to destabilize the entire International Red Cross.

Communist attacks against the ICRC

This was, however, precisely the danger faced by a foundering International Red Cross at the beginning of the Cold War. In

---

[24]'Statuts du Comité international de la Croix-Rouge,' Art. 4.b, in CICR/LSCR, *Manuel*, pp. 174–175.
[25]'Statutes of the International Red Cross,' Art. 7, in ICRC/LRCS, *Handbook*, p. 307.

1945 the USSR and Yugoslavia began to make virulent attacks on the ICRC regarding its conduct during World War II, attacks which the USSR had been leading up to since 1943.[26] The Communist countries as a group, through their aid societies, accused the ICRC of having abandoned the Soviet prisoners of war, of having failed to find ways to alleviate the suffering of the partisans, resistance fighters, and victims of Nazi barbarism, and of having remained silent in the face of Hitler's crimes against the Slavic and Jewish peoples – a silence which, in Communist eyes, made the ICRC an accomplice by omission in the crimes of the Fascists.[27]

The ICRC responded through various channels: personal letters from members, articles published in the *Revue internationale de la Croix-Rouge* (RICR),[28] white papers, and reports on its yearly activities.[29] Its defense was substantially as follows (I have italicized the points it considered most important). During World War II, the ICRC, a neutral intermediary among belligerents, had fulfilled its *statutory mandate* by acting in accordance with the international humanitarian conventions. From that standpoint, it considered assisting *prisoners of war* as its primary obligation, *in*

---

[26] See on this subject Ernest Gloor, *Le Comité international de la Croix-Rouge et les prisonniers de guerre soviétiques. Réponse à un étranger* (Renens: L'Avenir, Dec. 1943), 19 pp.

[27] See, for example, *Jugoslovenski Crveni Krst* 1 (Aug.-Sept. 1946), Ibid. 2 (Nov.-Dec. 1946); *Borba* [Belgrade] (Nov. 26 1946); *Jugoslovenski Crveni Krst* 3 (Jan.-Feb. 1947); Drago Marusic, Croix-Rouge Yougoslave, 'Lettre ouverte au Comité international de la Croix-Rouge,' Belgrade, April 26, 1947 (AICRC CR/0052). See also François Achille Roch, 'La vie internationale, le CICR pris à partie par la Croix-Rouge yougoslave,' *Tribune de Genève* (Oct. 18, 1946).

[28] The official organ of the Red Cross movement, which is sent to governments that have signed the conventions.

[29] See, for example, Carl Burckhardt, President of the ICRC, telegram to Stettinius, Chairman of the Conference of San Francisco, Geneva, May 11, 1945, in *RICR* 317 (May 1945): 344–345; Martin Bodmer and Ernest Gloor, open letter to Dr Drago Marusic, Vice-President of the Yugoslav Red Cross, Geneva, July 9, 1947, appended to CP 153 [press release] (AICRC, CR 00/52, and ICRC Library); Frédéric Siordet, *Inter Arma Caritas, The Work of the International Committee of the Red Cross during the Second World War* (Geneva: ICRC, 1947), a translation of the 1947 French edition; and ICRC, *The Work of the ICRC for Civilian Detainees in German Concentration Camps from 1939 to 1945* (Geneva: ICRC, 1975) pp. 3–13, originally published in 1946, in French. For a complete account of ICRC actions during World War II and ICRC commentary on them, see ICRC, XVIIth International Red Cross Conference, Stockholm, August 1948, *Report of the International Committee of the Red Cross on Its Activities during the Second World War (September 1, 1939–June 30, 1947)*, 3 volumes (Geneva: ICRC, May 1948). Vol. I: *General Activities*; Vol. II: *The Central Agency for Prisoners of War*; Vol. III: *Relief Activities*.

accordance with the conventions in force. For this purpose it established the Central Prisoners of War Agency in Geneva, which employed more than 3,000 volunteers. Using its right to initiate humanitarian action, the ICRC monitored the treatment of prisoners of war to ensure that it conformed with the Prisoners of War Convention, making more than 11,000 visits to prisoner-of-war camps in the capacity of a *neutral intermediary* and sending reports on them to the detaining power and to the government of the prisoners' country of origin. On the basis of these reports and its delegates' observations, it negotiated improvements in the detention conditions of the prisoners in the camps visited. For those prisoners who lacked a protecting power, such as the Yugoslavs in Germany and the Yugoslavs and Greeks in Italy – among others – the ICRC had done its best to act as a *surrogate protecting power for humanitarian purposes*. It had also provided substantial aid by dispatching individual and collective Red Cross parcels to prisoners, who were entitled to them under the Prisoners of War Convention.

The ICRC admitted that it had done very little for Soviet prisoners of war held by the enemies of the USSR; but it claimed that the main responsibility for that situation lay with the USSR itself, which, although a signatory of the Geneva Convention for the Amelioration of the Condition of the Wounded and Sick in Armed Forces in the Field, had not acceded to the Prisoners of War Convention. The ICRC had in fact tried to remedy this deficiency by proposing to the USSR the establishment of an official information bureau which would be furnished with lists of the enemy prisoners of war held by the Soviets.[30] The ICRC could then have persuaded the USSR's adversaries to reciprocate, and in this way perhaps have been in a position to assist the Soviet prisoners of war. But the USSR – whether it was in the person of Molotov, the Soviet foreign minister, or through the Alliance of Red Cross and Red Crescent Societies of the USSR – had consistently rejected any intervention by the ICRC; no ICRC representatives ever managed to enter Soviet territory.

The ICRC also asserted that it had intervened on behalf of the partisans and resistance fighters, but with no tangible results; their prisoner-of-war status was subject to interpretation under

---

[30] This proposal was implicitly based on the 'Annex to the Hague Convention of October 18, 1907,' Art. 14, in ICRC/LRCS, *Handbook*, p. 31.

the terms of the Prisoners of War Convention, and the governments approached by the ICRC had refused to heed the latter's arguments.[31]

As for *civilians* in the main, argued the ICRC, they were not covered by *any humanitarian convention* – and not for lack of proposals by the ICRC, either. In fact, every four years representatives of the various arms of the International Red Cross met together with representatives of the governments that had signed the Geneva Convention to discuss the humanitarian issues of concern to the Red Cross movement. At the fifteenth conference of this kind – the XVth International Conference of the Red Cross held in Tokyo in 1934 – the ICRC had *submitted a draft international convention concerning the conditions and the protection of civilians of enemy nationality in international wars, known ever since as the Tokyo Draft*.[32] The Tokyo Draft could not be a legal instrument in due form until it had been adopted by a diplomatic conference, and the task of convening such a conference was entrusted to the Swiss government. The outbreak of World War II, however, prevented this, with the result that civilians of enemy nationality (and, by the same token, all other civilians) were unprotected by any international convention during the war.

The ICRC had nonetheless tried to persuade the belligerent countries to apply the Tokyo Draft on an ad hoc basis, on condition of reciprocity, or even to give interned civilians the same treatment accorded to prisoners of war. *The warring states agreed,*

---

[31]The Prisoners of War Convention does not define a prisoner of war, but refers the reader to The Hague law, another branch of international humanitarian law governing the laws and customs of war on land. Prisoners of war are defined as all the persons captured by the enemy and referred to in Articles 1, 2 and 3 of the Regulations annexed to the Hague Convention of Oct. 18, 1907, Concerning the Laws and Customs of War on Land. These persons consist in members of the army, militias, and organized volunteer corps led by a commander and manifestly bearing arms and wearing uniforms, as well as civilian populations of occupied territories who openly take up arms at the approach of the enemy. See 'Convention of July 27, 1929, Relative to the Treatment of Prisoners of War,' Part I, 'General Provisions,' Article I, in ICRC/LRCS, *Handbook*, p. 71, and 'Annex to the Hague Convention of Oct. 18, 1907, Regulations Concerning the Laws and Customs of War on Land,' in ICRC/LRCS, *Handbook*, p. 28.

[32]'Projet de convention internationale concernant la condition et la protection des civils de nationalité ennemie qui se trouvent sur le territoire d'un belligérant ou sur un territoire occupé par lui,' in CICR/LSCR, *Manuel*, pp. 490–499; for English translation, see 'Tokyo Draft, Draft International Convention Concerning the Condition and the Protection of Civilians of Enemy Nationality in the Territory of a Belligerent or in a Territory Occupied by It,' mimeographed working document (341.3/44 bis, ICRC Library).

in part: They were willing *to offer treatment similar to that reserved for prisoners of war to civilians of enemy nationality* who, present on their territory at the beginning of the hostilities, had been interned simply because of their nationality. These people were designated as *'civilian internees.'* But the belligerent powers *refused to apply* the section of the Tokyo Draft that covered *civilians of enemy nationality in occupied territories* – to the ICRC's regret, since that section forbade in particular deportations and the taking of hostages. Without the Tokyo Draft, *the ICRC had no legal grounds to intervene* on behalf of these civilians, even in an ad hoc capacity. ICRC delegates made 3,000 visits to civilian internee camps to monitor conditions there, but it could do nothing for civilians in occupied territories.

Regarding the treatment of nationals by their own governments and the Jews made *stateless* by the 1941 racial laws in Germany and, later, in other countries following Germany's example, the ICRC maintained that these people could not be protected by the Tokyo Draft, which covered only civilians of enemy nationality. *The ICRC had no legal basis for intervening on their behalf.* Nevertheless, it had not stood idly by, but had given them practical assistance in a purely humanitarian spirit. Still, it did not consider this action as one of its traditional tasks.[33]

The ICRC brought out the fact that it had begun by sending parcels to some 50 concentration-camp inmates whose names and places of internment it knew. The acknowledgements of receipt that came back to it often showed, besides the name of the addressee, other names and information. The ICRC was thus able to keep expanding the number of people benefiting from this operation, organized with the particular support of the American Joint Distribution Committee. By the end of the war, the ICRC's list of recipients had grown to some 93,000 names and the number of parcels sent to about 400,000.

At the very end of the war, in March, 1945, the president of the ICRC, Carl Burckhardt, obtained from the Nazis – represented by Kaltenbrunner, head of the Central Security Office of the Third Reich – permission to repatriate the Belgian and French inmates of concentration camps, and to post ICRC delegates in some of the camps, on condition that they remained there to the end

---

[33]In my view, the ICRC did not consider this action as part of its tradition because at the time there was no prospect of a legal instrument that would protect nationals and stateless people in the future.

of the war. Their presence helped protect the camps from destruction as the Allied forces advanced, thereby saving tens of thousands of lives. *The ICRC admitted, however, that it had been cautious about intervening on behalf of civilians in concentration camps, especially Jews, to avoid antagonizing Hitler and endangering the activities it was able to conduct lawfully and effectively to help prisoners of war.* It pointed out, moreover, that its headquarters were in a country hemmed in by the Axis countries.

Why, in fact, did the ICRC remain silent in the face of the crimes committed by Hitler and the Fascists in general? It explained that beginning in September 1939, in order to maintain its freedom of action, it had informed all the belligerents that it would not apportion blame *should allegations be made regarding violations of international law,* to avoid being blamed itself. Accordingly, it would not spontaneously assume the role of a commission of enquiry. At most, at the request and with the consent of all the parties, it would agree to appoint neutral experts from outside the ICRC. *The ICRC made a point of never denouncing, never acting as a judge,* censor or arbiter of belligerents. And although it might report conventional violations by a particular state, it did so only on the basis of its own delegates' observations and by means of confidential contacts with the government in question. The ICRC underlined the fact that it was under no obligation to monitor the belligerents' application of international conventions, that task being, strictly speaking, the responsibility of the protecting powers. It visited prisoner-of-war camps only to appeal for possible improvements in the material conditions of detention, and it mentioned the terms of the international conventions only to remind the signatories of the Prisoners of War Convention of their obligations. For ultimately, the ICRC emphasized, *the success of its own actions depended on how faithfully the belligerents respected their conventional commitments, and, in the final analysis, on the political will of the power holding the prisoners.* Where prisoners of war and civilian internees were concerned, the ICRC could invoke the obligations undertaken by the belligerents, but for the civilian victims of the concentration camps, particularly the Jews, the ICRC had little chance of success since their fate depended essentially on Hitler's wishes.

Red Cross impartiality: a source of misunderstanding

These arguments did not convince the ICRC's Communist detractors. What were those conventions, authored – they believed – solely by the ICRC and basing the principle of impartiality on non-discrimination between war victims of different nationalities? They thought that the principle of impartiality should be understood as the obligation to assist first of all those who most needed help, as had been the case with the Slavic peoples subjected to Nazi atrocities and the Jews systematically massacred by the German people. Was it impartial to aid *Fascists*? they asked. Nor could the ICRC's silence be justified, according to the Communists, even by the fear of Hitler engendered by Switzerland's enclosed situation; the Yugoslav Red Cross, for example, pointed out that the ICRC's silence in the face of Fascist crimes had begun well before World War II. The Committee had not protested when the Japanese bombed Shanghai in 1932, nor had it reacted when, during the war in Abyssinia, the Italians had attacked a Swedish Red Cross ambulance. The source of this attitude was the Swiss nationality and *bourgeois outlook* of the ICRC members, said the Yugoslav Red Cross, which in 1946 was the spearhead of Communist propaganda against the Committee. The ICRC needed to be liberated from the *ideological tutelage of the Fascists*.[34] The International Committee of the Red Cross *did not deserve the adjective 'international.'*

The situation was all the more critical for the ICRC because, obeying the behest of the IRC Statutes to relieve the misery engendered by war, it was at the time focusing its main efforts on the plight of German prisoners and citizens of Axis countries held by the Allies. In so doing, it was applying, with some delay, the principle of impartiality that, under the Prisoners of War Convention, demands the uniform application of the convention's provisions to all prisoners, whatever their nationality. Deviating somewhat from its usual policy, it was also lending material assistance to displaced populations, including the *Volksdeutsche*

---

[34] Arguments of the type expressed by the Yugoslav Red Cross can be found, for example in ICRC, *Conférence préliminaire des Sociétés nationales de la Croix-Rouge pour l'étude des conventions et de divers problèmes ayant trait à la Croix-Rouge, Genève, 26 juillet-3 août 1946*, stenographic procès-verbal, Geneva, non-consecutive numbering. Session of Saturday, July 27, 1946. See also CICR, procès-verbal, Bureau meeting of July 25, 1946 (AICRC, no file number).

refugees (German minorities in Eastern European countries).[35] The Communist countries felt that Red Cross aid should not go to 'fascist' peoples,[36] since even disarmed or noncombatant enemies could do ideological harm. What was more, the peoples of Yugoslavia and Poland, among others, were still suffering terribly from the consequences of the war, and deserved prior attention from the Red Cross.

The ICRC's record of assisting civilians was another weak point. On its own initiative it had created, in 1941, the Joint Relief Commission of the International Red Cross to aid civilian populations, taking as its partner the League of Red Cross Societies, which was paralyzed by its multinationality. During World War II the Joint Relief Commission – a legal entity distinct from the League and the ICRC – concentrated on improving conditions for civilian populations, mainly in the territories occupied or annexed by Nazi Germany.[37]

The Joint Commission could have continued its operations on a massive scale after the war, concentrating on the Balkans from the winter of 1945 on. But the ICRC realized this too late. In mid-May, 1945,[38] responding to a suggestion made by the American Red Cross in 1944,[39] the ICRC announced its withdrawal from the Joint Commission, which meant the Commission's demise. This was the beginning of what the press called 'the war of philanthropists,'[40] which pitted the ICRC against the League as rivals in aiding civilian populations. In the summer of 1946, the League Board of Governors, chaired by the American Basil O'Connor, met in Oxford and resolved that the Joint Relief Commission of the International Red Cross should be liquidated in

[35]ICRC, XVIIth International Red Cross Conference, Stockholm, August 1948, *Report of the ICRC on Its Activities during the Second World War*, Vol. 3, pp. 387–388.

[36]Petrovska Boris, 'Après la conclusion de la Conférence régionale de la Croix-Rouge,' *Politika* [Belgrade] (Oct. 4, 1947), ICRC translation (AICRC, CR 00/52).

[37]ICRC/LRCS, *Report of the Joint Relief Commission of the International Red Cross, 1941–1946* (Geneva, 1948), pp. 276–299. The Joint Relief Commission transmitted donations from not only National Societies, but also governments and private sources to recipient groups or communities; sometimes the target of the aid was designated by the donor, and sometimes it was not.

[38]Letter from Carl J. Burckhardt, President of the ICRC, Geneva, to Albert Lombard, Chairman of the Joint Relief Commission of the International Red Cross, May 18, 1945, in ICRC/LRCS, *Report of the Joint Relief Commission*, Appendix IV, p. 445.

[39]CICR, procès-verbal, Bureau meeting of Nov. 1, 1944 (AICRC, no file number).

[40]E.S., 'La Croix-Rouge va-t-elle se faire hara-kiri?' *Servir, Grand Hebdomadaire romand* [Lausanne] 42 (Oct. 17, 1946): 1.

six months, and until then should do nothing more than transfer aid sent by the Red Cross Societies.[41] At that point, the Alliance of Red Cross and Red Crescent Societies of the USSR, which wanted to eliminate American influence on relief operations involving Eastern Europe,[42] demanded the immediate dissolution of the Joint Commission. The League asserted that once the Joint Commission had been dissolved, aid would have to pass directly from one Red Cross Society to another.

In the ICRC's view, such an arrangement posed great danger for the impartial spirit of Red Cross operations. National Societies had no real independence vis-à-vis their respective governments, yet they would be able to select the beneficiaries of donations, which would be contrary to the goals of the International Red Cross. It also meant that Germany, deprived of statehood and with its Red Cross Society in abeyance, and such countries as Romania and Hungary, which no longer had functioning National Red Cross Societies, would receive no more aid. In fact, the League's decision at Oxford, which the Americans, British, and Soviets all supported, would have the effect of cutting the ICRC off from all future relief operations benefiting civilians – regrettable both in view of the current situation and for the sake of the ICRC's future humanitarian policy. Besides the fact that no international convention as yet offered any significant protection to civilian populations and the ICRC was working to promote such a convention, the organization had another compelling reason for assisting this category of victims: In areas where the ICRC was little known or not well accepted, aiding civilian populations earned it valuable points, being a way of demonstrating its good intentions. Once the ICRC had won the trust of the relevant authorities, it could ask, and perhaps be permitted, to visit detention centers, thereby performing its

---

[41]Resolution adopted at the nineteenth session of the Board of Governors of the League of Red Cross Societies, Oxford, July 8–20, 1946, 'Joint Relief Action,' in ICRC/LRCS, *Report of the Joint Relief Commission*, Appendix VIII, p. 450.

[42]ICRC, procès-verbal, Bureau meeting of Aug. 29, 1946 (AICRC, no file number). 'Work of the Red Cross. Supreme Authority to Replace Swiss?' *The Manchester Guardian* (July 16, 1946): 6, annexed to letter from Paul Ruegger, Minister of Switzerland in London, London, to Max Petitpierre, Federal Councilor, head of Federal Political Department, Bern, July 19, 1946 (IZG, Zurich, Fonds Ruegger).

primary function of neutral intermediary or protector of prisoners of war.[43]

The ICRC feared losing the possibility of conducting relief operations all the more because it believed there would be another war. Anticipating a conflict involving the Soviets[44] in which civilians would be the main victims,[45] it was anxious that its operations among civilian populations should not cause additional misunderstandings with the USSR. Its relations with the Soviets would be crucial to its role as neutral intermediary in the world war that, it was certain, would break out sooner or later.

Consequently, the ICRC did not want to give up its relief activities among civilians in general just because the Joint Relief Commission was being eliminated, even if it had to conduct such operations on its own. Yet, even in theory, it could not contemplate taking responsibility for the whole world. Therefore, the criteria determining which countries would benefit from its material aid would be not only the actual need of the civilians in the countries concerned, but also whether the ICRC could play a role there as neutral intermediary.[46] It had set its sights in particular on Greater Berlin, where it was the only humanitarian organization allowed to send parcels by the local Soviet authorities.[47]

To carry out such operations over the long term, however, the ICRC needed money; between 1946 and 1947, it did not have the funds to implement its policy.[48] The Joint Relief Commission

---

[43]Edouard Chapuisat, circular to delegation heads and ICRC correspondents, 'Liquidation de la Commission mixte de la Croix-Rouge internationale,' Geneva, Sept. 24, 1946 (AICRC, G.3/00).

[44]ICRC, procès-verbal, Bureau meeting of Sept. 12, 1946 (AICRC, no file number).

[45]Ibid.

[46]ICRC, procès-verbal, Bureau meeting of April 18, 1946 (AICRC, no file number).

[47]ICRC, procès-verbal, Committee meeting of Oct. 3, 1946 (AICRC, no file number). ICRC, procès-verbal, Bureau meeting of Sept. 3, 1946 (AICRC, no file number).

[48]For what the ICRC considered a reliable analysis of the reasons for the dissolution of the Joint Relief Commission of the International Red Cross, see E.S., 'La Croix Rouge va-t-elle se faire hara-kiri?' *Servir, Grand Hebdomadaire romand* [Lausanne] 42 (Oct. 17, 1946): 1; E.S., 'La Croix-Rouge va-t-elle se faire hara-kiri, un autre son de cloche,' *Servir, Grand Hebdomadaire romand* 43: 1 and 2. According to ICRC, procès-verbal, Bureau meeting of Oct. 17, 1946 (AICRC, no file number). See also ICRC, procès-verbal, Bureau meeting of Oct. 24, 1946 (AICRC, no file number).

was dissolved in November, 1946, and Switzerland created an International Center for Relief to Civilian Populations, which took over the distribution of aid from donors other than the Red Cross Societies. Now the ICRC was alone and without means to carry out the work it wanted to do for civilian populations.

In July, 1946, while the dissolution of the Joint Relief Commission was being discussed,[49] the ICRC faced an additional problem, with even greater implications. During the Oxford meeting of the League Board of Governors, the Alliance of Red Cross and Red Crescent Societies of the USSR proposed that the ICRC be eliminated and replaced with the League. Ten days after the Oxford congress, during a conference of National Red Cross Societies[50] that the ICRC had convened a long time previously to debate issues regarding the future of both humanitarian law and the International Red Cross, the Yugoslav Red Cross (the Alliance had refused to come) reopened the debate on the ICRC's priorities during World War II. Swept up in the argument, the entire International Red Cross began to object to the ICRC's all-Swiss membership and the fact that the headquarters of the organization were in Switzerland.

Count Folke Bernadotte, president of the Swedish Red Cross – who would have been happy to see Sweden take Switzerland's place in humanitarian issues – proposed this plan for internationalizing the Committee's membership: In peacetime, the ICRC would be multinational, its members elected by a procedure yet to be determined; in wartime, members from the

---

[49]For a synthesis of the conditions of liquidation of the Joint Relief Commission, see ICRC, XVIIth International Red Cross Conference, Stockholm, Aug. 1948, *Report of the ICRC on Its Activities during the Second World War*, Vol. III, pp. 384–400.

[50]ICRC, *Report on the Work of the Preliminary Conference of National Red Cross Societies for the Study of the Conventions and of Various Problems Relative to the Red Cross* (Geneva, 1947). The National Red Cross Societies of the following countries participated in the conference: Albania, Argentina, Australia, Austria, Belgium, Brazil, Bulgaria, Canada, Chile, China, Colombia, Cuba, Czechoslovakia, Denmark, Egypt, Ecuador, Finland, France, Great Britain, Greece, Guatemala, Hungary, the Indies, Iraq, Iran, Ireland, Italy, Lichtenstein, Luxembourg, Mexico, Norway, Netherlands, New Zealand, Panama, Poland, Portugal, Romania, Siam, Sweden, Switzerland, Turkey, Union of South Africa, United States, Venezuela, Yugoslavia.

warring countries would be replaced by members from neutral countries.[51]

Bernadotte enjoyed special prestige in the Red Cross. In the spring of 1945, shortly before the contacts between Burckhardt and Kaltenbrunner, he had managed to persuade Himmler to approve the liberation of 15,000 Scandinavians from concentration camps, and they were repatriated under his aegis.[52] He was a man people listened to. His proposal resulted in the creation of the Special Commission to Study Ways and Means of Reinforcing the Efficacity of the Work of the ICRC. It was made up of representatives from the Alliance of Red Cross and Red Crescent Societies of the USSR – whose participation was desired despite its absence from the conference called by the ICRC in 1946 – together with representatives of the American, Belgian, Brazilian, British, Chinese, Egyptian, French, Swedish, and Czechoslovakian National Societies.

The ICRC preferred not to take part in the Commission's work, since it was itself to be the object of study. If it participated, it would not be able to react with the necessary objectivity and independence when the time came for conclusions.[53] Wanting to be well-informed, however, it appointed two observers to the Commission, Jean Pictet and Roger Gallopin.[54] Both of them held important positions in the ICRC: Pictet was in charge of general affairs, while Gallopin was responsible for directing the ICRC's humanitarian operations from Geneva.

Following the Commission's discussions from a distance, the ICRC progressively analyzed the implications of Bernadotte's

---

[51]'Allocution par le Comte Folke Bernadotte, Président de la Croix-Rouge suédoise, concernant les relations du CICR avec les sociétés nationales de la Croix-Rouge,' Geneva, July 30, 1946 (AICRC, CRI 26); and CICR, *Conférence préliminaire des sociétés*, session of July 30, 1946, 'Rôle du CICR et de son financement.' Non-consecutive numbering. (This idea was not new; it had been considered when the League of Red Cross Societies was established in 1919, together with various other plans to restructure the International Red Cross. It had been in reaction to the 1919 debate, in spirit very different from that of 1946–1948, that Max Huber and the vice-chairman of the League of Red Cross Societies had conceived the Statutes of the International Red Cross, which were adopted in 1928. D.-D.J.).

[52]Comte Folke Bernadotte, *La fin, mes négociations humanitaires en Allemagne au printemps 1945 et leurs conséquences politiques* (Lausanne: Marguerat, 1945), 140 pp.

[53]ICRC, procès-verbal, Bureau meeting of Oct. 24, 1946 (AICRC, no file number).

[54]ICRC, procès-verbal, Committee meeting of Oct. 3, 1946 (AICRC, no file number).

plan for its activities and spheres of action. A multinational ICRC would be unable to perform the function of neutral intermediary which it saw as its raison d'être. It could not, in fact, break the link between its own image of neutrality and that of Switzerland's perpetual neutrality.[55] If it were internationalized, it would lose its ability to decide and act swiftly, as well as its right to initiate humanitarian operations – essential, in its view, since that right of initiative allowed it to direct its own development. Moreover, as an international body it would no longer be neutral enough to act as the guardian of the uniform principles of the Red Cross. In short, by attacking the ICRC's Swiss, uninational character, the Red Cross movement was depriving itself of its best guarantee of unity and permanence.[56]

To change the make-up of the ICRC, the Statutes of the International Red Cross had to be revised, since they laid down the ICRC's composition. These Statutes had been adopted by the XIIIth International Conference of the Red Cross in The Hague, in 1928. They could be reviewed by the XVIIth International Conference of the Red Cross, the first since the war. Since 1946[57] this conference had been scheduled for Stockholm in the summer of 1948, and it was at the Stockholm Conference that the Special Commission to Study Ways and Means of Reinforcing the Efficacity of the Work of the ICRC (hereafter 'Special Commission') was to present its conclusions and submit its proposals to a vote. The rules of procedure required that the Special Commission complete its study six months before the conference began – that is, in the spring of 1948.

In the meantime, the Standing Commission of the International Conference would rule – subject to the conference's final approval – on any differences that might arise between the League and the ICRC, and would set the conference's agenda. The Standing Commission was composed of five members appointed by the conference, together with two ICRC representa-

[55]ICRC, *Report of the International Committee of the Red Cross on Its Activities during the Second World War*, Vol. I, pp. 28 ff. Switzerland's perpetual neutrality, the basic principle of that country's foreign policy, was recognized by the 1815 Treaty of Vienna, among others, together with the inviolability of its borders.

[56]For an example of this line of reasoning, see ICRC, procès-verbal, Bureau meeting of Nov. 18, 1946 (AICRC, no file number).

[57]Standing Commission, procès-verbal, meeting of July 30, 1946, at 17:00. Unsigned (AICRC, no file number).

tives and two League representatives, for a total of nine members. Entitled to appoint its own chairman, it chose Bernadotte for the post in July, 1946.[58]

The threat of schism

The reverberations of the dawning Cold War within the International Red Cross soon forced Bernadotte to abandon his plan to internationalize the ICRC membership. Indeed, at a regional conference of European Red Cross societies that met in Belgrade in the fall of 1947[59] and which the ICRC attended as an observer, the International Red Cross narrowly avoided rupture. The Alliance of Red Cross and Red Crescent Societies of the USSR[60] expressed the indignation of the Polish and Yugoslav Red Cross societies over the tragedy of the displaced persons in the occupied zones in Germany and over the dilatoriness of the American and British Red Cross societies in seeking out the child victims of the Nazi 'Germanization program' (*Germanisierung*). At the Alliance's instigation the Belgrade conference denounced these societies. The Alliance also made accusations about the anti-Soviet attitude shown by these two societies, which, it said, used the Swedish Red Cross as an intermediary to support Baltic organizations that spread propaganda against the USSR.[61] The American, British, and Swedish Red Cross societies were accused of withholding aid from Soviet displaced persons wishing to return home.[62] The Swedish Red Cross was also accused of transferring American aid to 'pro-Fascist' directors of displaced persons' camps, and of assisting antidemocratic centers in the Baltic countries.[63]

As president of the Swedish Red Cross, Bernadotte was caught in the crossfire of this dispute, and he drew a number of con-

---

[58]Ibid. Although instituted by the Statutes of the International Red Cross, the International Conference of the Red Cross and its Standing Commission are not, properly speaking, components of the Red Cross like the League (now called 'Federation') and the ICRC. They are rather cogwheels that keep the movement functioning.
[59]Croix-Rouge yougoslave, *Conférence régionale des Croix-Rouges européennes, Belgrade, 24 septembre-1er octobre 1947, compte rendu* (Belgrade, n.d.), 118 pp.
[60]Ibid., speech by Vasili Vaneiev, Sept. 25, 1947, p. 38.
[61]Croix-Rouge yougoslave, *Conférence régionale*, speech by Vasili Vaneiev, Sept. 25, 1947, pp. 39–41.
[62]Ibid.
[63]Ibid.

clusions from it. The principal one was that the membership of the ICRC must remain Swiss,[64] since that averted any serious internal dissension. Although the ICRC's effectiveness in wartime still needed improvement, it was even more important to prevent the International Red Cross from breaking up.

The Communist East and the Czech Red Cross continued to favor the idea of an internationalized ICRC, while the Committee worried about the Alliance of Red Cross and Red Crescent Societies of the USSR, which, denigrating the ICRC, was refusing to participate in the meetings of the Special Commission. Meanwhile, Bernadotte lent his support to an alternative plan for structural reform, conceived by Pierre Depage, president of the Belgian Red Cross and a member of the Standing Commission of the International Conference of the Red Cross.

Under Depage's plan, the Standing Commission, which at the time had the sole function of providing an administrative bridge between one Red Cross international conference and the next, would become a high council governing the International Red Cross. It would supervise both the ICRC and the League, whose purposes would be merged.[65]

The Depage plan would have almost the same effects on the ICRC as internationalizing it. Should members be absent, the power of the Standing Commission, in its new identity as high council of the International Red Cross, might very well fall into the hands of a single person.[66] Another possibility was that only one of the two Cold War blocs would be represented in the high council. In such circumstances, even if the ICRC were allowed complete freedom of action, it would not be able to appear as neutral and independent. Once it was subordinate to an international body that itself was vulnerable to internal disputes, the ICRC would no longer have the independence and neutrality necessary for its role of neutral intermediary. Moreover, if it had

[64]Count Folke Bernadotte, *Instead of Arms* (London: Hodder and Stoughton, 1949), p. 131.

[65]'Observations concernant l'avant-projet de Statuts de la Croix-Rouge internationale établi par Pierre Depage, Président de la Commission spéciale.' Unsigned, Geneva, March 10, 1948 (AICRC, CP 273).

[66]If this happened immediately, it would be Bernadotte, as chairman of the Standing Commission of the International Conference.

to submit its initiatives to the high council, its ability to respond on the spot to emergencies would be diminished.[67]

The Depage project, which implied sacrificing the ICRC in its traditional form, would probably not, in any case, have prevented a schism in the International Red Cross. At the end of 1947, the British Red Cross realized the danger the Depage plan might pose for both the ICRC and the entire International Red Cross. It believed that during that difficult period any revision of the Statutes of the International Red Cross should be avoided, since it could only increase the risk of schism in the organization. It was imperative that the International Red Cross present a united front in dealing with the victims of the ravages of war in Europe.

At the request of the British society,[68] Bernadotte, Depage, Bonabes de Rougé (the secretary-general of the League), and O'Connor (both the chairman of the League and the president of the American Red Cross) met quietly in London on January 5, 1948, to seek a way of resisting the process that had begun. The ICRC was invited, but preferred to stay away from a meeting to which not all the experts of the Special Commission had been invited. However, one of the ICRC's vice-presidents, Gloor, and its director of operations, Gallopin (who was also an observer on the Special Commission), were in London to negotiate other matters with the British government, and under the circumstances, they agreed to an informal consultation with the little group that the British Red Cross had called together.

This 'think tank' that met in London at the beginning of January 1948 came up with a new plan for running the Red Cross organization, one which did not require a revision of the 1928 Statutes; they could be merely amended. The plan would be backed by the British Red Cross, which would present it to the Special Commission. Under this proposal, the League and the ICRC would be maintained, but would have to undertake to consult each other regularly. The Standing Commission could be given a greater role in coordinating the activities of the two

---

[67]Commission spéciale, 'Quelques idées sur la position du CICR,' March 17, 1948 (AICRC, CRI 26).
[68]Telegram from Susan J. Warner, British Red Cross, London, to ICRC Geneva, Dec. 27, 1947, (AICRC, G.85).

organizations.[69] Bernadotte, who accepted this plan only with reservations, took the initiative again. In the name of the Swedish Red Cross, he proposed a structure almost identical to that suggested by Pierre Depage, but which could be codified in the International Red Cross Statutes in the form of a provisional amendment, to be replaced eventually by a revision.[70] The French Red Cross later made a proposal along the same lines.[71]

From that point on, the ICRC faced two great threats: that its membership would be internationalized, an option favored by the USSR and its allies, and that it would be subordinated to the Standing Commission of the International Conference of the Red Cross, an idea supported in principle by Bernadotte, the Belgians, and the French.

All the plans examined by the Special Commission, even those it subsequently rejected, could be discussed or even adopted by the XVIIth International Conference of the Red Cross, which was to meet in Stockholm in the summer of 1948 – including the scheme to internationalize the Committee. That particular idea might well be proposed for debate by the USSR – if, as the ICRC half hoped, half feared, the latter came to Stockholm at all – or else by Czechoslovakia, a fervent supporter of the plan.

A difficult financial situation

While the ICRC faced these dangers to its character and raison d'être, its financial situation made it even more vulnerable. During World War II, Swiss donations and contributions to its budget represented 55% of its income. At the end of the war, the ICRC was short of funds. German assets to which it had a claim were blocked by Switzerland, and although the Emperor of Japan had given it a donation of 10 million Swiss francs on the eve of Japan's surrender, the Allies had frozen the money and the United States and Great Britain were examining ways of deduct-

---

[69]Susan J. Warner, British Red Cross, 'Memorandum presented by the British Red Cross Society to the Special Commission for the Reinforcement of the Work of the International Red Cross Committee,' London, February 23, 1948 (AICRC, CRI 010).

[70]'Propositions présentées par le Comte Bernadotte, Président de la Croix-Rouge suédoise, à la Commission spéciale d'étude.' Unsigned. Geneva, March 18, 1948 (AICRC, CRI 26).

[71]Paul Kuhne, 'Substance des différentes propositions soumises à la Commission spéciale,' March 18, 1948 (AICRC, CRI 26).

ing reparations from it.[72] Then, in 1946, several governments informed the ICRC that they were going to stop their payments. To make ends meet, the ICRC again had to request assistance from Switzerland. On April 5, 1946, the Swiss government allocated it an emergency fund[73] in case generalized hostilities should break out.[74] The ICRC could borrow on the strength of the fund,[75] though that would be impolitic – if its financial dependence on Switzerland increased, it would merely be adding grist to the mill for those who already accused it of an excessively Swiss orientation.[76]

Without money, the ICRC could not keep up its activities, and it was essential to do so in the period leading up to the Conference of Stockholm. To deal with this emergency, once the remains of German wartime contributions had been exhausted, the ICRC took up discreet collections in the German colonies abroad for the time being, in order to raise the wherewithal to assist German prisoners of war.[77] It also requested funds from the Americans, the British, and the French; but the fate of German prisoners of war meant little to them, and the ICRC could no longer render them any services as a neutral intermediary. Struggling with their own postwar budget problems, they made no significant response to the ICRC's requests. The ICRC also appealed to the National Red Cross Societies, who undertook to pay it a total of 15 million Swiss francs, 10 million of that by the end of 1947.[78]

---

[72] Jean-François Golay, *Le financement de l'aide humanitaire, l'exemple du Comité international de la Croix-Rouge* (Bern, Frankfort, New York, Paris: P.U.E., Peter Lang, 1990), pp. 71–72. See also ICRC, procès-verbal, Bureau meeting of Aug. 15, 1946 (AICRC, no file number).

[73] ICRC, circular letter to governments and central committees of National Red Cross Societies, 'Financial Situation of the International Committee of the Red Cross,' Geneva, June 25, 1946, in *Circulaires non-numérotees du C.I.C.R., 1916–1951* (Circulars Collection, ICRC Library).

[74] According to a letter from Paul Ruegger, President of the ICRC, Geneva, to Max Petitpierre, Federal Councillor and head of the Federal Political Department, Geneva, May 8, 1949 (AICRC, CR 59).

[75] Ibid.

[76] ICRC, procès-verbal, Bureau meetings of Sept. 12, 1946, and May 8, 1947 (AICRC, no file number).

[77] ICRC, XVIIth International Red Cross Conference, Stockholm, Aug. 1948, *Report of the ICRC on Its Activities during the Second World War*, Vol. III, pp. 103–105.

[78] 'Resolution VIII, The Role of the International Committee of the Red Cross and its Finances,' in ICRC, *Summary Report of the Work of the Preliminary Conference of the National Red Cross Societies, Geneva, July 26–August 3, 1946* (Geneva, 1946), p. 30.

But they were slow to pay,[79] perhaps because the ICRC's future was still uncertain.

The development of a strategy

Under the double threat represented by the projected structural changes and its own financial difficulties, the ICRC gradually developed a strategy to reestablish and reinforce its position before the XVIIth International Conference of the Red Cross which was to meet in Stockholm in August 1948. The process of forging this strategy, which spanned the years from 1946 to 1948, had nothing Machiavellian about it, but rather consisted in a series of reactions to circumstances. Undeniably, to the men and women of the Committee, safeguarding a neutral, independent, Swiss ICRC was synonymous with safeguarding its work and ideals; they saw preventing essential change in the ICRC as preserving the means of perpetuating Henry Dunant's gesture towards wounded soldiers. Moreover, a principle essential to this work had to be protected, that of Red Cross impartiality. The Committee was aware that these objectives depended on the maintenance of its integrality, which insured its independence and neutrality.

To insure its financial health while reducing its dependence on Switzerland,[80] the ICRC planned, between June and August, 1947, to propose to the International Conference in Stockholm that the participating governments and National Societies adopt the principle of financing the Committee on a regular, universal basis. This principle would then have to be formalized in either a statute or a convention. At the same time, the ICRC would take all necessary steps to set up a fund of its own to tide it over in peacetime.[81] To maintain the fund, it would press its claims to the German assets and the Japanese donation. Ideally, it would be able to back up these steps with new and useful activities as a neutral intermediary, since it was actions that attracted funds

[79]Jean-François Golay, *Le financement*, p. 74.
[80]ICRC, procès-verbal, Bureau meeting of Sept. 12, 1946 (AICRC, no file number).
[81]CICR, Commission spéciale pour l'étude du financement du Comité international de la Croix-Rouge, procès-verbal, June 15, 1947. See also the procès-verbaux for the meetings of June 11 and 18, 1947 (AICRC, CRI 26). See also Jean-François Golay, *Le financement*, pp. 74–9.

and not the other way around.[82] Thus, the Committee's financial recovery was closely linked to the continuation of its activities and their possible extension.

Revising and completing the Geneva Convention

Considering ways to improve its effectiveness, the ICRC decided to promote the reinforcement of international humanitarian law, taking its previous experiences as a guide but also trying to foresee future situations.[83] The ICRC members were convinced that it was their organization's independence and neutrality that had allowed it to accomplish what it had during World War II – accomplishments that had gone far beyond the international conventions. Those qualities were guaranteed by its Swiss membership, its autonomous recruiting procedure, and its Swiss headquarters, all of which allowed it to act as a credible neutral intermediary. Its failures were due to a lack of legal grounds for intervention, and the Red Cross needed to work on reinforcing that legal basis, rather than attacking the structure of the movement and the composition of the ICRC.[84] Such reinforcement would involve revising existing conventions and adopting new ones, a task the ICRC had begun even before the end of World War II.[85]

The ICRC's general objective was that conventions should cover the largest possible categories of civilians, beginning with those defined by the Tokyo Draft – that is, foreign civilians on territory belonging to or occupied by a belligerent. This was an essential if incomplete lesson learned from the ICRC's experience during World War II; for conceptual reasons, linked to limits inherent in the philosophy of the Geneva Convention,[86] the Tokyo Draft did not provide for stateless people, or citizens detained

---

[82]ICRC, procès-verbal, Bureau meeting of Dec. 5, 1945 (AICRC, no file number).
[83]See, for example, CICR, 'Pourquoi il faut réviser les conventions,' in *Les Nouvelles du Comité international de la Croix-Rouge* [Geneva] 46–47 (May 1–15) Unnumbered. In bound volume: CICR, *Les Nouvelles du Comité international de la Croix-Rouge, 1945–1947.* Stenographic transcript, unnumbered pages (ICRC Library).
[84]'Observations sur l'avant-projet' (AICRC, CP 273).
[85]CICR, 'Mémorandum adressé par le Comité international de la Croix-Rouge aux gouvernements des Etats parties à la Convention de Genève et aux Sociétés nationales de la Croix-Rouge,' Geneva, Feb. 15, 1945. In *RICR* 510 (Feb. 1945): 85–89.
[86]See pp. 35–6.

by their own governments for 'political' or 'security' reasons – those two large categories of people who were thrown into Hitler's camps and, for the most part, exterminated there. Nonetheless, until the beginning of 1948, the ICRC, eager as it was, did not see a way to go beyond the provisions of the Tokyo Draft, or other similar instruments.

Laws were also needed to protect civilian populations against bombardments and other war actions, a matter the ICRC had been considering since World War I but which had taken on new urgency after Hiroshima. The urgency was compounded by the fact that France, Sweden, and the United Nations had already begun to draft conventions for the protection of civilian populations, conventions which could have the disadvantage of diverging from the philosophy of the Geneva Convention and thus fostering a disorganized development of international humanitarian law.

To protect civilian populations against bombing, the ICRC went back to a prewar proposal dating from 1938, the application of which it had advocated unsuccessfully during the war. It involved adding a provision to the Geneva Convention that would allow states, at the approach of hostilities, to agree upon the establishment of hospital zones or localities offering a safe refuge – especially from bombing – to wounded and ill soldiers and, by extension, to the civilians living in those areas.[87] It was the only way the ICRC and the governmental experts could find to include the protection of civilian populations in the philosophy of the Geneva Convention.

From 1946 onward, noting the beginnings of internal conflicts in various countries throughout the world, the ICRC also sought to continue 'the study of problems raised by civil war in the sphere of the Red Cross,'[88] drawing on its own practical experience. Ideally, the ICRC wanted the application of the international conventions to be extended to civil war. The main

[87]The text of this draft is quoted without a title in CICR, *Rapport du Comité international de la Croix-Rouge sur le projet de convention pour la création de localités et zones sanitaires en temps de guerre, adopté par la Commission d'experts réunie à Genève les 21 et 22 octobre 1938* (Geneva: ICRC, 1939), p. 9.

[88]Meylan, in-house note, 'Rôle et action de la Croix-Rouge en cas de guerre civile,' April 29, 1946 (AICRC, CR 211). [Translation: M.G.]

precedent for this was its own experience in the Spanish Civil War, when it obtained the written agreement of both sides to respect the Geneva Convention,[89] despite the absence of any draft convention or provision.[90]

Recalling the precedent of the war in Spain, in July, 1946, the ICRC proposed that the parties involved in civil wars should be asked to apply the principles of the Geneva Convention, on condition of reciprocity.[91] In April, 1947, the participants in the Conference of Government Experts for the Study of Conventions for the Protection of War Victims, taking up the 1946 formula, agreed on a draft article to be inserted in revised or new conventions, making their principles applicable 'in case of civil war, in any part of the home or colonial territory of a Contracting Party'[92] by the parties at war, on condition of reciprocity.[93] The same article also proposed an arrangement for cases of territory occupied during international wars.[94] But the Conference's suggestion implied a conceptual evolution: How could the first Geneva Convention, which covered only wounded and sick military personnel of regular armies, be made applicable to civil wars, which involved other categories of fighters?

On January 16, 1948, the ICRC found the solution: A distinction should no longer be made between military personnel and civilians, but rather between combatants and noncombatants. All wounded, sick, and imprisoned noncombatants would be

---

[89] Frédéric Siordet, 'Les Conventions de Genève et la guerre civile,' *RICR* 374 (Feb. 1970): 113.

[90] The ICRC could, however, invoke the resolutions of the International Red Cross Conference: 'Résolution XIV, Guerre civile,' in CICR, Xème Conférence internationale de la Croix-Rouge tenue à Genève du 30 mars au 7 avril 1921, *Compte rendu* (Geneva, ICRC), pp. 217–218; and 'Résolution XIV, Action de la Croix-Rouge en temps de guerre civile,' in CICR, XVIème Conférence internationale de la Croix-Rouge tenue à Londres du 20 aù 24 juin 1938, *Compte rendu* (Geneva, ICRC), p. 104.

[91] ICRC, Preliminary Conference of National Red Cross Societies for the Study of the Conventions and of Various Problems Relative to the Red Cross, Geneva, July 26 to August 3, 1946, *Documents Furnished by the International Committee of the Red Cross*, Vol. 1, in Conférence préliminaire des Sociétés nationales de la Croix-Rouge, Genève, 26 juillet au 3 août 1946, *Rapports et Documents*, mimeographed, n.d., non-consecutive page-numbering, p. 25 (ICRC Library).

[92] ICRC, *Report on the Work of the Conference of Government Experts for the Study of the Conventions for the Protection of War Victims, April 14–26, 1947* (Geneva: ICRC, 1947), pp. 8, 103, and 272.

[93] Ibid.

[94] Ibid.

'protected persons' under the revised conventions the ICRC hoped would be adopted in 1949. The traditional definition of 'enemy civilian' also seemed to be too narrow if the conventions were to be applied to occupied territories as well – including a new convention for the protection of enemy civilians which the ICRC was trying to formulate along the lines of the Tokyo Draft. The ICRC did not want to limit the concept of 'enemy civilian' to 'civilian of enemy nationality,' since in some cases occupation led to the disappearance of a state, whose citizens thereby lost their nationality. Accordingly, on January 16, 1948,[95] the ICRC abandoned the concept of 'civilian of enemy nationality' in favor of an opposite line of reasoning: The future convention would protect civilians who were not nationals of the power under whose dominion they found themselves. This covered stateless people, but still excluded the nationals of the country where the conflict was taking place, who remained subject to their own government's exclusive sovereignty. This conceptual limitation reflected the wishes of the government experts, who wanted to maintain the states' complete sovereignty over their own nationals.

In addition to these changes, the ICRC wanted future conventions to expand its own legal grounds for intervention by assigning to it every foreseeable task that could be performed by a neutral intermediary, by confirming its role as a substitute for the protecting power, and by extending its right of initiative – hitherto limited to operations involving prisoners of war – to all categories of victims covered by international humanitarian law.

Uniting East and West over the updated Geneva Conventions

From January to March, 1948, the ICRC was busy putting the finishing touches on convention drafts embodying all these ideas, which it planned to submit to the Stockholm Conference for preliminary approval. If the drafts were accepted by the representatives of both the Western and Soviet camps,[96] the diplomatic

---

[95]ICRC, procès-verbal, Legal Commission meeting of Jan. 16, 1948 (AICRC, CR 211).
[96]See ICRC, procès-verbal, Bureau meeting of Nov. 14, 1946 (AICRC, no file number).

conference required to adopt them could be quickly convened, under the aegis of the Swiss government, in Geneva.[97]

Clearly, in reinforcing the humanitarian conventions the ICRC was applying what it had learned from World War II and giving itself more extensive grounds for intervention in the hypothetical third world war that it could not help envisioning. It felt obliged to remain in constant readiness for such a war, but it kept these worries to itself – it did not want the reputation of a Jeremiah, nor did it want to fuel the Communists' claims that it had an interest in preferring war to peace. For historical and functional reasons, the ICRC's sphere of action was the battlefield, and it kept to that. In any case, however it might wish for peace in absolute terms, it was careful not to refer to it too often at a time when the concept of peace was subject to interpretation and used by the Communist countries for purposes of propaganda.[98]

ICRC administration and operation between 1945 and 1952

Appointing the president of the ICRC

The ICRC was handicapped for the diplomatic game it was preparing to play – and on which its future depended – by the absence of a strong president. Max Huber, who had assumed the difficult post during most of World War II, had retired at the end of 1944, at the age of 70. Carl Burckhardt, the former high commissioner of the League of Nations at Danzig, took over for just long enough to negotiate with Kaltenbrunner for the few concessions obtained from the Nazis in the spring of 1945. Shortly afterwards, he accepted the position of minister of Switzerland[99] in Paris, and was not replaced. On February 24, 1945, Max Huber, appointed honorary president, agreed to hold the post for the interim, but in January, 1947, exhaustion obliged him to resign. In the meantime, the ICRC had appointed two vice-presidents: Martin Bodmer, a Genevan Protestant, and, more significantly,

[97]In light of the tense atmosphere of 1947, the ICRC and many government experts even considered hastening the adoption of the conventions by holding the diplomatic conference before the Stockholm Conference. ICRC, *Report on the Work of the Conference of Government Experts*, p. 332.

[98]ICRC, procès-verbal, Bureau meeting of Dec. 5, 1946 (AICRC, no file number).

[99]In Switzerland at that time, the title of 'minister' was equivalent to 'ambassador.'

THE IMPERILED RED CROSS

the Socialist Ernest Gloor, Committee advisor on relations with the Soviet bloc. Gloor's appointment was a way of expanding the Committee's circle, culturally if not internationally, since up till then its membership had been co-opted from among the liberal Protestant bourgeoisie. Neither Gloor nor Bodmer, however, had the caliber and political profile necessary for an ICRC president.

Meanwhile, in the Swiss government, Max Petitpierre, head of the Federal Political Department,[100] and Edouard de Haller, Federal Council's Delegate for Mutual International Aid at the Federal Political Department and a former ICRC member, anxiously followed the developments that would affect the organization's future. In October, 1947, just after the Belgrade conference of European Red Cross societies, de Haller observed that it was 'supremely important for the ICRC and indirectly so for Switzerland, given the significance of the Committee's fate for Swiss foreign policy,'[101] that the Committee appoint, by the end of the year, a 'president who could not equal Bernadotte in caliber, but who would effectively assume his role'[102] in amalgamating the different trends in the International Red Cross. There was some talk of reappointing Burckhardt, but this idea was speedily rejected. He was not familiar enough with the Committee's recent problems, and, most important, he would not be a popular candidate with the Communists due to his past in Danzig,[103] where in the course of his duties he had often been in the company of Nazi party members.

Thoughts then turned to Paul Ruegger, minister of the Swiss Confederation in London, a Roman Catholic.[104] Ruegger had a long legal and diplomatic career behind him. In 1936 he had been appointed minister of Switzerland in Rome, where he earned a solid reputation. For reasons unclear at the time, Italy asked

---

[100]In Switzerland, the Federal Political Department was in charge of the country's foreign affairs.
[101]Report of the meeting of Oct. 23, 1947, in Bern between Huber, Bodmer, van Berchem, and de Haller concerning the presidency of the International Committee of the Red Cross (AFPD 2800–1967/61). [Translation: M.G.]
[102]Ibid.
[103]Ibid.
[104]Ibid.

the Swiss government to recall him in January, 1942.[105] Since Switzerland did not find him another diplomatic post that suited him, Ruegger joined the ICRC in 1943, where for several months he performed legal tasks alongside Max Huber, whom he had known since his youth. Subsequently appointed minister of Switzerland in London, he attempted to foster closer relations between Switzerland and the Soviet Union. In London he provided constant support for the steps the ICRC took to deal with the problem of its financing and the risks involved in revising the 1928 Statutes of the International Red Cross. He realized that the ICRC needed a president able to guide it through the delicate and fateful days ahead.[106]

When Switzerland and the ICRC decided to offer him the post, Ruegger was on a diplomatic mission in New Delhi. He received the Committee's official request on December 21, 1947, having been formally co-opted on December 18.[107] Unable to make up his mind, he consulted Lady Mountbatten, who at the time held a senior position in the British Red Cross, and her husband, Lord Mountbatten. The notes that Ruegger himself made at the end of these consultations indicate that Lady Mountbatten believed the ICRC could be more acceptable in some areas – unspecified by Ruegger – than the United Nations.[108] Given the date, Mandatory Palestine comes irresistibly to mind; the UN had been unpopular there in Arab and Moslem circles since the General Assembly had voted for the partition plan, and the discontent engendered threatened to spread to the Moslem communities in the Commonwealth.

Identifying with the ICRC and with the cause of active neutrality, Ruegger accepted the appointment, even though it meant giving up any real political career: 'In this critical hour,' he wrote to the head of the Federal Political Department, Max Petitpierre,

[105] According to a report from Louis Micheli at the Swiss legation in Rome to Pilet-Golaz, Federal Councilor, on Jan. 26, 1942 (IZG.17.1, Zurich, Fonds Ruegger). See also Stephan Winkler, *Die Schweiz und das geteilte Italien bilaterale Beziehungen in einer Umbruchphase. 1943–1945* (Basel, Frankfurt am Main: Helbling und Lichtenhahn, 1992), 647 pp.

[106] Paul Ruegger, 'Briefe zu Prof. Dr. Med. H. Zangger, Mitglieg des IKRK,' no place given, July 1, 1946. See also Paul Ruegger, 'Briefe zu Herr Legationsrat Alfred Escher, Zurich,' no place given, July 19, 1946 (IZG, Zurich, Fonds Ruegger).

[107] Intercroixrouge radiogram, Geneva, Dec. 20, 1947, to Paul Ruegger, Government House, New Delhi (28.2.1. IZG, Zurich, Fonds Ruegger).

[108] Paul Ruegger, 'Tagebuch,' unnumbered, handwritten pages, Dec. 22 and 23, 1947 (23.7.3.IZG, Zurich, Fonds Ruegger).

'we must make every attempt to maintain the institution to which our country is so closely tied and on which much of Switzerland's prestige depends.'[109] Paul Ruegger officially took up his duties as president of the ICRC on May 20, 1948.

Switzerland and the Committee saw Ruegger as the right man to rally the East and the West together around the ICRC and its values – a feat which first required the establishment of trust with the Soviet Union. In the course of his duties as minister of Switzerland in London, he had spent time with USSR diplomats. Politically, then, he was the man for the job.

The question was, however, whether his conduct would give the lie to the Soviet propaganda that accused the ICRC of putting Switzerland's interests before those of Hitler's victims. Were Ruegger's humanitarian propensities strong enough so that in exceptional circumstances he would be able to defend humanitarian principles in the face of political considerations contrary to his ideals? Apparently, neither Switzerland nor the ICRC asked this question, but a choice that Ruegger had made in the past might have made it difficult to answer. The incident occurred in December, 1938, after the *Anschluss*, the Conference of Evian, and *Kristallnacht*. At the time Ruegger was minister of Switzerland in Rome. The German and Austrian Jews had thought to find in Italy a refuge, albeit a temporary one, from Nazi persecution. In December, however, the Swiss police learned from the Swiss consul-general in Milan that the Italian police intended to 'pass these persons into Switzerland by night, in order to be rid of them by a practical, inexpensive means,'[110] just as the Gestapo had done for a time at Switzerland's northern border. Moreover, the Italian Jews would be made stateless in March 1939, and might well seek asylum in Switzerland. The Swiss authorities, fully aware of their decision's consequences for the cruel fate of Jews in Nazi territory during this period, resolved – not without qualms – to turn back the 'non-Aryans,' a term they had borrowed from the Nazi vocabulary. To identify these refugees, Switzerland managed to persuade the Germans, after rather

---

[109] Letter from Ruegger to Petitpierre, New Delhi, Dec. 27, 1947 (AFPD, 2800–1967/69).

[110] 'Le Ministre de Suisse à Rome, P. Ruegger, au Chef de la Division des Affaires étrangères du Département politique P. Bonna,' Dec. 10, 1938. Document no. 472.E 2991 (D)I/95, *Documents diplomatiques suisses*, Vol. 12, 1937–1938 (Bern: 1994), pp. 1083–1085.

extended negotiations, to stamp the passports of Jews from the Reich with a 'special sign,' the letter J. The various reasons for this decision are well-known, and I will not repeat them here.[111]

In Switzerland and abroad, the measures taken by the Federal Council provoked criticism and accusations of racism. Switzerland sent its representatives in the countries under Nazi influence, where there was no provision for marking Jews' passports with a special sign, restrictive instructions regarding the granting of visas to Jews. Here and there some of the representatives acted according to their consciences, whether by openly disregarding their government's orders or by showing no haste to carry them out.

Ruegger, however, was not one of them. Zealously reacting to Italy's measures to expel foreign Jews and the prospect that Italian Jews would very soon be deprived of their citizenship, on December 10, 1938, he sent his government a 'very urgent' message concerning the possible 'Entry into Switzerland of Israelites coming from Italy.'[112] He pointed out to the Swiss authorities that negotiations to persuade Italy to mark Italian Jews' passports with a special sign (NA for 'Non-Aryan') would take too long to do any good. He therefore proposed that the Swiss government and police adopt a different procedure: They could check at the Swiss border all persons bearing Italian passports and demand that the Italian Jews among them – who would become stateless as from March 1, 1939 – either undertake in writing to leave Switzerland before the said date or obtain a visa allowing them to return to Italy. Ruegger stated that he was aware of the fact that it would be almost impossible to obtain such documents. He also proposed, in the event that Jews should be 'evacuated' to Switzerland, that the Swiss authorities could make a visa obligatory for all Italians until the decree rendering Italian Jews stateless came into force. In Ruegger's mind, the visa obligation had the advantage of being in conformity with Switzerland's

[111]On this subject, see Carl Ludwig, *La politique pratiquée par la Suisse à l'égard des réfugiés au cours des années 1933 à 1935* (report addressed to the Federal Council for the benefit of legislative councils) (Bern: 1955), pp. 61–147. For a short but very solid study, see Daniel Bourgeois, 'La porte se ferme, La Suisse et le problème de l'immigration juive en 1938,' *Relations internationales* 54 (summer 1988): 181–204.

[112]'Le Ministre de Suisse à Rome, P. Ruegger, au Chef de la Division des Affaires étrangères du Département politique P. Bonna,' Dec. 10, 1938. Document no. 472.E 2991 (D) I/95, in *Documents diplomatiques suisses*, Vol. 12, pp. 1083–1085.

laws and constitution, since it was non-discriminatory, and therefore would not give rise to further accusations in the press that the government was following racial policies. Once the date of March 1, 1939 – a fateful one for Italian Jews – had passed, 'everything would return to normal', the Swiss authorities could withdraw the visa obligation, and the 'peril' to which Ruegger referred would be avoided.[113]

Nothing in Ruegger's proposal indicated that the minister of Switzerland in Rome gave a thought to the very cruel plight of the innocent people his plan would affect. This serious incident shows that in exceptional circumstances[114] where a person might be called upon to choose between 'reasons of state' – or any comparable 'reasons' – and 'humanitarian reasons,' Paul Ruegger was capable of opting for the former.

For reasons that were unclear at the time, Italy insisted that the Swiss government recall Ruegger in January 1942. Mussolini's rejection of Ruegger on the eve of World War II was undeniably good for the image of the new president of the ICRC. Moreover, none of the documents I consulted in the archives of Switzerland or the ICRC indicates that either entity was aware of or took into consideration the episode described above at the time of Ruegger's appointment to head the ICRC.

Ruegger was the Swiss government's candidate, but he was not unknown to the ICRC, either. A friend of Max Huber, he had been appointed by the Committee as adviser to the president during the years 1943–1944. These factors naturally greatly facilitated his co-optation by the International Committee of the Red Cross.

The Committee and the directors

When Ruegger accepted the presidency, the ICRC was already operating in an established mode. At the head of the organization was the Committee itself, numbering up to 25 members, the maximum permitted by the Committee's own Statutes. Many of the members had been active since before World War II. The Committee met every month, in a plenary session, to debate

---
[113]Ibid.
[114]And in the absence of a specific study on Ruegger's attitude towards Jews or the Fascist and Nazi doctrines.

THE RED CROSS IN PERIL AND THE ICRC

General Organization of the Committee's Departments

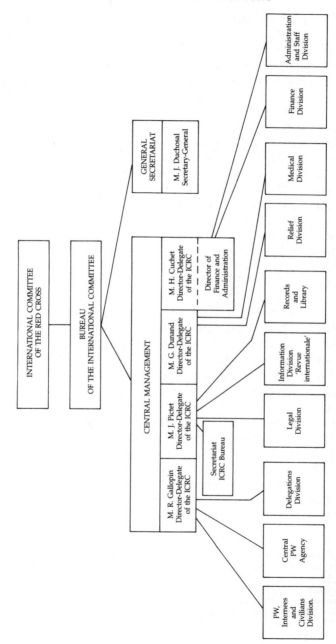

and decide the general orientation of the ICRC's activities and administration. Every week members of the Committee and directors of the ICRC met in an executive council, called the 'Bureau,' which supervised current operations.

Among the directors, the names most relevant to the present study are Roger Gallopin, who dealt with operational matters, and Paul Kuhne, his assistant. Gallopin, it may be recalled, was immersed in the problem of revising the 1928 Statutes, since along with Jean Pictet he was an observer in the Special Commission. It is hard to believe that he mentally dissociated that task from the work of conducting the operations under his control.

The ICRC delegates operating in the arena of the Palestine-EY conflict reported to Gallopin and Kuhne up until Ruegger took office in mid-May 1948. In fact, from the minute he arrived at the ICRC, Ruegger took direct control of ICRC action in the Palestine-EY conflict, which had begun six months earlier. This can be interpreted as a sign of the particular significance this operation held for the ICRC, since in general the president of the ICRC does not direct the conduct of operations himself.

Another protagonist was Max Wolf, who at the beginning of 1948 had joined the Committee at Ruegger's request, with the title of 'special adviser' to the president. This Swiss from abroad, a former correspondent of the *Manchester Guardian* and other newspapers in Berlin and London, had married Anita Warburg, the third daughter of Max Warburg, a well-known Jewish banker.[115] He was introduced into veteran Zionist society, meeting Chaim Weizmann, among others.[116] His appointment as an adviser was undoubtedly connected with the accusations made against the ICRC and its desire to improve its image and financial situation. In fact, the Committee believed that the criticisms leveled against it were largely due to the fact that, overly modest, it had not sufficiently publicized its principles, its criteria for action, and its activities.[117] Since it was expecting a future war,

---

[115] Jacques Attali, *Un homme d'influence, Sir Siegmund G. Warburg, 1902–1982* (Paris: Fayard, 1985), p. 212.

[116] According to a letter from Kahany, Delegate of the Provisional Government of Israel to the European Office of the United Nations and to the International Committee of the Red Cross, Geneva, to Moshe Shertok, Foreign Ministry, Tel Aviv, June 18, 1948 (ISA/MEA 2406.6).

[117] ICRC, procès-verbal, Bureau meeting of May 16, 1947 (AICRC, no file number).

the Committee was concerned about public opinion.[118] It set up an information service, called a 'Propaganda Service' at the time, and published many reports describing and explaining the organization's work.

The responsibilities and values of the leaders

The members of the Committee were linked to Switzerland, whose neutrality insured that the ICRC could fulfill its vocation, but they were also conscious of serving indirectly that unique principle of Swiss foreign policy, active neutrality.[119] The Red Cross was a sacred calling for them.[120] These men and women did, of course, see their commitment to the ICRC as a way of serving Swiss values, and more precisely, the 'spirit of Geneva'; but through it they were also embracing the cause of war victims, without necessarily coming in actual contact with them. Far from the realities of the 'field,' they felt they were helping those victims by fostering the development of humanitarian law and promoting its principles.

That is why, during the critical period encompassed by this study, they devoted their energies to safeguarding the ICRC's character and position. They assumed responsibility for the acts of their predecessors as for their own. Whether or not they had been with the ICRC during World War II, they all defended a common position: that the ICRC had acted for the best in the circumstances prevailing at the time – which goes to show how uncritical their perception was.

The Committee was very anxious to emphasize its link with the 1929 Conventions, because they were all that obliged the states to protect actual and potential war victims; but another, particularly significant reason was that the conventions relieved it of much of the responsibility for its failures or successes, since these always depended ultimately on the consent of the belligerents. It sought to gain the protection of future conventions as well, by ensuring that new conventions made formal provision

---

[118]ICRC, procès-verbal, Bureau meeting of Sept. 12, 1946 (AICRC, no file number).
[119]ICRC, procès-verbal, Bureau meeting of Nov. 18, 1946 (AICRC, no file number).
[120]Information provided over the telephone by Jean Pictet (the notes have gone astray – D.-D.J.).

for its traditional, essential tasks. Such provision would help deflect any attack on the Red Cross's work, to which it devoted itself in the belief that in this way it was serving the general cause of war victims, in the short and long term.

Although its frame of reference was in a fragile state – since the old conventions were in the process of being revised – the Committee had set itself up as a moral authority, a guardian of the humanitarian principles underlying the Geneva Convention that it had originated: the principles of impartiality and of respect for the unarmed or noncombatant. Nonetheless, although it was vulnerable to competition, the Committee had no desire to monopolize humanitarian activities in wartime. It only wanted to conserve the means of operating in situations where it alone, by virtue of its neutral, independent character, was in a position to act.[121]

ICRC documents and the testimony of the people involved indicate that the members and directors of the ICRC considered their work to have a civilizing mission. This little Committee of Geneva, made up of cultivated people with varied interests, occasionally translated its ideals into lyric terms, especially in public documents; their tone contrasted with the very prosaic one of the debates the members conducted in pursuing the goals they had set with respect to the Stockholm Conference. Caution was the watchword in the internal, well-regulated expression of political intentions. Occasionally, at moments of crisis, these intentions appeared clearly; but for the most part they remained hidden. To those who served the ICRC, being 'political' was suspect; and if they were constrained to maintain an internal policy, such as the one establishing a relation between actual practice and its codification in law, it was with a sort of reluctance; better to talk about it as little as possible and keep it in the form of 'ulterior motives.'[122] Only humanitarianism in its pure, essentially noble state deserved to be formulated, highlighted, and retained for posterity.

The ICRC thus presented a contradictory character. On one hand, it claimed to be concerned for all war victims – that was its true vocation, where its heart lay, and accordingly no pain

---

[121]ICRC, procès-verbal, Bureau meeting of Oct. 24, 1946 (AICRC, no file number).

[122]Information provided over the telephone by Jean Pictet. (The notes have gone astray.)

caused by war could leave it indifferent. On the other hand, it explained that it could not take all war victims into account, and that it must adhere to the categories of victims defined by international humanitarian law or implicit in the philosophy of the Geneva Convention. Such divergent messages gave the ICRC a paradoxical image: The big-hearted 'Red Cross' could be expected to provide unconditional aid; but, at the same time, one had the impression that for the ICRC members in Geneva, the victims were a theoretical notion rather than human beings whose suffering must arouse, as it had in Henry Dunant, indignation and emotion. For the ICRC leaders, even indignation over the plight of the victims could be too 'political.' This can be attributed to various factors: the distance between the Committee in Geneva and the battlefield, the fear of censure, and perhaps the Calvinist culture, which considered emotion as a sign of weakness.

The delegates

While the Committee in Geneva concerned itself with the ICRC's general orientations, the organization's delegates were the closest to the victims, and therefore more deeply affected by their plight. It was their responsibility to watch over them, as dictated by the Committee's role of neutral intermediary and the conventions – which they nevertheless did not have to know by heart. ICRC delegates of the time enjoyed considerable freedom of initiative, mainly because communication between Geneva and the countries at war was apt to take some time. What the Committee expected of them was not clearly defined. There was no occupation known as 'ICRC delegate'; the *'metier du terrain'* ('fieldwork'), an expression used at the ICRC, was learned by experience, but it was actually a talent: The field worker had to be able under all circumstances to adapt the rules deriving from the general spirit of the conventions and the ICRC's role as neutral intermediary to whatever situations arose in the unpredictable course of war. The ICRC's envoys in the field were usually amateurs. Their actions, which the ICRC counted as its own – while reserving the right to repudiate them – were therefore all the more strictly a function of their individual personalities.

The men and women who served the ICRC might be tempted

to forget, for the term of their employment, their own consciences as individuals and let themselves be swept along by an ideal to which they sacrificed themselves, by which they felt transcended and surpassed. They might be convinced that if the ideal was perfect, the actions performed in its service were performed in a laudable spirit, and conclude that the principles the ICRC promoted entitled it to exercise the moral authority it invoked. Adhering to the ideals and identifying with the institution were apt to replace the individual conscience, or weaken its function of vigilance.

These thoughts prompt some remarks about the ICRC and anti-Semitism – an issue that cannot be ignored in a study of this type, since much of it is about Jews. I will do no more than touch on the subject in the course of this book, however, because my main purpose is to examine the relation between the beleaguered Red Cross and the Palestine-EY conflict; in this perspective, the problem of anti-Semitism cannot take center stage. I will say, however, by way of introduction, that ICRC documents show that the Committee did not react – as will be seen – to evidence of anti-Jewish or anti-Semitic attitudes in the reports of certain delegates.[123] This is difficult to explain, especially since the ICRC's principles obliged those who accepted them to fulfill their mandate without discrimination as to nationality, race, religion, or political affiliations. Whatever any of them might think privately, they were required to act in accordance with this rule, which lies at the very core of the Red Cross ideal.

Interpreting an ICRC operation: a challenge for the historian

In my view, the ICRC's operations in the period under consideration, including the one it was conducting in Palestine, can be truly understood only as the product of a dialectic between the Geneva-based Committee, which defined the ICRC's major policy lines, and the reactions and achievements of the delegates in the field. The history of an ICRC operation is actually the history of the interactions between the two poles of Geneva and the battlefield.

Interpreting an ICRC operation is a true challenge for the historian, however, due to the great deal that is not said in ICRC

---

[123]See in particular pp. 122, 168, 175, 177, 222.

documents. The reason is that the members and directors of the ICRC knew each other well. They had developed a mutual understanding, and crucial discussions were often held outside the walls of the organization – hence the absence of written evidence of many choices and decisions. Those documents that exist are in many cases elliptical: The ICRC's public documents, like most of the in-house ones, are products of a neutralist mentality – one affected, moreover, (especially the internal papers) by a fear of 'the eye of Moscow.'[124]

ICRC members expressed themselves in a neutral, impartial language, making skillful use of litotes, euphemisms, omissions, allusions, extrapolations, and abstractions. The result was a wooden dialect that tried to blend ideals with neutrality. With rare exceptions, it expressed no clear political intentions, emotions, personal feelings. Historians must therefore show intuition and a certain boldness in interpreting these papers. Comparing documents, they must, in a word, decode these archives and take the corresponding risks.

The documents produced by ICRC delegates in the field usually offer a different set of problems. Although ICRC delegates used the same wooden language in their official statements, they did not always do so when communicating with ICRC headquarters in Geneva. They related events more directly than Committee members. Under the pressure of their work, they often wrote their reports in haste, subjectively and impulsively. Reports by ICRC delegates could transmit emotion. The delegates themselves often seemed to appreciate this outlet, for in the field they were not, in theory, permitted to show the least political partiality in their local negotiations with the belligerents. In fact, they had to maintain the greatest discretion in any circumstances that might endanger the accomplishment of their mission.

---

[124]According to Jean Pictet, in a conversation with the author in Geneva, ICRC, 1985.

Chapter Two

ACTING IN MANDATORY PALESTINE: MOTIVES AND STRATEGIES

In May, 1948, three months before the beginning of the Stockholm Conference, the ICRC published its first article in the *Revue internationale de la Croix-Rouge* on its overall activities in the Palestinian conflict. It dated its decision to act to December, 1947, the time of the first clashes between Arabs and Jews in Palestine following the United Nations vote in favor of partition. At that time the ICRC reportedly decided 'to examine to what extent it could offer its good offices to assist the victims of the nascent conflict, basing such action on article VII, paragraph 2, of the International Red Cross Statutes, which stipulate that the ICRC "shall continue to be a neutral intermediary whose intervention is recognized as necessary, especially in time of war, civil war or civil strife." '[125]

The ICRC archives show, however, that the organization did not wait for the disturbances following the UN vote on the partition plan to decide to intervene as a neutral intermediary on behalf of the victims in the Palestine conflict.

1945: a distant conflict

Appeal on behalf of Jewish Palestinians deported to Eritrea

In February, 1945, a small Zionist organization based in Washington, the Hebrew Committee of National Liberation (HCNL), informed the ICRC that the British had deported some 300 Jewish Palestinian citizens from British 'concentration camps' (sic) in Mandatory Palestine to Asmara, Eritrea, which was then under

---

[125]CICR, 'Le Comité international de la Croix-Rouge en Palestine (décembre 1947 au 1er mai 1948),' *RICR* 353 (May 1948): 329. [Translation: M.G.]

ACTING IN MANDATORY PALESTINE: MOTIVES AND STRATEGIES

British administration. According to the HCNL, the deportees had first been interned in Palestine and subsequently been exiled to Eritrea, where they were imprisoned without trial or due process of law, merely on the suspicion that they might have been maintaining contacts with violent Jewish resistance organizations in Palestine.[126] The HCNL was alluding to the Irgun Zva'i Le'umi, or IZL (National Military Organization), and to the Lohamei Herut Yisrael, or Lehi (Fighters for the Freedom of Israel) – also known as the Stern group, from the name of its founder. These two groups opposed the British presence in Palestine, where they wanted to establish a Jewish state by force, and their terrorist attacks were notorious. They were considered dissidents by the Jewish Agency, the organization that officially represented the Jewish community in Palestine; it, too, favored the establishment of a Jewish state in the near future, but by legal, political means.

The political convictions of the IZL and Lehi members – which derived from the Revisionist school of Zionism founded by Vladimir Jabotinsky in 1923 – were reinforced by the systematic massacre of the Jews of Europe, as well as by Chamberlain's White Paper, a document issued by Great Britain on May 17, 1939, and still in force in 1945, when more than 100,000 Jewish survivors were languishing in displaced-person camps in occupied Germany. The White Paper provided that Palestine would become an independent state with an Arab majority after a period of ten years. It limited Jewish immigration in the coming five years to a total of 75,000 people,[127] thus preventing Jewish survivors from legally entering Palestine at the end of the war, and favoring Arab opposition to a Jewish national home on the territory of the Mandate.

The HCNL, led by Hillel Kook (alias Peter Bergson), devoted itself to making the aims of the IZL known and understood in

---

[126]Letter from Peter Bergson, Hebrew Committee of National Liberation, Washington, to ICRC Geneva, Feb. 10, 1945. Annexed to note from Marc Peter, ICRC Washington, to ICRC Geneva, Feb. 12, 1945 (AICRC, G.59/7).

[127]For the text of the White Paper, see 'Document no. 17, The White Paper of 1939,' in *The Israel-Arab Reader. A Documentary History of the Middle East Conflict*, ed. Walter Laqueur and Barry Rubin, revised and updated edition (1st ed. 1969) (New York, Harmondsworth, Victoria, Markham, Auckland: Penguin Books, 1984), pp. 64–77.

the United States through public relations.¹²⁸ In February, 1945, the ICRC was apparently not familiar with the HCNL and did not take an interest in armed Jewish resistance groups. At the time, it saw Palestine as a colonial territory where it visited prisoners and foreign civilian internees – many of them Germans – held by the British.

When the ICRC received the HCNL's request, it was just on the point of asking the governments that had signed the Geneva Convention to look into the possibility of adopting the Tokyo Draft as a new convention protecting civilians of enemy nationality on territory belonging to or occupied by a belligerent. Its memorandum on the subject was sent out to the various states on February 15, 1945. The president of the ICRC, Carl Burckhardt, was preparing to negotiate with the Nazi Kaltenbrunner for the repatriation of Belgian and French deportees, a proceeding he considered compatible with the spirit of the Tokyo Draft, since Part III forbade a belligerent to deport foreign civilians present on its territory unless they threatened the security of the inhabitants.¹²⁹

Having got wind of these negotiations, the HCNL wrote to the ICRC again at the end of February, 1945 and drew its attention to the fact that by its reckoning an estimated one million Jews made technically stateless by the Axis countries of which they had formerly been citizens were being submitted to inhuman horrors by the Nazis. Presenting itself as a temporary mouthpiece for the Hebrew nation, the HCNL considered that nation to be at war with Germany; Germany, it said, had declared war on the Jews and committed acts of total, unrestricted war against them.¹³⁰ The HCNL rejected the argument the ICRC had handed to Jewish organizations for several years when asked to intervene officially on behalf of the Jews: namely, that there was no humani-

---

¹²⁸Israel Gutman, ed., *Encyclopedia of the Holocaust* (New York, London: MacMillan Publishing Co., 1990), vol. 1, pp. 190–192; also author's interview with Hillel Kook (Israel, Dec. 24, 1988).

¹²⁹'Projet de convention internationale concernant la condition et la protection des civils de nationalité ennemie qui se trouvent sur le territoire d'un belligérant ou sur un territoire occupé par lui, adopté par la XVème Conférence internationale de la Croix-Rouge à Tokyo en 1934,' Titre III, 'Des civils ennemis qui se trouvent sur le territoire occupé par un belligérant,' Art. 18.A), in CICR/LSCR, *Manuel*, p. 495.

¹³⁰Letter from Bergson, HCNL, 'Subject: status of civilian prisoners from French and Belgian territories,' Washington, Feb. 26, 1945, annexed to note from Peter, ICRC Washington, to ICRC Geneva, Feb. 28, 1945 (AICRC, G.59/7).

tarian convention or even a draft of one to provide a basis for intervention, since the Jews in question were stateless rather than of enemy nationality. The HCNL then underlined the cruelty of such restrictions, and said that the Jews should be considered as nationals of the Hebrew nation so that Germany could be asked to treat them as prisoners of war,[131] their representation as a nation to be provisionally assumed by the Hebrew Committee itself.

Bergson's letter may have reminded the ICRC of similar suggestions already made to it by Jewish organizations or individuals. They had proposed reinterpreting the definition of enemy civilian so that instead of being limited to enemy nationals, as it was in the Tokyo Draft, it would take into account the fact that Germany had declared the Jews as 'enemies.' On that basis, the ICRC could 'declare' the Jews as 'prisoners of war' or 'civilian internees.' The ICRC had tried to explain to these organizations that it did not have the power to declare who was a prisoner of war and who was not, that this was a matter that depended on conventions and governments. It could request only that a civilian detainee be *treated* as a prisoner of war, his situation being analogous to that of prisoners of war. It had made such requests successfully on an ad hoc basis for civilians of enemy nationality on the territory of a belligerent, in the spirit of Part II of the Tokyo Draft, which provided for this situation. The Tokyo Draft also envisaged another situation, that of foreign civilians in occupied territory, but for such individuals the ICRC had achieved nothing.[132]

Was the ICRC's attitude ascribable to its desire to remain within the meaning of the Tokyo Draft, which it was seeking to promote at the time? It had refused to heed the arguments of the Jewish organizations during the war, and it was equally unresponsive to the HCNL's request at the end of the war. From that point on, however, it was at least familiar with the point of view of this support organization for Jewish resistance fighters in Palestine.

The case the HCNL had raised concerning the Palestinian Jews

---

[131]Ibid.
[132]For details on these negotiations, see Arieh Ben Tov, *Facing the Holocaust in Budapest. The International Committee of the Red Cross and the Jews in Hungary, 1943–1945* (Geneva: Henry Dunant Institute, and Dordrecht, Boston, London: Martinus Nijhoff Publishers, 1988), pp. 43–59, 103–106, 213–235.

deported to Eritrea did not at once capture the ICRC's attention. In fact, the ICRC did not respond at all until May 29, 1945, three months after the HCNL's request, when the war in Europe had ended.[133] During the Conference of the United Nations in San Francisco, Carl Burckhardt sent a telegraph to the chairman of the conference, Edouard Stettinius, on May 11, explaining to the United Nations the priorities the ICRC had set for itself during the war. He used the arguments with which the ICRC usually refuted criticism[134]: The ICRC had chosen to concern itself first of all with prisoners of war, since it had legal grounds for intervening on their behalf, but nevertheless it had not neglected the needs of civilians. It had succeeded in securing for civilians of enemy nationality present on the territory of a belligerent when hostilities broke out the right to be treated as prisoners of war, since their situation was analogous. It had not, however, achieved the equivalent for foreign civilians in occupied territory. For the other civilians, the ICRC had done what it could, on a practical basis.

An atypical case for the ICRC

This was the background, in terms of ambiance and mood, to the ICRC's first step on behalf of the Jewish Palestinian detainees in Eritrea. For the ICRC, their case was atypical; strictly speaking, there was no armed conflict in Mandatory Palestine, and these detainees were not victims of a war, but prisoners of a category known as 'political detainees,' who were not covered by any convention or draft convention.[135] However, they were also foreign civilians vis-à-vis the authority detaining them in Eritrea; that authority, although British, was not the same as the government of Palestine. In this respect, then, their case resembled the situation envisaged in the Tokyo Draft. Yet the draft was applicable only in cases of armed conflict. Consequently, the case of the Palestinian deportees in Eritrea did not conform to any of the situations analyzed and provided for in draft laws in 1945. This

---

[133] Note from Paul Kuhne, ICRC Geneva, to ICRC Cairo, May 29, 1945 (AICRC, G.59/7).

[134] See Chapter 1, pp. 15 ff.

[135] On the ICRC's traditional policy regarding political prisoners, see Jacques Moreillon, *Le Comité international de la Croix-Rouge et la protection des détenus politiques* (Geneva, Lausanne: Institut Henry Dunant, L'Age d'Homme, 1973).

ACTING IN MANDATORY PALESTINE: MOTIVES AND STRATEGIES

may be partly why the ICRC was slow to take an interest in the plight of these prisoners.

Nonetheless, on May 29, 1945, the ICRC forwarded the HCNL's request to its delegate in Cairo, asking him to negotiate with the local British military authorities for authorization to visit the Palestinians imprisoned in Eritrea, and to send a detailed report on their conditions of detention to the Committee in Geneva.[136] The ICRC actually had no legal grounds to request permission for such a visit, for which there was no very firm precedent; ICRC actions on behalf of individuals detained for political or security reasons were still in their infancy.

A pragmatic approach, and a pragmatic, laconic response: On July 23, 1945, the ICRC delegate in Cairo strongly advised the ICRC in Geneva to abandon the project, due to the 'delicate situation prevailing in Palestine.'[137] He gave no details and the ICRC asked for none; but it was doubtless a question of treading carefully with Great Britain, which was conducting a policy of repression in Palestine and trying to prevent the situation from degenerating, since it wanted to retain the mandate the League of Nations had conferred on it in 1922.

At the end of July, 1945, the HCNL returned to the attack. The internees at the Asmara camp had decided to begin a hunger strike; someone had to come to their assistance, for it was a matter of life or death.[138] The internees' distressing situation apparently was not enough to galvanize the ICRC, however. It did not react until five weeks after the HCNL's SOS, and even then only in the context of its work to promote international law.

At the beginning of September, 1945, having had no response to its memorandum of February 15 to the various states, the ICRC invited the British, Chinese, French, American, and Soviet governments – the victors of the war and the permanent members of the United Nations Security Council – to meet in the summer of 1946 to study ways of bringing the old conventions up to date and to look into the possibility of drafting a new

---

[136]Note from Paul Kuhne, ICRC Geneva, to ICRC Cairo, May 29, 1945 (AICRC, G.59/7).

[137]Telegram from von der Mühll, ICRC Cairo, to ICRC Geneva, July 23, 1945 (AICRC, G.59/7). [Translation: M.G.]

[138]Letter from Samuel Merlin, Secretary-General, HCNL Washington, to Charles Huber, ICRC Washington, July 27, 1945, annexed to note from Matthey, ICRC Washington, to ICRC Geneva, Aug. 2, 1945 (AICRC, G.59/3/43).

convention covering civilians of enemy nationality, along the lines of the Tokyo Draft.[139] If these governments agreed, the ICRC planned to consult additional states. The invitation to Britain was sent directly to Ernest Bevin, the foreign secretary, on September 5, 1945.[140]

Given these circumstances, the ICRC was interested in creating precedents. Since the era of the Komintern, however, Britain had traditionally shown certain misgivings[141] about the trend towards conventions protecting civilians; it did not want to risk creating obligations – even humanitarian ones – for states towards rebels, and during World War II, it had been unenthusiastic about the Committee's wish to aid the German civilian internees in British hands.

Two days after writing to Bevin, on September 7, the ICRC decided to do something about the detainees at Asmara, against the recommendation of its Cairo delegate.[142] It informed its London delegate of the HCNL's request, asking him to contact the Foreign Office directly, and gave him a general outline of the negotiations he was to conduct: The delegate was to stress that the ICRC was not taking the initiative in this matter, but was intervening only by request, and would serve the function of a neutral intermediary. The ICRC delegate was to request authorization to visit the internees, but he was to insist that the ICRC's intentions were strictly humanitarian. A visit from one of the ICRC's representatives could not, in any case, affect the future legal status of the internees, the delegate was to explain in his contacts with the British.[143] By using all this diplomatic delicacy, the ICRC may have been trying to avoid giving the Foreign Office the feeling that it was being forced in the direction of adopting a convention for the protection of enemy civilians.

---

[139]Letter from Max Huber, Acting President, ICRC Geneva, to Ernest Bevin, Secretary of State, Foreign Office, London, Sept. 5, 1945 (AICRC.G.85), annexed to note from Jean Pictet, ICRC Geneva, to ICRC London, Sept. 5, 1945 (AICRC, G.85.G.3/3b).
[140]Letter from Huber, Acting President, ICRC Geneva, to Bevin, Secretary of State, Foreign Office, London, Sept. 5, 1945 (AICRC, G.85. G.3/3b).
[141]ICRC, procès-verbal, Bureau meeting of Nov. 14, 1946 (AICRC, no file number).
[142]Note from Kuhne, ICRC Geneva, to ICRC Cairo, Sept. 7, 1945 (AICRC, G.59/3/43).
[143]Note from Kuhne, ICRC Geneva, to ICRC London, Sept. 7, 1945 (AICRC, G.59/3/43).

ACTING IN MANDATORY PALESTINE: MOTIVES AND STRATEGIES

Britain is reluctant

The Foreign Office referred the ICRC to the Colonial Office, which warned it not to expect authorization to visit the detainees. At most, it might be permitted to send them material aid, but the Colonial Office wanted time to consider the matter.[144] The ICRC waited for months. Nothing in its archives indicates that it worried about the fate of the detainees during this time.

In January 1946, the ICRC delegate in the US sent the Committee a note, to which was attached a clipping from the *New York Times*,[145] saying that on January 17, 1946, two of the detainees in Eritrea had been killed and twelve wounded by their Sudanese guards, and that the Hebrew Committee of National Liberation was asking the ICRC to pay an urgent visit to Special Camp No. 119 in Asmara, where the events had taken place, and to send relief parcels to the internees.[146] Geneva asked its London delegation to take over the negotiations and give them priority,[147] and the delegate complied.

On March 25, 1946, the Colonial Office sent the ICRC a letter referring it to British military headquarters in Cairo. The Asmara special camp in Eritrea, it argued, was a military installation under the control of the commander-in-chief of the British army in the Near East; the ICRC should apply to him.[148] Prudently, the Colonial Office also made it clear that although the Palestinian deportees were being held by the army, they should not be considered prisoners of war in the sense intended by international humanitarian law. Their deportation and subsequent detention had been ordered by the British High Commissioner in Palestine under the Palestine Defence Emer-

---

[144]Note from Jean Cellérier, ICRC London, to ICRC Geneva, Oct. 22, 1945 (AICRC, G.59/3/43).

[145]Note from Matthey, ICRC Washington, to ICRC Geneva (Jan. 28, 1946 (AICRC, G.49/3/43). Gene Currivan, '2 Interned Jews in Eritrea Slain, Killed in a Disturbance in a Camp,' Jan. 18, Jerusalem, *New York Times* (Jan. 19, 1945) (AICRC, G.59/3/43).

[146]According to a telegram from Matthey, ICRC Washington, to ICRC Geneva, Jan. 23, 1946 (AICRC, G.59/3/140).

[147]Note from Kuhne, ICRC Geneva, to ICRC London, Feb. 4, 1946 (AICRC, G.59/3/140). Note from Kuhne, ICRC Geneva, to ICRC Cairo, Feb. 7, 1946, for information (AICRC. G.59/3/43).

[148]Letter from J.M. Martin, Colonial Office, London, to ICRC London, March 25, 1946 (AICRC, G.3/3b).

gency Regulations,[149] which permitted such measures in dealing with individuals suspected of disturbing the public order by supporting violent organizations.[150] Nonetheless, Britain had just recently allowed a chief rabbi from Palestine to visit the internees. He had reportedly declared himself satisfied with their conditions, and was able to confirm that they were allowed to practice their religious and cultural way of life in the camp.[151]

Three days after receiving this missive from the Colonial Office, on March 28, 1946, the ICRC received another letter from Britain, this one concerning the development of the law. The foreign secretary would be happy to send an expert to the meeting the ICRC was planning to hold in the summer of 1946 to revise the old conventions and possibly draw up new ones, but he expressed misgivings about the idea of a convention to protect enemy civilians, preferring to postpone any examination of the subject.[152]

A comparison of the dates and contents of the two British letters suggests that the British did not forget the link that could be established between the ICRC's practices and the evolution of international law, and that in the case of the Jewish Palestinian civilians in Eritrea, the ICRC could not expect too much of London.

The ICRC did not yield, however, in its concern for the future of humanitarian law. In its contacts with Bevin, it insisted that the convention for the protection of enemy civilians could not be eliminated out of hand from the agenda. It recalled the fate of civilians in the two world wars, and stressed the precedent the belligerents had established during World War II when they

[149]The Palestine Defence Emergency Regulations were issued by the High Commissioner in Palestine on Sept. 22, 1922, based on the Palestine (Defence) Order in Council, which stipulated in Article 6(1) that the High Commissioner could take exceptional measures 'for securing public safety, the Defense of Palestine, the maintenance of public order and the suppression of mutiny, rebellion and riot, and for maintaining supplies and services essential to the life of the community.' See Susan Hattis Rolef, ed., *Political Dictionary of the State of Israel* (New York: MacMillan Publishing Co.; London and Jerusalem: Collier MacMillan Publishers, 1987), p. 99.
[150]Letter from J.M. Martin, Colonial Office, London, to ICRC London, March 25, 1946 (AICRC, G.3/3b).
[151]Ibid.
[152]Letter from O. Davidson, Foreign Office, London, to the Acting President of the ICRC, Geneva, March 28, 1946 (AICRC, CR 240).

agreed to implement part of the Tokyo Draft for the protection of enemy civilians on an ad hoc basis, by treating civilian internees as prisoners of war.[153]

Meanwhile, in Cairo, ICRC delegate Jean Munier approached the British military command with no other aim than the humanitarian one of obtaining permission to visit the Asmara detainees. He was apparently unaware that a rabbi had already accomplished this; he, too, procured the authorization he sought. He visited the detainees in Special Camp No. 119 on June 12 and 17, 1946, and sent in his report to the ICRC on July 22, 1946.[154] According to Munier, the internees' living conditions were difficult, but not unreasonably so. In his view, what the Asmara detainees needed most was moral support; they were worried about their families and were suffering from uncertainty as to their own fate, since they had not been tried or even interrogated since their arrest, and did not know how long they were to be held. Munier proposed to Geneva that it take this problem under consideration and that it also provide the internees with books and a typewriter, at the expense of the Hebrew Committee of National Liberation. Munier had taken it upon himself to voice this suggestion to the Palestinian government, and the latter had offered no objection as long as the HCNL did not appear as the donor of the funds.[155]

On the same date that Munier submitted his report to Geneva – July 22, 1946 – the IZL blew up a wing of the British administration building in Jerusalem, the King David Hotel. The situation in Palestine was very tense during the following month – and the ICRC was having a difficult time as well. From July 26 to August 3, 1946, the Preliminary Conference of National Red Cross Societies for the Study of the Conventions and of Various Problems Relative to the Red Cross took place, providing a platform for an onslaught of criticism from the Communists regarding the ICRC's weak reactions to Nazi crimes. In the course of the debate on diversifying the ICRC's sources of financing, which was linked to the criticism concerning the organization's depen-

[153]Letter from Huber, Acting President, ICRC, to Bevin, Secretary of State for Foreign Affairs, Foreign Office, London, May 23, 1946 (AICRC. CR 240).
[154]Report by Jean Munier, ICRC Cairo, July 22, 1946 (AICRC, G.59/3/140).
[155]According to a letter from Roger Gallopin, ICRC Geneva, to ICRC London, Sept. 24, 1946 (AICRC, G.3/eb).

dence on Switzerland, Bernadotte suggested internationalizing the composition of the Committee. The British Red Cross expressed the view that the timing was bad for such a move, leading the ICRC to see the British society as an ally in the difficult period it was undergoing.

Was the ICRC trying to appease Great Britain? The fact remained that the ICRC was not doing anything about Munier's report. Munier himself, passing through Geneva, was concerned, and tried several times, without success, to see Gallopin, who directed ICRC operations. He was finally received by Gallopin's assistant, Kuhne, to whom he explained how much it was in the ICRC's interest to help these victims. Geneva gave him no answer – in fact, it did not react at all. On September 23, 1946, worried by his superiors' inertia, Munier wrote a letter to Gallopin, insisting that Geneva follow up on his report of July 22, 1946, 'in the interest of the International Committee, of our work here, and the concerned parties whom we have undertaken to assist.'[156] Munier did not explain in his letter what he meant by 'the interest of the International Committee,' although he placed it first.

In September, 1946, the ICRC was deeply concerned about the public attacks being made on it by the Yugoslav Red Cross, which accused it of conniving, through its silence, at Hitler's violations of international law. The ICRC felt unjustly accused, an outlook that also had a certain influence on its humanitarian approach in the case of the Asmara detainees.

Eligible and ineligible victims

At the end of September, 1946, having received Munier's letter begging for a follow-up to his June visit in Asmara, the ICRC decided to stop making allowances for Britain's difficulties in maintaining order in Palestine, and to pay serious attention to the question of the deported Palestinian Jews in Eritrea. It forwarded Munier's report to the Foreign Office, through the agency of its delegate in London, and at the same time, after some hesitation, sent a summary of the report to the HCNL. The ICRC was a little cautious in its contacts with Jewish organizations; it did not

[156]Letter from Munier, ICRC Cairo, concerning 'internés politiques juifs en Erythrée,' to Gallopin, ICRC Geneva, Sept. 23, 1946 (AICRC, G.8/43). [Translation: M.G.]

ACTING IN MANDATORY PALESTINE: MOTIVES AND STRATEGIES

want them to be too obvious,[157] perhaps because it feared losing Britain's trust.

In a letter to the Colonial Office on September 27, 1946, the ICRC did not ask to repeat the June 1946 visit to the Asmara camp; according to Munier's report, it explained, the material conditions of detention there were adequate. Sending parcels to the internees would be sufficient. The ICRC had one express request, however: that the detainees be tried by due process of law. If nothing could be proved against them, it suggested, they should be released or placed under house arrest.[158] For the first time during this affair, the ICRC brought up the fact that it had no legal basis to negotiate. Its members were intervening, it emphasized, solely in the name of 'purely humanitarian principles which, for so many years, have guided them in all they have undertaken in behalf of civilians of all nationalities, detained on the ground of public safety.'[159]

The formula was vague, but Frédéric Biéri, the ICRC's delegate in London, was instructed to back up the negotiations in person. The ICRC told him generally what he should say to the British: that although the ICRC's request had no basis in law, it was founded on the same humanitarian grounds that during the war had led the ICRC to approach the German authorities on behalf of the inmates of the concentration camps. The ICRC hoped the British authorities would give its request a more favorable reception than the Nazis had.[160] It thus based its negotiations on behalf of the Jewish detainees in Asmara on the same line of argument that it offered in response to the criticisms concerning its weak reactions to the plight of the concentration-camp victims.

The influence of the Committee's reasoning was also felt in the treatment of other victims of the Palestine conflict, but this time negatively. Here, instead of using its arguments as motives for acting, the ICRC used them as reasons not to act. In November, 1946, a Revisionist prisoners' aid organization, the Assire Zion Committee ('Prisoners of Zion,' in Hebrew), hopefully asked the

---

[157]According to note from von der Mühll, ICRC Cairo, to ICRC Geneva, Oct. 26, 1945 (AICRC, G.59/3/43).
[158]Letter from Gallopin, ICRC Geneva, to Secretary of State, Colonial Office, Sept. 27, 1946 (AICRC, G.59/3/43; CZA.14901).
[159]Ibid.
[160]Note from Gallopin, ICRC Geneva, to ICRC London, Sept. 24, 1946 (AICRC, G.3/3b).

ICRC to visit 36 Jewish women in Bethlehem prison, some of whom had been held since 1941. They, too, were suspected by the British of activism or collaboration with terrorists. The Assire Zion Committee was worried about their prison conditions, which it had reason to believe were deplorable; the Jewish women in the Bethlehem prison were mixed in with Arab criminal offenders.[161]

The ICRC proceeded to analyze the status of the Jewish prisoners in terms of the state of the draft laws, which at the time, following the example of the Tokyo Draft, covered only civilians of enemy nationality. The Jewish women in Bethlehem prison, of course, were Palestinian subjects and not civilians of foreign nationality. The ICRC therefore decided at the outset that the fate of the Jewish detainees in Bethlehem was not its concern, since they were citizens of the detaining country. It believed that if it were to intervene, the government of Palestine could accuse it of interfering in the country's internal affairs, especially since there was no international conflict. If these women had been foreign nationals, like the Jewish Palestinians interned in Eritrea, the ICRC might have been obliged to take a hand.[162] Although both Eritrea and Palestine were under British authority, the governments of those territories were two different entities, and therefore the Palestinians in Eritrea had to be considered as aliens in the hands of a foreign power – if not an 'enemy' power in the classic sense, since Palestine and Eritrea were not at war with each other.

---

[161]Letter from (Mrs.) F. Brickman, Assire Zion Committee, London, to Gallopin, ICRC Geneva, Nov. 14, 1946 (AICRC, G.59/7). The Assire Zion Committee also informed the ICRC that after Munier's visit to Asmara, on June 26, 1946, 54 detainees had escaped; of those, 34 had been recaptured and were going to be tried. It asked the ICRC to attend their trial and on that occasion to do its best to have the status of the internees clarified with regard to the type and length of their sentences. The ICRC refused; from the moment a regular procedure had been instituted, the matter was no longer the Red Cross's concern. According to note from ICRC London to ICRC Geneva, Oct. 24, 1946 (AICRC. B.59/3/140). See also note from ICRC Geneva to ICRC Cairo, Nov. 1, 1946 (AICRC, G.59/3/140).

[162]Note from ICRC Geneva to ICRC Cairo, Nov. 1, 1946 (AICRC, G.59/3/140). Also note from Munier, ICRC Cairo, to ICRC Geneva, Nov. 20, 1946 (AICRC, G.59/3).

ACTING IN MANDATORY PALESTINE: MOTIVES AND STRATEGIES

The criteria for action in the absence of a juridicial frame of reference

The ICRC's decision to aid the Palestinian detainees in Eritrea but not the Palestinian internees in Palestine illustrates the ICRC's confusion in dealing with so-called 'political' or 'security' detainees when it lacked a legal basis that might serve as a frame of reference. It was perfectly willing to aid political prisoners, but it was unwilling to stray too far from the Tokyo Draft. Conditioned by the reasoning of that draft convention, it continued to differentiate between foreign civilians and others, an orientation it retained until January 16, 1948, when, adapting new draft conventions to a preamble that provided for their application in civil wars and occupied territories, it finally dropped the distinction between aliens and nationals in cases of armed conflict or disturbances, putting them all into the category of 'protected persons' or civilians who were not nationals of the power under whose dominion they found themselves.[163] It must be admitted, too, that if the ICRC had agreed to protect these women, who were nationals of the detaining power, it would have been taking a position it did not take on behalf of those of the victims of the concentration camps who were in a similar legal situation; this would have weakened the arguments it used to defend itself against its critics.

The ICRC's perspective on both its mediation on behalf of the Jewish Palestinians in Eritrea and its refusal to intervene in favor of the Palestinian prisoners in Bethlehem was doubtless influenced by its crisis of credibility regarding the victims of Nazi camps and by its intention to use the precedent it had created during World War II – when it had achieved the partial, ad hoc application of the Tokyo Draft – in order to promote a future convention for the protection of enemy civilians.[164]

Trafford Smith of the Colonial Office, receiving the ICRC's solemn note of September 27, 1946, asking that the Eritrea

[163]See Chapter 1, p. 35.
[164]The choices the ICRC made in this respect indicate, in my interpretation, the limits the organization could impose on itself – despite the right of humanitarian initiative it reserved for itself in its own Statutes – when faced with categories of victims who were not potentially eligible for protection under the evolving international humanitarian law, such as the Jews under Nazi control in Germany or the countries allied or subordinate to the Reich during World War II.

detainees be tried, did his best to distinguish his government from the Nazis, rejecting the parallel the ICRC delegate had drawn between the deportees and the concentration-camp inmates in respect to the absence of legal grounds for ICRC intervention. Smith conveyed his government's pleasure that a humanitarian organization as impartial and neutral as the ICRC was had been able to report, following Munier's visit to Asmara in June 1946, that the detainees were being properly treated physically. The ICRC's evaluation came at an opportune moment, since, according to Smith, Britain was currently the target of attacks in the US press comparing the British camps where Jews were being held to the Nazi camp of Bergen-Belsen.[165]

Smith next admitted that the Jewish Palestinian prisoners were being held without any solid legal basis; for the most part, they had been thrown into the camps merely as suspects, and no valid evidence could have been produced against them in a court of law. They could not, however, simply be released, because – again according to Smith – the release of Jewish suspects would immediately arouse protests from the Arabs; they would demand the release of an equal number of Arab internees, which would put Britain in a very difficult position.[166] The Colonial Office asked the ICRC to be patient, but promised that its demands concerning the internees' right to trial would be studied.[167] By now it was October, 1946.

The ICRC waited five months to raise the issue again with the British government. In the meantime, from October, 1946 to March, 1947, the ICRC spoke to the Mandate authorities about the Asmara prisoners only for specific purposes. For example, after two detainees were murdered by Sudanese guards on January 17, 1946, the ICRC succeeded in having all the Sudanese guards in the camp replaced by English ones. In September, 1946, however, the Sudanese guards were reinstated.[168] The prisoners lived in fear. The ICRC again asked the British to replace the Sudanese guards with more trustworthy ones, and to permit its

---

[165]Note from Biéri, ICRC London, to ICRC Geneva, Oct. 23, 1946 (AICRC, G.59/3/140).
[166]Ibid.
[167]Ibid.
[168]Letter from Fowler V. Harper, HCNL Washington, to ICRC Geneva, Jan. 8, 1947 (AICRC, G.59/3/140).

delegate to make a second visit to the camp.[169] The Colonial Office prevaricated, just as it had over the question of the internees' legal status. The ICRC finally lost heart, as indicated by the message it sent its Cairo delegate at the beginning of February, 1947: 'For our part, we think the current situation in Palestine is too tense for us to take any more steps for some time, unless of course new incidents should occur that would justify such an intervention.'[170] The ICRC did not want Munier to visit the Asmara camp again until it received an answer to its note of September 27, 1946,[171] to the British authorities insisting on the internees' right to a trial.

1947: the ICRC changes course

At the end of February, 1947, the ICRC in Geneva began to change its policy. It decided there was no longer any need to wait for a response from the Colonial Office; it must, without hesitation, ask to make another visit to the Asmara camp.[172] I found no mention in the ICRC archives of any particularly serious incident at Asmara that would explain why the ICRC in Geneva changed course at this point. Another month passed, and on April 2, 1947, Geneva resumed its negotiations. The Committee urged Munier, its delegate in Cairo, to request permission to visit the detainees in Asmara. Biéri, its delegate in London, was instructed to demand the British government's response to the ICRC's note of September 27, 1946, asking that the detainees be tried with due process of law.

The ICRC's volte-face was not limited to the case of the Palestinian prisoners in Eritrea. The organization also wished to visit the Jewish men, women, and children who had been arrested and imprisoned in the British camps in Cyprus for having attempted to immigrate to Palestine in violation of the restrictions imposed by the White Paper of 1939. Finally, it decided to instruct one of

[169]Note from Munier, ICRC Cairo, to ICRC Geneva, Jan. 4, 1947 (AICRC, G.59/3/140), and note from Kuhne, ICRC Geneva, to ICRC Cairo, Feb. 4, 1947 (AICRC, G.59/3/140).
[170]Note from Kuhne, ICRC Geneva, to ICRC Cairo, Feb. 4, 1947 (AICRC, G.59/3/140). [Translation: M.G.]
[171]Ibid.
[172]Note from Kuhne, ICRC Geneva, to ICRC Cairo, Feb. 27, 1947 (AICRC, G.59/3/140).

its itinerant delegates, Charles Helbling, who was in Cairo, to try to visit the Jewish Palestinians interned for so-called 'reasons of security' in Palestine proper.[173] The ICRC was thus no longer limiting itself to the provisions of the Tokyo Draft, which offered protection only to foreign detainees, but had decided to expand its activities to include aid to Palestinian nationals, even though there was not even a draft convention to cover them.

Clearly, something new had happened since November, 1946, when the ICRC had been afraid to attempt any assistance to the Jewish Palestinian women imprisoned in Bethlehem. Something must have induced the ICRC suddenly, in March, 1947, to abandon the criterion of enemy nationality and come to the aid of Jewish Palestinian civilians imprisoned in Palestine by their own government, in addition to the foreign civilian detainees in Eritrea that it was already helping.

Mandatory Palestine on the brink of civil war

On February 18, 1947, Bevin announced Great Britain's intention of giving up its mandate for Palestine and handing the Palestine problem back to the United Nations. The confrontations between Britain and the Jewish extremists intensified. On March 2, 1947, the British high commissioner, Sir Alan Cunningham, imposed martial law on those regions of Palestine with a Jewish majority. On March 3, the Hebrew Committee of National Liberation called the ICRC's attention to the consequences of the British repression for the Jewish civilian population: theft, pillage, rape, economic asphyxiation. The HCNL compared the situation to that prevailing in Nazi Germany at the beginning of Hitler's persecutions, and asked the ICRC to send an official delegation to Mandatory Palestine.[174]

This, then, was what had changed the ICRC's outlook. Up until then, Peter Bergson, the president of the HCNL, had not requested the dispatch of an ICRC delegation to Palestine. The British army had not yet intervened on a massive scale to subdue the Jewish population on Palestinian territory; the situation could not really be described as armed conflict within the territory of

[173]ICRC, procès-verbal, Bureau meeting of March 27, 1947 (AICRC, no file number).
[174]Letter from Bergson, HCNL Paris, to ICRC Paris, March 3, 1947 (AICRC, G.59/7, G.59/I/G.C).

a state. From here on, however, the ICRC was dealing with a civil war or something close to it – the difference between 'civil war' and 'internal strife' was only a question of degree for the ICRC, and the way the organization defined the conflict did not affect the nature of the conflict in law. And, in a war within a sovereign territory – the main characteristic of a civil war – the combatants, and hence the potential victims, are not, for the most part, of enemy nationality.

Creating a precedent: acting in a civil war

On March 27, 1947, at a Bureau meeting devoted mostly to the subject of offering the ICRC's services in Indochina and Greece – both prey to 'civil wars' – Gloor declared that it 'would be a good thing if the intervention of the Hebrew Committee of National Liberation gave rise to an action on behalf of the victims of the civil war.'[175] It was not long now until April 14, when the Conference of Government Experts would begin work on revising the old conventions, drawing up a new one, and formulating an article which would extend the application of existing conventions to situations of civil war or any other internal war that might break out in the home or colonial territory of a contracting party. Meanwhile, the ICRC was already seeking to act in situations of civil war, partly for humanitarian reasons, but also, undoubtedly, in order to enrich its tradition in this field and create precedents that would facilitate the adoption of an article allowing the application of future conventions to civil war.

This was not always easy, however. In Greece, the Metaxas government was unwilling to authorize the ICRC to aid the partisans of General Markos.[176] In Indochina, the French High Commissioner in Saigon was willing to let it intervene in favor of French hostages taken by the Viet Minh, but not in favor of the Viet Minh.[177] The ICRC never made enough progress in either case to act as a neutral intermediary. However, given the calls for its internationalization or subordination to a multinational

---

[175]ICRC, procès-verbal, Bureau meeting of March 27, 1947 (AICRC, no file number).
[176]Letter from Tsaldaris, Government of Athens, to ICRC Geneva, March 8, 1947 (AICRC, G.44/53).
[177]ICRC, procès-verbal, Bureau meeting of March 27, 1947 (AICRC, no file number).

body, the ICRC could only be very eager to reaffirm the usefulness of its role as a neutral intermediary, a role it would no longer be able to play if the measures intended to reinforce its effectiveness should be adopted. In this context, the hope Bergson's letter aroused at the ICRC and its stimulating effect were all the more understandable.

Up to the end of February, 1947, when letters from the HCNL were filed in the ICRC archives they were given a file code that dated from World War II and signified 'Jews, deportees, hostages.' It was accompanied by one number indicating the category of the victim or petitioner and another number denoting the delegation concerned. Bergson's letter of March 3, 1947, requesting the dispatch of an ICRC delegation to Palestine was given a new file code, G.59/G.C., indicating 'war, Jews, civil war' (*guerre, Juifs, guerre civile*). That letter was the first item deposited in the account of the humanitarian enterprise the ICRC hoped to develop in the 'civil war' between Jews and British that was taking place in Mandatory Palestine. It was thus from March, 1947, on – not November, the date given by the *Revue internationale de la Croix-Rouge* – that the ICRC sought to act in the Mandatory Palestine conflict, which by its criteria was a civil war.

Aiding the Palestinian deportees

From then on, the ICRC made an increasingly greater distinction between the steps it was taking on behalf of the Jewish exiles and the measures it planned to take in the context of the 'civil war' in Palestine. In March, 1947, Great Britain transferred the Asmara prisoners to the Gil Gil camp in Kenya. The ICRC never did achieve its aim of getting them tried by due process, despite many appeals to the Colonial Office and the government of Palestine. The British kept citing the difficulty of determining the competent judiciary authority.

Munier visited the Gil Gil camp from October 9–29, 1947.[178]

---

[178]Letter from Munier, ICRC Cairo, to Government of Palestine, and annexed report, Nov. 10, 1947 (AICRC, G.59/3/140). Letter from Kuhne, ICRC Geneva, to HCNL Paris, Dec. 29, 1947 (AICRC, G.59/3/140). Letter from Kuhne, ICRC Geneva, to Assire Zion Committee, London, Jan. 5, 1948 (AICRC, G.59/3/140). Letter from Kuhne, ICRC Geneva, to ICRC Paris, Jan. 5, 1948 (AICRC, G.59/3/140).

ACTING IN MANDATORY PALESTINE: MOTIVES AND STRATEGIES

He had various cultural supplies sent to the internees, aid which at first was discreetly subsidized by the HCNL, as arranged with the government of Palestine. Later, other Jewish groups contributed as well, including Assirenu (Hebrew for 'our prisoners'), an organization for aid to Jewish prisoners which answered to the Va'ad Le'umi.[179] The latter body was the national council of the Palestinian Jewish community, composed of representatives of all the Jewish political factions in Palestine.

In May, 1948, the ICRC wrote in the *Revue internationale de la Croix-Rouge* that, following the United Nations vote on November 29, 1947, in favor of partition, it had begun to seek ways to act within the framework of the Palestine conflict.[180] It was then in the process of supporting an appeal by the Gil Gil detainees to the UN and the Mandatory authority so that those deportees might be allowed to return to their country before May 15, 1948, the date the British would probably leave, for strictly humanitarian reasons.[181] Since March, 1947, however, the protagonists of the war had changed: The struggle of the Jewish partisans against the Mandatory power had given way in December, 1947, to a bloody conflict between the Arabs of Palestine, who refused to share a land they considered their own, and the Jews, who agreed to partition in order to found a Jewish state.

At the beginning of April, 1948, the ICRC began its official activity, under circumstances that will be described shortly.[182] In May, 1948, the same month that the article in the *Revue internationale de la Croix-Rouge* was published, the ICRC's moral support for the claims of the Jewish Palestinian exiles was best concealed from the Arabs; such knowledge would undoubtedly have jeopardized the Arabs' trust, which the ICRC required in order to carry out its mission properly. This may help to explain why the ICRC did not publicly attribute its decision to act in Palestine to its relations with the HCNL. Indeed, in the years between 1945

---

[179]Letter from Kahany, Jewish Agency, Geneva, to ICRC Geneva, Aug. 20, 1947 (AICRC, G.59/3/140).

[180]CICR, 'Le Comité international de la Croix-Rouge en Palestine (décembre 1947 au 1er mai 1948),' *RICR* 353 (May 1948): 329.

[181]Letter from David de Traz, ICRC Geneva, to Secretary of State, Colonial Office, May 5, 1948 (AICRC, G.59/3/140). See also Letter Jewish Political Detainees in Exile, Gil Gil, Kenya, to United Nations Palestine Commission, Lake Success, USA, March, 19, 1948 (AICRC, G.59/3/140). Letter from Ralph J. Bunche, Principal Secretary, United Nations Palestine Commission, to Jewish Exiled Detainees, Gil Gil, Kenya, March 25, 1948 (CZA.S.25.7730).

[182]See Chapter 3, p. 128.

and 1948 the *Revue internationale de la Croix-Rouge* had no ambition to serve as a reference for historians. At the time it was above all an organ of 'propaganda' – to use the modern term – which allowed the ICRC, in particular, to convey selected messages illustrated by a vindicatory account of its actions to the readers of the publication: the National Red Cross Societies and the governments that had signed the humanitarian conventions.

The Jewish Palestinian exiles were not to see Palestine again before the end of the Mandate, despite the ICRC's support. They left Kenya via Sudan, with a British escort, in July, 1948. They feared for their safety in the wake of a rumor that Major Roy Farran, an Englishman who had assassinated Jewish extremists, was in Kenya, so at their request they were accompanied by an ICRC delegate, Nicolas Burckhardt.[183] He did not make the entire journey with them, however, for fear the Arabs should hear of the ICRC's role in organizing their repatriation,[184] but left them at Tobruk. The 254 exiles arrived in Tel Aviv on board the *Ocean Vigour* on July 11, 1948. The ICRC learned of it from the newspapers.[185] The Committee's actions on behalf of the exiled Jewish detainees, first in Eritrea and then in Kenya – which had begun the process leading up to the ICRC's decision to undertake a more generalized operation in Mandatory Palestine when the situation there developed into civil war – had finally reached their end, on the fringe of the Arab-Israeli war of 1948.

Objective: neutral intermediary

Upon receiving the HCNL's request in March, 1947, to establish an official delegation in Palestine, the ICRC sought the means to act as a neutral intermediary in the 'civil war' in Palestine, in the sense of Article VII of the International Red Cross Statutes. It began, that same month, by wondering whether the HCNL

[183]Nicolas Burckhardt was an ICRC delegate in London during World War II, and during the period that concerns us he represented the ICRC in the British zone of occupation in Germany.

[184]Note from David de Traz, ICRC Geneva, to ICRC Cairo, May 14, 1948 (AICRC, G.59/3/140).

[185]'Kenya Detainees Freed,' *The Times* [London] (July 8, 1948); 'Kenya Detainees Come Home, 254 Men Reach T.A. During Air Raid,' *Palestine Post* (July 13, 1948): 3 (AICRC, G.49/3/140).

ACTING IN MANDATORY PALESTINE: MOTIVES AND STRATEGIES

was truly representative of the Jewish community in Palestine, enough to negotiate for it in the contacts with Britain that the ICRC wanted to referee as a neutral intermediary. It therefore instructed its delegate in France, William Michel, who was a relation by marriage of Pierre Mendès-France and had a large Jewish acquaintance, to find out from the latter who the HCNL's sympathizers in Palestine were. He learned that this little organization in the US supported the IZL and Stern dissident movements in Mandatory Palestine, which were described to him as being 'of communist inspiration.'[186]

Since the HCNL appeared to be a very marginal organization, the ICRC decided to establish contact with the Jewish Agency, which was an official, representative body. It explained the matter very openly to the vice-president of the HCNL, Samuel Merlin, who was staying at the Lutetia Hotel in Paris.[187] Merlin promised to convey the ICRC's wishes to the Jewish Agency, and in mid-April, 1947, he brought back the response: The Jewish Agency refused to make common cause with the HCNL.[188] Consequently, Merlin advised the ICRC to take up the issue of the detainees in Cyprus – such a matter would be likely to interest the Jewish Agency.[189]

On May 14, 1947, Andrei Gromyko declared in the United Nations that the USSR would follow with great interest the decisions taken in respect of Palestine. The fact that Palestine was attracting attention from both sides of the Cold War spurred the ICRC's efforts to intervene there as a neutral intermediary. Since Biéri, the ICRC's London delegate, Michel, the Paris delegate, and Helbling, the Near East delegate, all happened to be in Geneva at the time, the ICRC seized the opportunity to devise a concerted plan of action. On May 16, 1947, it decided to send Helbling to the Near East. Helbling was to try to visit the camps for illegal immigrants in Cyprus and the camps for Jewish Palestinian detainees in Palestine itself. He was also supposed to go to see the British high commissioner in Palestine, Sir Alan

---

[186]ICRC, procès-verbal, Bureau meeting of March 27, 1947 (AICRC, no file number).

[187]Procès-verbal (March 26, 1947) of meeting between Roth, ICRC Paris, and Merlin, HCNL Paris, March 26, 1947, Paris (AICRC, G.59/I/G.C.).

[188]Procès-verbal (undated) of meeting between Roth, ICRC Paris, and Merlin, HCNL Paris, April 15, 1948, Paris (AICRC, G.59/I/G.C.).

[189]Ibid.

Cunningham, and ask him whether ICRC intervention would be desirable, and if so, in what form.[190]

The matter was all the more urgent to the ICRC because in Greece one of its delegates, who had been striving to intervene on behalf of the Communist partisans, had been questioned about what the ICRC was doing in Palestine.[191] Moreover, in May, 1947, the ICRC was in a better position than it had been in March to undertake measures in the context of a civil war: The Geneva Conference of Government Experts of April 14–30, 1947 had recommended the insertion of an article in the revised and the new conventions that would extend the application of their principles, on condition of reciprocity, to civil wars and other internal wars on the home or colonial territory of a contracting party.[192]

During the second trimester of 1947, while the ICRC awaited news from Helbling, the situation in Palestine continued to deteriorate. Since 1946, when the British had captured IZL member Dov Gruner, condemning him to death in January, 1947, Britain and the Jewish extremists had been locked in a cycle of reprisals. Britain had pronounced death sentences on several other Jewish combatants, and the IZL had managed, by dint of taking hostages, to get them postponed. The IZL asked the British to grant their captives the status of prisoners of war, but to no avail. On April 14, 1947, while the IZL was preparing to attack the Jerusalem prison and liberate the condemned men, Britain forestalled the rescue by quietly transferring four prisoners to the Saint Jean prison in Acre and hanging them there on the night of April 15–16. The reprisals resumed with all the more ferocity, culminating on July 12, 1947, with the IZL's capture of two British sergeants, whom it threatened to kill if the death sentences against several other IZL members were not revoked. At the HCNL's request, the ICRC considered intervening, but it was too late: On July 29, Britain hanged two members of the IZL, and on July 30 the IZL hanged the two British sergeants.

---

[190]ICRC, procès-verbal, Bureau meeting of May 16, 1947 (AICRC, no file number).
[191]Ibid.
[192]ICRC, *Report on the Work of the Conference of Government Experts for the Study of the Conventions for the Protection of War Victims*, Geneva, April 14–26, 1947, p. 8.

ACTING IN MANDATORY PALESTINE: MOTIVES AND STRATEGIES

Reasons to approach the Jewish Agency

Between mid-June and mid-July, still without news from Helbling, the ICRC decided to approach the Jewish Agency directly – and not only because of the dramatic escalation of tension in Mandatory Palestine. During that period the ICRC had been considering the problem of expanding its sources of funds and the solutions it would propose in Stockholm. It had to be able to continue its activities, and sought money from all sides, wanting to escape from its financial dependence on Switzerland. It was no longer willing to undertake new operations without having funds at its disposal in advance. Through its delegation in Paris, it contacted the HCNL and offered to visit the detainees in Gil Gil, but requested financial assistance, since it could not expect any from the British. On July 9, 1947, the HCNL refused the offer.[193]

The ICRC – in the person of Kuhne, who was assisting Gallopin with matters relating to prisoners – next turned to the representative of the Jewish Agency Executive in Geneva, Menahem Kahany. Unaware – probably deliberately – of the divisions in the Palestinian Jewish community, Kuhne told Kahany about the ICRC's intervention on behalf of the Palestinian exiles interned in Kenya, and explained that the organization would like to send a delegate to visit Gil Gil, but lacked the necessary funds. He went on to ask whether the Jewish Agency would make a contribution to the ICRC or else put it in touch with 'an Israelite organization' that could assist it in its efforts to 'improve the lot of the Israelite victims of the current events.'[194]

Kahany answered that the Jewish Agency had protested repeatedly to the British government in Palestine and in London against the deportation of Palestinian citizens 'whatever the offense of which they are suspected or have been convicted.'[195] The Jewish Agency considered that these deportations violated the constitutional law of the Mandate; Palestinian citizens should

---

[193] According to note from Kuhne, ICRC Geneva, to William Michel, ICRC Paris, July 9, 1947 (AICRC, G.8/51).
[194] Confidential letter from Kuhne, ICRC Geneva, to Kahany, Jewish Agency, Geneva, July 10, 1947 (AICRC, G.59/3/140 and B.59/7). See also note from Kahany, JA Geneva Office, 'strictly confidential,' to Executive of the JA, Jerusalem, July 14, 1947 (CZA.S.25.3933). (Translation: M.G.)
[195] Letter from Kahany, Jewish Agency, Geneva, to Kuhne, ICRC Geneva, July 14, 1947 (AICRC, G. 3/143 and CZA.S.25.3933). (Translation: M.G.)

be tried in their own country. According to Kahany, however, the Jewish Agency was afraid to take part in an action, even a humanitarian one, that would implicitly recognize an illegal deed committed by the British administration. It also could not risk associating itself in any way with the IZL or the Stern group.[196] For these reasons, the Jewish Agency preferred not to assist the ICRC with its action in aid of the Gil Gil detainees – even though, Kahany assured Kuhne, the Agency sympathized with the Red Cross's aim. He proposed to put the ICRC in touch with the Va'ad Le'umi.[197]

Thus began the relationship of trust that the ICRC had wished to establish with an official Jewish authority in Palestine in order to achieve its ultimate objective of acting as a neutral intermediary on all the territory of the Mandate; but now that relationship had to be consolidated. The results of the Helbling mission were not helpful. Helbling had inspected the Latrun camp for Jewish Palestinian detainees in Palestine, but he had been accompanied by a British officer and had been unable to follow the preferred ICRC practice of speaking with the detainees alone.[198] In Cyprus, he had received permission from a British army officer to make an informal tour of the Famagusta internment camp for illegal immigrants, but had managed to get only a quick look around.[199] At the end of November, 1947, the ICRC decided not to take any further action regarding the Cyprus detainees, since it could not act as a neutral intermediary in the matter.[200] This, however, was undoubtedly not its only reason; in the meantime, an opportunity had arisen for the ICRC to undertake a new operation likely to involve all the Jewish interests and Britain as well.

The tragedy of the *Exodus 47*: an opportunity for the ICRC

In mid-July, 1947, when the ICRC was still worrying about Helbling's mission, of which it had had no news, a drama took place which increased tension in Palestine still more: the saga of the

[196]Ibid.
[197]Ibid.
[198]ICRC, procès-verbal, Bureau meeting of July 24, 1947 (AICRC, no file number).
[199]Ibid.
[200]Note from Munier, ICRC Cairo, to ICRC Geneva, Nov. 15, 1947 (AICRC, G.59/3/140).

ACTING IN MANDATORY PALESTINE: MOTIVES AND STRATEGIES

Exodus 47. A group of refugees who had survived the systematic massacre of European Jews had embarked for Palestine on the ship *Exodus 47*, seeking a free life. Their voyage had been organized secretly by the Mossad le-Aliyah Bet, which answered to the Jewish Agency and the armed forces under its control. After harassment by British warships during the voyage, the *Exodus 47* was attacked off the Gaza coast by six British destroyers and then boarded. The passengers of the ship, after vain attempts to resist with the pathetic means at their disposal, were taken under British escort to Haifa, where they arrived on July 18, 1947. The 4,500 Jewish passengers – including old people, women, and children – were brutally transferred to three Liberty ships of the British navy, the *Runnymede Park*, the *Ocean Vigour*, and the *Empire Rival*, and shipped back in the direction of the French Mediterranean coast where they had embarked.[201]

Several boatloads of Jewish refugees had already tried, during and since World War II, to reach the safety of Palestine, but had been prevented from doing so by the British, who faithfully implemented the provisions of Chamberlain's White Paper. Many potential immigrants met their deaths as a result. In 1947, the pathetic and courageous attempt of the *Exodus 47* immigrants and their inhuman deportation stood out in particular. Both the local and international press were interested in the story, especially since the future of the British Mandate in Palestine might be at stake: The members of the United Nations Special Commission of Palestine (UNSCOP) had been present when the British turned the Jewish survivors back at Haifa. In the meantime, while all this was happening, the escalation of executions in Palestine was about to culminate in the IZL's reprisals against the two British sergeants taken hostage on July 12, 1947. Politically Britain was at a delicate juncture; to public opinion, it seemed to be incapable of maintaining order in the territory for which it was responsible.

At sea, spokesmen for the immigrants declared that the latter would not set foot on any shore but that of Palestine. Bevin tried to persuade the French to make the Jews disembark on French soil, but on July 24, 1947, François Mitterand, the minister of war veterans, publicly announced his government's position: France

---

[201]For a detailed account of this episode, see, for example, Jacques Derogy, *La loi du Retour: la secrète et véritable histoire de l'Exodus* (Paris: Fayard, 1970), 439 pp.

would take in the immigrants, but not against their will. He made this declaration while the immigrants were still at sea and no one yet knew where they were to land. The press and the general public waited with bated breath.

Such was the atmosphere when, that same July 24, the HCNL asked the ICRC in Paris to send delegates to the as yet unknown port where the rejected immigrants would make land. The ICRC delegation in Paris requested Geneva's approval, and since an immediate decision was necessary, Gallopin gave his authorization without consulting his colleagues.[202] At the same time, in the French capital, William Michel contacted the French foreign minister, who agreed to an ICRC mission – without, however, telling the organization where the ships were expected to land.[203] Two days later, on July 26, it was the turn of the British ambassador in Paris to endorse an ICRC aid operation to help the refugees.[204]

The ICRC already had a representative for Bouches-du-Rhône in Marseilles, René Porchet. He was immediately mobilized for the mission, together with a colleague, Max-Henri Huber, called in from Bordeaux, where he was in charge of organizing convoys of German prisoners of war released by the French for repatriation. The ICRC was expecting to receive the immigrants on French soil and escort them to the reception centers that France had set aside for them. René Roth, an ICRC delegate in Paris, joined his colleagues in Marseilles and assumed the leadership of the operation.

Many charitable organizations, Jewish and otherwise, were already on the spot, and the ICRC was thus, at that juncture, neither the only one that could act by the rules it set for itself, nor a neutral intermediary. It joined together with Entr'aide française, the French relief society officially in charge of arranging accommodation, food, and medical care for the immigrants.[205]
On July 28, 1947, the ICRC delegates learned that the ships were

---

[202]ICRC, procès-verbal, Bureau meeting of July 24, 1947 (AICRC, no file number).

[203]Letter from Michel, ICRC Paris, to Raymond Bousquet, Minister of Foreign Affairs, Paris, July 24, 1947 (AICRC, G.59/5/ex).

[204]Letter from Coulson, British Embassy, Paris, to Michel, ICRC Paris, July 26, 1947 (AICRC, G.59/5/ex).

[205]Roth, 'Procès-verbal de la réunion à la Préfecture des Bouches-du-Rhône le 27 juillet 1949 à 15 heures,' Marseilles, July 28, 1947 (AICRC, G.59/5/ex).

ACTING IN MANDATORY PALESTINE: MOTIVES AND STRATEGIES

expected the following day[206] at Port de Bouc, chosen because the design of the harbor did not allow ships to dock; they were obliged to lie at anchor offshore. This was supposed to prevent the ships from being assailed by journalists or infiltrated by Mossad agents.

The head of the ICRC mission, Roth, immediately went to see the British consul-general at Marseilles. He took it upon himself to try to dissuade the consul from having the immigrants disembarked by force, if that was indeed what he had in mind; if the British were to elect such a course of action, Roth warned, the ICRC would be obliged to protest.[207] Roth also asked permission to board the ships, but the consul could not authorize this, since, he claimed, it was not up to him, but rather the captain, Colonel Gregson.[208]

On July 29, 1947, as soon as the ships arrived, the French authorities reiterated their offer of asylum for the immigrants, but the latter declined, and requested a visit from the ICRC.[209] Roth reacted with caution. The ICRC was not in the habit of responding directly to appeals from the victims themselves; it usually approached the belligerents, generally on its own initiative, in order to offer its services as a neutral intermediary. This permitted it to preserve its neutrality and to exercise some control over the possible political implications of its proceedings. Roth feared that boarding the ships in the capacity of delegation head would make whatever he said binding on the ICRC; he preferred to reserve enough room to maneuver so that he could refer questions back to Geneva as necessary.[210]

Thus it was Porchet, Roth's subordinate, who boarded the leading ship, the *Runnymede Park*. There he was told that the captain, the only person who could authorize him to make an official inspection of the premises, was absent. He therefore made an informal visit, and noted that the immigrants were being treated

[206]Roth, 'Procès-verbal d'entretien de la réunion à la Préfecture du Rhône à Marseille, le 28 juillet 1947 à 17–neuf heures' (sic), n.p., erroneously dated Aug. 28, 1947. Probable date July 28, 1947 (AICRC, G.59/5/ex).

[207]Roth, 'Procès-verbal d'entretien du 28 juillet 1947 au Consulat général de Grand Bretagne à Marseille entre M. Kay, Consul général, et M. Roth, délégué du CICR,' Marseilles, Aug. 28, 1947 (AICRC, no file number).

[208]Ibid.

[209]Ibid.

[210]Roth, 'Rapport sur la mission du CICR à Port de Bouc les 29 et 30 juillet 1947, en relation avec les immigrants illégaux israélites du SS Exodus 1947,' n.p., Aug. 28, 1947 (AICRC, no file number).

like captives in bad camps, with a cruelty unjustified by security requirements. Men, women, and children were locked in cages, packed in behind barbed wire in unbearably crowded conditions. The summer sun of southern France overheated the metal interior of the ships. The immigrants had no mattresses – nothing but a blanket apiece to sleep on. To pressure them into leaving the ships, the British had informed them that the meal served to them that day, July 29, 1947, would be the last. But the immigrants were unshakable: They would disembark only in Palestine.[211] In the face of their determination, Roth sent Huber, the delegate from Bordeaux in charge of repatriation convoys, back to Geneva to report to the ICRC.

On July 31, 1947, Huber arrived in Geneva and reported to Gallopin, the ICRC official in charge of matters involving civilian prisoners and internees (and also, as noted, an observer on the Special Commission). That same evening Gallopin telephoned Kahany to brief him on the activities of the ICRC delegates. Kahany had already been informed by an envoy of the American Joint Distribution Committee who was at Port de Bouc. The envoy had suggested that the ICRC dispatch neutral doctors, preferably Swiss, to the ships as quickly as possible, in case they put out to sea again for a new destination. Kahany endorsed this idea, and asked the ICRC to consider it. Gallopin promised to act quickly.[212] The ICRC had finally achieved its aim, a mandate from an official body representing the Jews of Palestine; and from the moment it received the Jewish Agency's request, it cut its ties with the Hebrew Committee of National Liberation, except in matters pertaining to the Kenya internees.

In order to act as a neutral intermediary and to carry out the mission desired by the Jewish Agency, the ICRC required British consent. Gallopin wasted no time in instructing Biéri, in London, to request permission from the British authorities. It was now August 1, the Swiss national holiday. But Biéri exerted himself, and was able to inform the ICRC that same day that the Foreign Office and the Colonial Office had both given their consent. However, the British wanted to be sure of the ICRC men; they

[211]Ibid.
[212]According to letter from Kahany, JA Geneva, marked 'confidential,' to Shertok, JA Tel Aviv, Aug. 1, 1947 (CZA.S.25.3893).

were afraid to let strangers go on board, because members of the Haganah might seize the opportunity to infiltrate the immigrants and encourage them to persist in their refusal to disembark in France.[213] Biéri reassured the London officials and promised in addition that the written reports of the delegates authorized to visit the ships would be addressed exclusively to the ICRC in Geneva, and would not be leaked to the press.[214]

The British then imposed a condition that demanded a great concession on the ICRC's part: If the new destination of the ships – which were soon to leave Port de Bouc – did not suit the Jews, the ICRC delegates were not to mediate between the Jewish Agency and Great Britain.[215] At the price of renouncing that cherished role of the ICRC, Biéri seized on the desired authorization and, in order not to lose any time, informed Paris even before reporting back to Geneva.[216] The smooth working relationship between all the ICRC employees was evident.

Now three doctors had to be found to carry out the mission. Pierre Gaillard, the Geneva official responsible for recruiting delegates and allocating them among the various ICRC delegations, chose Roland Marti, head of the ICRC's medical and relief divisions. Marti was one of the rare ICRC administrators who had had experience 'in the field' and who knew how to reconcile the operations in aid of victims with the demands of ICRC doctrine and tradition. He had carried out his first mission in the Spanish Civil War, and he had subsequently directed ICRC activities in Berlin during World War II. A fervent exponent of the Red Cross principle of impartiality, he had just finished raising funds among the Germans for the ICRC operation on behalf of German prisoners of war, relying on his own personal reputation.[217] Marti was aware of the ICRC's general objectives, but he was not a diplomat.

Two other doctors, Drs. Georges Dubois and Pierre Ducommun, who had never worked for the ICRC before, completed the team, but only for the short term. The arrangement was therefore

---

[213]Note from Biéri, ICRC London, to ICRC Geneva, Aug. 1, 1947 (AICRC, G.59/5/ex).

[214]Ibid.

[215]According to letter from Gallopin, ICRC Geneva, to ICRC London, Aug. 6, 1947 (AICRC, G.59/5/ex).

[216]Note from Biéri, ICRC London, to ICRC Geneva, Aug. 1, 1947 (AICRC, G.59/5/ex).

[217]On this subject, see AICRC, G.8/51.

temporary, but on Aug. 1, the ICRC was still able to respond affirmatively to Kahany's request, formulating its acceptance in such a way as to cast the Jewish Agency in the role of petitioner, on the one hand, and to emphasize the ICRC's quick reaction time, on the other: 'In accordance with the measures you have formulated in the name of the Jewish Agency,' the ICRC 'has taken emergency measures to obtain the assistance of three Swiss doctors.'[218] By drawing attention to the ICRC's speedy response to the Jewish Agency's request, Gallopin reaffirmed an ability the organization would lose should any unfortunate changes be made in its composition, or in the structure of the International Red Cross.

Gallopin informed the Jewish Agency of the agreement reached with Britain: The ICRC delegates would have 'as their mission to board the ships carrying the Israelite refugees and to accompany them to the destination assigned to them by the British authorities.'[219] They would not be responsible for sanitary conditions on the ships. They would be able only to assist the passengers to the best of their ability.[220]

Despite the restrictions imposed by Britain, the ICRC was close to the position it had sought, that of a neutral intermediary mediating between the Jewish Agency and the Mandatory power on behalf of the victims of the 'civil war' in Palestine. It might win Britain's trust if its delegates scrupulously respected the rules the Colonial Office had laid down for their activities.

The ICRC delegates' mission in aid of the Jewish boat refugees – although in spirit as close as possible to the good Samaritan gesture Henry Dunant had made for the wounded and dying soldiers of the battle of Solferino – was an exceptional one for the ICRC, whose purpose was not to offer direct aid to war victims, but to act as a neutral intermediary between belligerents. It had decided to assist civilian populations solely in situations where it was the only agent able to act; yet in the *Exodus 47* case, Britain did not wish the ICRC to act as a neutral intermediary on behalf of the refugees, nor was the ICRC the only body able to help them. According to ICRC doctrine, the assistance to the *Exodus 47* refugees in Port du Bouc should have been provided

---

[218]Letter from Gallopin, ICRC Geneva, to Kahany, Jewish Agency, Geneva, Aug. 1, 1947 (AICRC, G.59/5/ex and CZA.S.25.3893). [Translation: M.G.]
[219]Ibid.
[220]Ibid.

by the League of Red Cross Societies. The Committee only raised this issue within the organization after the fact, during an internal meeting. Similarly, it pointed out that if the Depage plan had been in effect, the ICRC would have had to refer its decisions to a higher council and would never have been able to respond as quickly as it had to the Jewish Agency's request.[221] This was one more reason to resist any plan involving supervision of ICRC activities by an international body such as the Standing Commission of the International Conference of the Red Cross.

Despite the ICRC's haste to follow up the Jewish Agency's request, Gallopin did not forget to broach the question of financing the mission at the outset.[222] In his telephone conversation with Gallopin on July 31, 1947, Kahany promised financial assistance from the Jewish Agency in the form of a donation. It will be recalled that a month earlier, in June 1947, the ICRC had decided to diversify its sources of funding in order to reduce its dependence on Switzerland.

Between August 1 and 16, 1947, Britain sought a solution to the problem of what to do with the three boatloads of illegal immigrants. On August 21, 1947, Trafford Smith of the Colonial Office officially informed the Jewish Agency of Britain's decision: The illegal immigrants would be taken back to Germany, near Hamburg, in the British occupation zone.[223]

Meanwhile, the ICRC doctors, still unaware of the ships' destination, were evaluating the refugees' health needs, coordinating their activity with the local French and British authorities, as well as with other humanitarian organizations present in Port de Bouc. They prepared medicines and provisions. On August 5[224] Marti, the head of the mission, took his place on the leading ship, the *Runnymede Park*, where he shared a cabin with three British officers. Ducommun embarked on the *Empire Rival* and Dubois on the *Ocean Vigour*. The British then ordered the Jewish

---

[221]ICRC, procès-verbal, Bureau meeting of Aug. 13, 1947 (AICRC, no file number).
[222]According to letter from Kahany, JA Geneva, marked 'confidential,' to Shertok, JA Tel Aviv, Aug. 1, 1947 (CZA.S.25.3893).
[223]Derogy, *op. cit.*, p. 318.
[224]ICRC, 'Jewish Refugees at Marseilles,' press release no. 349, Geneva, Aug. 5, 1947 (Press Release Collection, ICRC Library).

doctors who had been allowed on board to get off the ships.[225] The ICRC was expecting its doctor-delegates' mission to be relatively short.[226]

Until the ships moved out into the open sea, Marti and his colleagues could move from one vessel to the next. But each of them was alone, confronting, in the name of the ICRC, the plight of the victims for whom they had accepted medical responsibility. Marti reported to Geneva from Port de Bouc. The food situation was acceptable, due mostly to the efforts of Entr'aide française. But sanitary conditions were disgraceful – so much so that they actually 'frightened'[227] the doctor, accustomed though he was in his profession to witnessing the suffering engendered by war. Despite 'attempts at cleaning and the emigrants' desire to keep in good health,'[228] Marti wrote, the refugees suffered from boils, impetigo, and abscesses caused by dirt and accumulated garbage. Some 60 percent of the patients had been stricken by dysentery, while the others suffered from constipation. The doctors also reported colds, long-standing intestinal and liver problems, gynecological complaints, eye infections, fevers of unknown origin. Yet – according to what Marti had been told on board – the Mossad had allowed only those emigrants healthy enough to withstand the voyage to embark on the *Exodus 47*.[229]

The ICRC doctors had nowhere to put their patients except the hold. On the *Empire Rival* and the *Ocean Vigour*, sick refugees lay on three-tiered 'beds',[230] with others sleeping on blankets between the bunks. It was difficult to isolate contagious patients; the doctors separated them from the other patients simply by hanging disinfected blankets between them. Assisted by Jewish nurses, the ICRC doctors went through the holds looking for sick refugees who had hidden in fear of being forced off the ship, and checked over the unceasing procession of patients, sending the serious cases to the 'hospital' in the hold.[231]

---

[225] Roland Marti, 'Rapport sur la mission médicale du CICR à bord de l'Exodus 47,' Marseilles, Aug. 12, 1947 (AICRC, G.59/5/ex).
[226] ICRC, procès-verbal, Bureau meeting of Aug. 14, 1947 (AICRC, no file number).
[227] Marti, 'Rapport sur la mission médicale.'
[228] Ibid.
[229] Ibid.
[230] The quotation marks are Marti's.
[231] Ibid.

ACTING IN MANDATORY PALESTINE: MOTIVES AND STRATEGIES

Should the *Exodus 47* refugees be abandoned?

At the beginning of August, while Marti and his colleagues were attending the suffering refugees of the *Exodus 47* – and having a very hard time of it themselves – in Geneva the ICRC was thinking about civilian populations, in particular those of Eastern Europe. The Regional Conference of Eastern European Red Cross Societies was soon to meet in Belgrade. The ICRC planned to send Ernest Gloor, one of its two vice-presidents, and Frédéric Siordet, the ICRC advisor on Soviet affairs, to the conference in the capacity of observers. Ideally, the two men would have liked to take the opportunity to tour the Balkan countries, in order to demonstrate the ICRC's concern for the suffering of the civilian populations of those regions. The ICRC hoped to assist the civilian inhabitants of states that had rejected the Marshall Plan.[232] For such a mission, however, it also required someone able to evaluate the local population's requirements in the way of provisions and medical aid. Naturally the ICRC thought of Marti in his capacity of head of the ICRC's relief and medical divisions. It had just heard that the British ships were going to set sail for 'somewhere in the antipodes,'[233] and it could not do without Marti for what might prove to be a long time, given the responsibilities of his office.[234]

On August 12, 1947, Gallopin telephoned Marti and told him to hurry back to Geneva so that he could prepare to leave for the Balkans.[235] The Balkan mission was very important to the ICRC in view of its relations with the Communists and the criticisms that had been leveled at it. Helping the Jewish refugees from the *Exodus 47* was politically much less important to the ICRC, since it could not play the role of a neutral intermediary on their behalf. In terms of the evolution of humanitarian law, the case of these refugees did not offer any particular interest. However, the consequences of Marti's departure would be particularly serious for the sick refugees, since Dubois and Ducommun were also obliged to return to Geneva because of private commitments.

[232]ICRC, procès-verbal, Bureau meeting of July 24, 1947 (AICRC, no file number).
[233]ICRC, procès-verbal, Bureau meeting of Aug. 14, 1947 (AICRC, no file number).
[234]Ibid.
[235]Ibid.

Marti understood the ICRC's political reasons, but he refused to return to Geneva. He emphasized the fact that he and his colleagues had made statements to the emigrants that were tantamount to promises made by the ICRC:

> We told them that our mission was purely medical, and we assured them of the sympathy the ICRC feels for them and of its regret that it was not able to assist them more in Germany, for most of them have been through concentration camps. What makes these people deserving of pity is their odyssey which has lasted for years, years of suffering, they've been killed, cremated, interned, from all the regions of the East. Absolutely piteous. And seeing them behind iron bars makes us absolutely dedicated. We have no need of stimulants. And despite everything, the emigrants are correct, clean, very disciplined. They are organized into groups, by schools, orphans put under the supervision of teachers. All day long you can see the schools studying on the decks, writing with chalk on the black parts of the ships, reciting, singing. An extraordinary example. . . .[236]

Marti was thus determined to continue what he had undertaken in the name of the ICRC, especially since, according to him, the emigrants did not want to disembark anywhere except in Palestine – which they spoke of constantly – and the sickest patients among them were likely to die if they did not get off the ship.[237] Yet by August 12, the date he wrote his letter to the ICRC, Marti had not managed to persuade a single patient to go ashore. Two serious cases arose, acute nephritis and acute appendicitis, but Marti was not able to have the patients evacuated to a hospital. In such situations, 'each case must be discussed with the ship committee, which imposes its decision on the family. There are hours of debate while they care for the patients. They want to wait to the last possible moment.'[238] Marti could not think of abandoning this mission:

> I began the one in Spain which lasted three years, the one in Germany which lasted six years. I would like to finish this one, which will not take long to resolve. I understand

---

[236]Marti, 'Rapport sur la mission médicale.' [Translation: M.G.]
[237]Ibid.
[238]Ibid.

very well the reasons calling me to Geneva, but despite everything I have the impression that this card is a good card, and we must work to the end, for problems will arise as soon as the weather changes and the emigrants find out that they are not leaving for Palestine.[239]

The ICRC was interested primarily in the political opportunities each action might offer it to serve as a neutral intermediary, promote the evolving international law, and improve relations with the Communist East; for the advancement of these ends, it could contemplate sacrificing a humanitarian operation already in progress. The ICRC delegate, in contrast, responded as the advocate of the victims and of the ideal he served. Generally speaking, the ICRC's action on behalf of the Jewish refugees of the *Exodus 47* was the result of the dialectic between headquarters and the field. This is not to say that this particular action was not carried out within the framework of a policy, as Marti indicated in his letter to the Committee: 'Our policy must be followed,' he wrote, 'and the internees must not be given the impression that the ICRC is already getting tired, that we are not in a position to give them doctors for more than two weeks.'[240]

Geneva gave in, but the Committee asked the Jewish Agency for an additional contribution, since the doctors' mission would last longer than anticipated.[241] The ICRC decided to postpone the mission to Central and Eastern Europe for a few weeks so that Marti could join it. Dubois and Ducommun returned to Switzerland and were replaced, on August 15, 1947, by two young doctors on their first mission, Michel Doret and Erwin Wildi. They set off on the adventure, apparently without knowing where the ships were bound.[242] In Geneva, according to Doret, there was talk of Cyprus or Kenya.[243]

[239]Ibid.
[240]Ibid.
[241]According to letter from Gallopin, ICRC Geneva, to Kahany, Jewish Agency, Geneva, Aug. 1, 1947 (AICRC, G.59/5/ex and CZA.S.25.3893). On Aug. 28, 1947, the Jewish Agency paid the ICRC the sum of 3,000 Swiss francs, specifying that it was a first installment. Subsequently, the ICRC demanded additional sums, stressing that the operation had taken longer than anticipated. The Jewish Agency was slow to pay, and when Israel became independent, the provisional government did not assume responsibility for the Jewish Agency's promises. It took the ICRC months to collect the anticipated payments – which aroused some resentment at the ICRC.
[242]Author's interview with Michel Doret, March 7, 1989, Geneva.
[243]Ibid.

From Port de Bouc to Hamburg

On August 22, 1947, in the presence of the ICRC doctors, an English officer boarded the ships and announced to the 'caged up' Jews (to use Doret's phrase) – men, women, children, elderly – that they could get off the boat in France. If they refused, they would be taken back to Germany, to Hamburg, where they would be interned in DP camps. Britain would give them 18 hours to decide. Doret, who was present, noted down the victims' reaction in his personal mission journal: 'No distress, but their singing at night on the deck is more richly charged [*fournis*] than ever.'[244] The ICRC doctors tried one last time to persuade the sickest refugees to let themselves be cared for in France. When the final moment came, only a few dozen people – ill, exhausted, or accompanying patients – debarked.

The British warships then put out to sea with some 4,500 Jews still on board, Jews who, after surviving the horrors of the Nazi camps, had endured in Port de Bouc stifling heat, overcrowding, uncertainty, imprisonment, armed surveillance, suspicion, illness. Now, in these conditions – inflicted by the British in order to assert the policy of the White Paper – they were on their way to Hamburg. Each ship carried an ICRC doctor (who could communicate with his colleagues by radio) and a British doctor. Restricted to a purely medical role, the ICRC doctors could make no objections of principle.

Doret is the only one who has provided us with a daily account written at the time the events took place. On board the *Empire Rival*, he kept a ship's log, drew the vessels, and apparently bore with fortitude the tension between his emotional response on one hand and the duty to remain neutral on the other. He asked himself no questions about the political implications of the adventure, but was content to set down a day-to-day account of misery, effort, fatigue, and the friendships he formed, especially with the Jewish nurses, in that wearing but cohesive environment. Wildi, on the *Ocean Vigour*, proved less resilient, and allowed himself to express indignation in his end-of-mission report to the ICRC. The only duty of the British soldiers on board, assisted by Arabs and Sudanese, he said, was to keep

---

[244]Doret manuscript, *Mission Croix-Rouge*, original, 43 pp., p. 8. See also Derogy, p. 350, who gives this quote, but has taken the liberty of replacing the word 'fournis' with 'pathétiques' (pathetic). [Translation: M.G.]

watch on the cages where the Jews were shut up, and their only other occupation was 'ironing and mending their clothes, biting their nails, and, the last three days before the ships arrived in Hamburg, getting their truncheons ready,' scraping them 'with old razor blades, sanding the metal blades on an old grindstone they had unearthed somewhere on board, and making the wooden part shine with shoe polish.' Among them, Wildi commented, 'there were some who reacted normally.'[245] Out of 'spite, jealousy, or anti-Semitism,'[246] he continued, bandages were thrown into the sea, medicines and syringes were stolen, and the infirmary was destroyed 'arbitrarily.'[247] As Biéri had promised the London authorities, the ICRC did not publicize its delegates' end-of-mission reports.

In Hamburg, Nicolas Burckhardt,[248] the ICRC delegate in Vlotho, awaited the ships' arrival in order to rendez-vous with his colleagues. When he heard from Wildi, on September 8, 1947, how the mission on the *Ocean Vigour* had gone, he reported to the ICRC in Geneva.[249] He also took it upon himself to protest, orally, to General Bishop, the adjutant of the military governor who commanded the local British forces, and pointed out to him that 'accusations made by the Jews who were aware of these facts could not be refuted' by the ICRC.[250] Geneva, for its part, considered the case serious enough to protest, orally, to the British consul in Geneva as well.[251]

The ICRC delegates observed the brutal way in which the British forced the Jews off the ships at Hamburg that overcast day, in front of a mob of reporters. According to Burckhardt, the Britons' task was a thankless one. He gave an example. On

---

[245]Wildi, 'Rapport concernant les conditions de vie, l'état sanitaire et l'activité médicale à bord du transport anglais de réfugiés israélites sur l'Ocean Vigour de Liverpool, parti de Port de Bouc le 22 août et arrivé à Hambourg le 7 septembre 1947,' Geneva, Oct. 3, 1947 (AICRC, G.59/5/ex). [Translation: M.G.]
[246]Ibid.
[247]Ibid.
[248]He was the same delegate who in July, 1948, would accompany the convoy of exiles from Gil Gil in Kenya to Tobruk. See p. 70.
[249]Report by Nicolas Burckhardt, ICRC Vlotho, to ICRC Geneva, Sept. 16, 1947 (AICRC, G.59/7.ex).
[250]Note from Nicolas Burckhardt, ICRC Vlotho, to ICRC Geneva, Sept. 16, 1947 (AICRC, G.49/5/ex). [Translation: M.G.]
[251]Note from Burckhardt, ICRC Vlotho, to ICRC Geneva, Nov. 26, 1947 (AICRC, G.59/5/ex), and note from Ribeaupierre, ICRC Geneva, to ICRC Berlin, Dec. 11, 1947 (AICRC, G.49/ex).

the *Ocean Vigour* there were some 200 children aged 6 to 16, accompanied not by their parents but by their Jewish schoolmasters, who did not allow them to eat – nor did they accept for themselves – the food the British offered them.

The ICRC delegate did not ask himself why they refused. Since it was his task to provide the victims with material assistance, he was put out because in order to persuade the Jews to eat that food, an ICRC doctor stationed at Hamburg had to go with them on the train that was to take them to a camp; it was only then, when the railcar with the barred windows had left the station, that the doctor managed 'to persuade the children's leader to have the food distributed, and the young people consumed it without resistance.'[252]

These children, and many other Jews from the *Exodus 47*, were forced to get on the train. They were accompanied by two of the ICRC doctors, Wildi and Monod, as far as the Poppendorf camp near Lübeck.

Marti remained on board the *Runnymede Park*. As a practitioner of ICRC neutrality, Burckhardt perceived the significance of this: If the head of the mission was not present, the ICRC would not have to give a verdict on the conditions of transfer by train, nor on the 'travelers' reception at the camp.'[253]

On September 9, 1947, Burckhardt went to meet his medical colleagues at Poppendorf, and took the opportunity to make a quick inspection of the premises. The camp was surrounded by barbed wire and rigged with electric lighting outside. Inside the camp, the administrative and medical personnel were Germans. The guards outside and around the camp were English soldiers. Physical conditions were satisfactory. No comment was made on the victims' mental anguish.[254] Before leaving Hamburg, Marti, Wildi, and Doret went to say goodbye to the sick and injured refugees at the Sainte-Marie hospital.[255]

The summary report that the ICRC in Geneva sent to the Foreign and Colonial Offices incorporated nothing from its delegates' individual reports but strictly medical data. It made no comment on the conditions on the ships, the attitudes of the

[252]Ibid. [Translation: M.G.]
[253]Note from Nicolas Burckhardt, ICRC Vlotho, to ICRC Geneva, Nov. 26, 1947 (AICRC, G.59/5/ex).
[254]Ibid.
[255]Ibid.

British on board or in Hamburg, or the camp facilities. It was a technical medical report, from which any moral or emotional overtones had been banished.[256]

This is perhaps the implication of the Red Cross's neutrality, a tactical principle of action that may tend to neutralize sensibility and the faculty of indignation, but without which, the ICRC believes from experience, it could not maintain the trust of belligerents. The ICRC balanced this coldness with an article in the *Revue internationale de la Croix-Rouge*[257] which combined sensitivity and neutrality, and by allowing Marti to give a journalist the controlled account of an experienced delegate.[258] Both articles appeared in October, 1947, just after the Belgrade conference of Eastern European relief societies.

Since May, 1947, the ICRC had been hoping that one day the Jewish Agency would spontaneously ask it to take action in Palestine[259]; in October of that year, in an article in the *Revue internationale de la Croix-Rouge*, it emphasized the request by the Jewish Agency and obscured the earlier one[260] by the Hebrew Committee of National Liberation.

The vote on the partition of Palestine: a new deal

When the United Nations voted on the partition plan on November 29, 1947, the United States and the USSR both pronounced themselves in favor of partition, for different but converging reasons. This development necessarily confirmed and reinforced the ICRC's desire to take a hand in the Palestine conflict as a neutral intermediary, in the meaning of Article VII of the International Red Cross Statutes – especially since the disturbances threatened to degenerate into generalized war. The declarations made by the League of Arab States and by the Arab

[256]ICRC, 'Report on the Work of the Delegates of the International Committee of the Red Cross in Behalf of the Emigrants of the Exodus,' unsigned and undated (CZA.S.41.525). French version dated Oct. 20, 1947 (AICRC, G.59/5/ex).

[257]'Action du Comité international de la Croix-Rouge en faveur des émigrants israélites de l'Exodus 47,' *RICR* 346 (Oct. 1947): 819–822.

[258]D., 'Le drame de l'Exodus. Un médecin suisse accompagnait les réfugiés du "Runnymede Park". Il nous a confié ses impressions,' *Servir, Grand hebdomadaire romand* [Lausanne] (Oct. 2, 1947): 8.

[259]ICRC, procès-verbal, Bureau meeting of May 16, 1947 (AICRC, no file number).

[260]'Action du Comité international de la Croix-Rouge en faveur des émigrants israélites de l'Exodus 47,' *RICR* 346 (Oct. 1947): 819–822.

Higher Committee, the Palestine Arabs' resistance organization, in response to the Zionist project left no doubt as to their bellicose intentions should the partition plan be put into effect. The ICRC stopped waiting for an invitation and took the initiative. On December 9, 1947[261] it asked Munier to try again where Helbling had failed – that is, to sound out the British high commissioner and the competent 'Israelite' authorities as to whether an ICRC intervention as a neutral intermediary would be welcomed. In light of the special value it attached to an operation in the Palestine conflict, however, the ICRC could not let Munier make the overtures for an offer of ICRC services all on his own. For this action the ICRC had intentions that it claimed it could not explain to its Cairo representative in writing, 'given the extreme difficulty of dealing with such a complex subject in a note.'[262] It therefore instructed William Michel, a former head of the Paris delegation (that same relative of Mendès France whose support it had sought for the Committee's various undertakings) to explain the Committee's plans to Munier, since he was due in Cairo on December 29. The ICRC was beginning a new phase in its approach to the Palestinian conflict.

---

[261]Note from Kuhne, ICRC Geneva, to ICRC Cairo, Dec. 9, 1947 (AICRC, G.59/I/G.C.).
[262]Ibid. [Translation: M.G.]

Chapter Three

THE ICRC ACHIEVES ITS AIM

The Palestine government's appeal to the ICRC
A welcome stroke of luck

As it turned out, neither Michel nor Munier would be needed to carry out the ICRC's mission. On December 31, 1947, Sir Henry Guerney, adjutant to the British high commissioner in Palestine, issued an appeal to the ICRC through the press, motivated by the recent armed clashes between the Jewish and Arab communities over the UN General Assembly's adoption of Resolution 181.[263] Was this a coincidence? The appeal was made a few days after Paul Ruegger met with Lady Mountbatten in New Delhi. On December 21, Ruegger wrote in his personal diary: 'We talk of Geneva and the ICRC's role. She attaches the greatest importance to it. The disappointments everyone has suffered with regard to the UN mean, according to her, that the International Red Cross remains almost the only institution that most of the states trust and whose work is apt to increase. . . .'[264] This view was shared by her spouse.[265] Sir Henry Guerney's appeal may have been a direct or indirect result of Ruegger's conversations with first Lady and then Lord Mountbatten; but nothing in the archives was found to confirm or exclude the possibility. In any case, the appeal came at just the right moment for the ICRC, which had long hoped to find an opportunity to carry out an

---

[263]The text of this appeal, taken from the *Daily Telegraph* (Dec. 31, 1947), was quoted by Biéri in his note from ICRC London to ICRC Geneva, Jan. 8, 1948 (AICRC, G.59/I/G.C.).

[264]Ruegger, 'Tagebuch,' original manuscript, unnumbered pages, entry for Sunday, Dec. 21, 1947 (IZG.23.7.3, Zurich, Fonds Ruegger). (Translation: M.G.)

[265]Ibid., Tuesday, Dec. 23, 1947.

operation as neutral intermediary in Palestine, in the spirit of Article VII (then in danger of revision) of the International Red Cross Statutes.

In an article in the *Revue internationale de la Croix-Rouge* on the subject,[266] the ICRC stressed that the British appeal had been unsolicited, proving that the ICRC's intervention could be 'recognized as necessary,' particularly in civil wars, as stipulated in Article VII of the 1928 Statutes. It undoubtedly hoped that Britain's request would serve as an example, since in other wars and disturbances the lawful powers showed a very prudent reluctance to accept ICRC intervention, as mentioned earlier in the examples of Greece and Indochina.[267]

On January 5, 1948, the Colonial Office approached the ICRC delegate in London and confirmed Guerney's appeal. Gloor and Gallopin happened to be in the British capital at the same time, to discuss post-war issues with the Foreign Office, and, not far away, a few members of the Special Commission were meeting unofficially. They were going to try to avoid a revision of the 1928 Statutes, since, in the prevailing political climate, revision would expose the International Red Cross to the danger of schism. In this respect Britain was an ally of the ICRC, opposed as it was to revising the 1928 Statutes and internationalizing the ICRC. But it remained unconvinced on another issue: the idea that the protection of an international convention should be offered to rebels and victims of civil wars. Given these factors, it was very important to the ICRC to gratify Britain.

The conditions posed

The Mandatory power, in turn, expected a great deal from the ICRC in Palestine. According to the Colonial Office, since the 'communal disorders'[268] that had broken out in Palestine at the end of December 1947, nearly 700 patients had been admitted to the hospitals of the Palestine government – most of them Arabs, since the Jews had hospitals of their own. The number of

---

[266] CICR, 'Le Comité international de la Croix-Rouge en Palestine (décembre 1947 au 1 er mai 1948),' *RICR* 353 (May 1948): 329.

[267] See Chapter 2, p. 67.

[268] Telegram from Colonial Office to ICRC Geneva, Jan. 5, 1948 (AICRC, G.59/I/G.C.). Letter from Fitzgerald, Colonial Office, London, to ICRC London, Jan. 5, 1948, quoted in note from Biéri, ICRC London, to ICRC Geneva, Jan. 8, 1948 (AICRC, G.59/I/G.C.).

patients had continued to grow, and the government hospitals, which contained only 1,800 beds in all – 900 of them reserved for infectious or mental illnesses – admitted about 50 people a day. For these patients the government of Palestine had only 600 beds. Despite improvised solutions, the hospitals were overflowing, and the situation was all the more serious since the medical staff did not want to continue working in such a risky situation.

For foreign-policy reasons, Britain could not simply leave Palestine and abandon the wounded and ill Arab Palestinians to their fate. But there was no organization other than the ICRC that could take over the health services of the Palestine government – certainly not the United Nations, which the Arabs rejected for having voted in favor of the partition plan. Britain wanted the ICRC to send medical teams and supplies to Palestine and to put them at the service of the Arab population. Aware that the Committee could not take action without receiving the necessary funds promptly – a fact it reiterated on every possible occasion – the Colonial Office declared that it was certain the Arabs would pay their financial contribution.[269]

To adhere to its general objectives, the ICRC needed to give Britain a rapid, independent reply, demonstrating the capabilities it would lose if it were internationalized or brought under the control of the Standing Commission of the International Conference of the Red Cross. The Committee members' state of mind and the presence in London of two senior ICRC officials should have expedited the ICRC's response, but two issues of principle gave the ICRC pause from the outset:

- Britain wanted the ICRC to confine itself to purely medical matters, as it had in the case of the Jewish refugees from the *Exodus 47*. This type of operation did not, however, correspond to the traditional role of neutral intermediary that the ICRC wanted to play, which consisted mostly in visiting prisoners and making sure they were treated in accordance with the conventions; direct care to the wounded was not, and never had been, its responsibility.

- Britain wanted the ICRC to give priority to the Arabs, who were cared for primarily by the Palestine government hospitals.

---

[269]Ibid. See also letter from Trafford Smith, Colonial Office, Jan. 6, 1948, cited in note from Biéri, ICRC London, to ICRC Geneva, Jan. 8, 1948 (AICRC, G.59/I/G.C.).

For the ICRC, however, working for the benefit of only one of the parties would be a betrayal of the cherished principle of impartiality – the same principle that had called down so much criticism on the organization when it aided German POWs after the war. The ICRC could only contemplate an action benefiting both parties in Mandatory Palestine, each according to its needs.[270] Moreover, the ICRC did not have the means to undertake a relief operation of this magnitude without financial support.[271]

The ICRC fulfilled the criterion of a rapid response by deciding immediately to send three delegates to Mandatory Palestine.[272] It met the criterion of independence through the instructions it gave them:

- to make contact with all parties involved, British, Arab, and Jewish;
- to obtain precise information on all current medical problems and all those that would arise with the departure of the British;
- 'to offer the Committee as a neutral intermediary in the case of one of the already existing conflicts or a more pronounced conflict'[273];
- to promote the creation of new National Societies wherever none existed;
- to examine the financial issues.[274]

At the last minute, just before the delegates left for Palestine, the ICRC began to wonder whether the Palestine conflict was still a 'civil war' in the ICRC's definition of the phrase, given the probable implementation of the partition plan sometime soon. The draft of the article that the ICRC proposed to insert in revised or new conventions in future defined a civil war as an armed conflict taking place on the home or colonial territory of a con-

---

[270]Note from Kuhne, ICRC Geneva, to ICRC London, Jan. 8, 1948 (AICRC, G.59/I/G.C.).
[271]Ibid.
[272]Note from Kuhne, ICRC Geneva, to ICRC Cairo, Jan. 9, 1948 (AICRC, G.59/I/G.C.).
[273]ICRC, procès-verbal, meeting of Jan. 19, 1948 concerning 'mission en Palestine du Dr Marti, de M. de Reynier, et de M. Munier.' Those present: Gloor, Odier, Chenevière, Dunand, Voegeli, Wolf, Kuhne, de Bondeli, Feller, Perret, Pilloud, Marti, and de Reynier (AICRC, G.59/I/G.C.). [Translation: M.G.]
[274]Ibid.

tracting party. According to this view, as long as Britain remained the Mandatory power and the two communities, Jewish and Arab, were in conflict on its territory, the Palestine conflict could be considered a civil war. In the period following the termination of the Mandate, however, several scenarios were conceivable, and the possibility of international war could not be excluded.

The ICRC delegates would have to take into account the possibility that two states might emerge. The delegates would have to think about preparing these states to adhere to the international conventions, and about creating two new national relief societies, one in the Jewish state and the other in the Arab state that could arise if Resolution 181 were implemented.[275] The ICRC would do everything possible to insure that the aid societies of these states adopted the red cross as their emblem. In this legalistic context and at this stage of the ICRC's reasoning, the political issue of a possible war between the two camps of the Cold War by means of 'interposed states' did not arise, although the Committee was not neglecting this aspect of the Palestinian conflict.

The choice of ICRC envoys

The ICRC's study mission was to begin on January 20, 1948, led by Roland Marti, who has already been mentioned. He demonstrated an undeniable understanding for the Jews of the *Exodus 47* – so much so that he may have conveyed the impression that the ICRC, in a much better position to carry out humanitarian actions since Hitler's defeat, felt relieved at finally being able to assist Jews who had suffered at the hands of the Nazis, as though this were a way of redeeming itself. The ICRC may have hoped that he would establish close ties with the Jewish Agency in Palestine. Marti was also experienced in situations of civil war, having worked for the ICRC in the war in Spain. Moreover, he was a doctor. He was therefore appointed to head the mission.

He was unfamiliar with the Arab world, however. The ICRC accordingly gave him the Arabic-speaking Jacques de Reynier as an assistant. An agricultural engineer from the Zurich Polytechnical School and a graduate of the Institut des Hautes études marocaines (Institute of Moroccan Graduate Studies) in Rabat,

---

[275]Note from Claude Pilloud, ICRC Geneva, to ICRC mission in Palestine, Jan. 15, 1948 (AICRC, G.59/I/G.C.).

he had lived in Tunisia and Morocco from 1929 to 1939. He had created and run rural enterprises. This past seemed likely to help him find the right approach to the Arab world. A reserve officer in the Swiss army, he had worked for the ICRC for a much shorter time than his colleague Marti, but he, too, had experienced civil war, in 1944, while carrying out an ICRC mission in the Greek civil war. Since August, 1947, he had headed the ICRC delegation at Baden-Baden, whence the ICRC called him to his new post. Eventually he was to take charge of all the ICRC activities in Mandatory Palestine.

Marti and de Reynier were to begin their mission by meeting Munier in Cairo, continuing on together from there. It may be recalled that Munier was the delegate who visited the Jewish Palestinian exiles interned first in Eritrea and later in Kenya. Like his colleagues, he was familiar with civil wars, and had carried out an ICRC mission on his own in 1944, in the Dodecanese Islands. The ICRC had subsequently appointed him to the Cairo delegation.

Ulterior motive as policy

The ICRC was well aware that Munier might feel undermined by the arrival of colleagues liable to diminish his own role, and took care to reassure him: He would be of invaluable assistance to Marti, and thus must take part in the mission, even if he would not be in charge of it. The ICRC had special plans for him in Mandatory Palestine, though it preferred not to divulge them in writing, telling him: 'It is difficult for us to develop our ideas in a note, as much as we could if it were possible to speak with you in person.'[276] What those ideas were is anyone's guess, and it can only be supposed that they had something to do with translating the Committee's general objectives, described in Chapter 1, to Palestine. They would not have been easy, psychologically or conceptually, to explain to Munier, since the ICRC's strategy bore more resemblance to an ulterior motive or a state of mind than an articulated political program. The Committee could not permit itself to draw attention, in a letter to its delegate, to the political advantage it would gain by performing the role

---

[276]Note from Kuhne, ICRC Geneva, to Munier, ICRC Cairo, Jan. 19, 1948 (AICRC, G.59/I/G.C.). [Translation: M.G.]

THE ICRC ACHIEVES ITS AIM

of neutral intermediary in Mandatory Palestine, by carrying out an ICRC operation in the framework of a civil war, by reasserting the principle of impartiality, and finally, most important, by attempting, through a large-scale operation, to re-establish both its prestige and its financial situation. The Committee members would certainly have felt they were betraying their ideals if they had openly admitted in a letter that they had such considerations in mind.

Scarcely had the delegates left for the Near East when the ICRC briefed all the delegations that were in a position to support the operation in Palestine or to derive some benefit from it: Rome, Athens, Algiers, Casablanca, London, Paris, and Berlin,[277] which was a point of contact between the ICRC and the Soviets. The ICRC also wrote to the Swiss legations in the same cities. It asked the Swiss Federal Political Department to commend the delegates to the Swiss delegations in Cairo, Jerusalem, Damascus, Beirut, Ankara, and Baghdad.[278] It informed one of its representatives, whom it had just sent to Bombay, of the Palestine mission so that he could 'follow the efforts of the International Committee of the Red Cross on behalf of the Arabs.'[279]

On January 27, 1948, a week after the delegates had left, the ICRC explained their mission to the Colonial Office. It referred to the British appeal and its main focus, the Arabs' health-care situation, which, of course, the ICRC envoys would examine. But the ICRC did not conceal from the Colonial Office its intention of giving first priority in Palestine to the traditional activities in which it could make a specific contribution: visiting both Jewish and Arab prisoners regularly and taking any humanitarian initiative that might seem indicated.[280] Of all the conflicts in which the ICRC sought to act during that period, the Mandatory Palestine conflict was the only one where it could pursue its

[277]Circular letter from Gaillard, ICRC Geneva, to ICRC Delegations in Rome, Athens, Casablanca, London, Paris, Berlin, Jan. 21, 1948 (AICRC, G.3/82, G.59/I/G.C.)

[278]Note from Voegeli, head of the Delegations Division, ICRC Geneva, to de Haller, Federal Councilor for Mutual International Aid, Bern, Jan. 20, 1948 (AICRC, G.59/I/G.C.).

[279]Letter from Gaillard, Delegations Division, ICRC Geneva, to Otto Wenger, Consulate-General of Switzerland, Bombay, British Indies, Jan. 21, 1948 (AICRC, G.59/I/G.C.). [Translation: M.G.]

[280]Letter from Bodmer and Gloor, ICRC Geneva, to Colonial Office, London, Jan. 27, 1948 (AICRC, G.59/I/G.C.).

specific objectives openly without fear that its services would be rejected – since, after all, Britain had requested them. Consequently, the ICRC risked little by making its intentions clear.

Evaluation: the first mission

Passing through Cairo

The ICRC delegates began their study mission in Cairo. Up until January, 1948, the ICRC had had little contact with the Arab world. In December, 1947, Geneva had asked Munier for advice on which Arab notables should be approached[281] and on January 8, 1948 the ICRC studied Munier's suggestions.[282] It decided that initially its representatives should arrange meetings with the Egyptian prime minister, Nukrashi Pasha; the secretary-general of the Arab League, Azzam Pacha; and the head of the Arab Higher Committee of Palestine, Hadj Amin el-Husseini.

Nukrashi Pasha, who received the ICRC delegates on January 26, 1948, was unreceptive to their declared intention of playing the role of a neutral intermediary – which would imply taking account of the Jews. This attitude was undoubtedly the corollary of the Arabs' refusal to accept the partition of Palestine. The only argument that the Egyptian prime minister welcomed was the idea that the ICRC might be disposed to offer material aid to the Arabs of Palestine.[283] Marti was nonplussed, and in subsequent interviews said nothing of the ICRC's intention to act as a neutral intermediary.[284]

When he met Azzam Pacha, he began by painting a general picture of the ICRC's recent traditional activities – essentially, its actions on behalf of prisoners of war from the countries defeated in World War II. He next told the secretary-general of the Arab League about the appeal from the British high commissioner in Palestine, and finally came to the object of his visit: that the ICRC would like information from the Arabs regarding their needs. He raised the possibility of obtaining Arab funds to finance the ICRC's activities, but without pressing the point, then demon-

---

[281]Letter from Kuhne, ICRC Geneva, to Munier, ICRC Cairo, Dec. 9, 1947 (AICRC, G.59/I/G.C.).
[282]ICRC, procès-verbal, Bureau meeting of Jan. 8, 1948 (AICRC, no file number).
[283]Note from Marti, Palestine mission, Cairo, to ICRC Geneva, Jan. 26, 1948 (AICRC, G.59/I/G.C.).
[284]Ibid.

strated the impartiality the ICRC meant to respect: If he was supposed to provide medical aid primarily to the Arabs, he still could not leave the Jews out. Marti also wanted to be certain that in Palestine he and his colleagues would enjoy complete freedom of movement so they could evaluate the needs of both sides in total independence.[285]

Azzam Pacha pointed out that charity was not the prerogative of Christianity, but declared that he could not be responsible for the behavior of the irregular Arab forces fighting the Jews in Palestine; the Arab League did not control them. He therefore advised the ICRC to accept a British escort until the Red Cross flag was familiar in Palestine. Once it was, it would no doubt be appreciated and respected for its Christian character, since in this conflict the Moslems considered the Christians as a neutral party. To maintain its credibility, the ICRC should avoid sending Jewish delegates to Palestine, he added, according to Marti's account.[286] The secretary-general of the Arab League gave the ICRC delegates letters of recommendation for the consuls of the Arab countries in Palestine and the local representatives of the Arab Higher Committee. He also introduced the delegates to Hadj Amin el-Husseini, the former Grand Mufti of Jerusalem and head of the Arab Higher Committee of Palestine, who was in Cairo, and whom the delegates, at Munier's suggestion (approved by Geneva), wished, of course, to win over, in view of his key position in the Arab resistance in Palestine.

Meeting the Grand Mufti

Since the delegates' departure, however, the ICRC had been reconsidering the proposed meeting with Hadj Amin el-Husseini, for the head of the Arab Higher Committee was a controversial figure. In 1941 he had approached Hitler and set up an alliance with him, calling upon the Moslems on the eastern front to support the Nazi war. The ICRC feared that public knowledge of a meeting between the ICRC delegates and Hadj Amin might damage the organization,[287] fueling the accusations regarding its alleged pro-German sympathies. On the other hand, if it ostra-

[285]Ibid.
[286]Ibid.
[287]Note from Kuhne, ICRC Geneva, to Marti, ICRC Cairo, Jan. 26, 1947 (AICRC, G.59/I/G.C.).

cized the Mufti, it could not hope to act effectively as a neutral intermediary between Jews and Arabs in Mandatory Palestine. Upon due consideration, it decided to warn Marti about the delicacy of the situation and its possible risks, and told him that it preferred he meet with lower-ranking members of the Arab Higher Committee, rather than the Mufti himself – although it left the final decision up to Marti.[288]

Geneva's prudent instructions arrived too late. Accompanied by the Arab press corps of Cairo, the ICRC delegates had already gone to visit the Mufti, by whom they were very warmly received. He was well-disposed towards them, he said, because when he had fled Germany, a 'Red Cross agent'[289] who preferred not to identify himself had offered to take the Mufti over the border in his car, on May 7, 1945, near Lake Constance.[290] The ICRC delegates did not dwell on this vague anecdote, and were happy enough, in view of the activities they hoped to pursue in Palestine, to benefit from a bias that worked in their favor – especially since the Mufti accepted the ICRC's strictures concerning the principle of impartiality. Marti also broached the question of money, but Hadj Amin put him off, saying he would discuss the matter with the ICRC envoys at a later date. He also voiced the same warning as Azzam Pacha: If the ICRC wanted to be able to rely on Arab cooperation in Palestine, it should not send Jewish delegates there. All ICRC personnel should be Christian and Swiss.[291] The Mufti and the delegates parted on good terms, and, as it turned out, the visit did not attract the attention or the criticism that the ICRC had feared.

The ICRC's study mission left Cairo and arrived in Lydda on January 29, 1948. It was met by the deputy director of the British health services in Palestine, Dr. Krikor Krikorian, who escorted the delegates to his superior, Dr. H.M.O. Lester. Lester was the representative appointed by the Palestine government to deal with the ICRC. Lester and Krikorian summed up the current situation from their point of view for the benefit of the ICRC envoys. On May 15, 1948, Britain would withdraw from the

---

[288]Ibid.
[289]Note from Marti, Palestine mission, Cairo, to ICRC Geneva, Jan. 28, 1948 (AICRC, G.59/I/G.C.).
[290]Ibid.
[291]Ibid.

territory of the Mandate, leaving behind the entire health-care infrastructure of the government of Palestine. According to Lester, the Jews were prepared for this, owing to their relations – which he considered privileged – with the World Health Organization. The Arabs, in contrast, were not organized either inside or outside Palestine, and their rejection of a UN role in Palestine, due to the vote for partition, put them in a weak position. The British government in London and in Palestine therefore considered that under these conditions the ICRC was the only organization suitable to take over the Palestine governmental health service when the British left.[292] Sir Henry Guerney confirmed Lester's summary.[293]

Marti and his colleagues tried to explain to the British officials that the ICRC did not intend to confine itself to medical aid. The ICRC was neither able nor willing to direct any country's health service; even if it had wanted to, asserted Marti, it did not have the financial, material, or human means to do so. Its role was that of a neutral intermediary, and that was the capacity in which it would seek a way of keeping the Mandatory government hospitals running after the British departed.[294] Some solution would have to be devised, but in the meantime, Marti would continue his local consultations.

In Tel Aviv, Marti met with Va'ad Le'umi officials: Itzhak Ben Zvi, the president; Abraham Katznelson, head of the health service; and a representative of the financial department of the Jewish Agency. In his report to Geneva, Marti mentioned these contacts only very briefly before going on to what seemed to him most important, his meeting with Leo Kohn, a legal expert in the Jewish Agency's political department.[295] From Kohn Marti obtained certain political information that could have repercussions for the future conduct of the ICRC's humanitarian operations, and passed it on to Committee headquarters.

[292]Note from Marti, Palestine mission, Jerusalem, to ICRC Geneva, Jan. 29, 1948 (AICRC, G.59/I/G.C.).
[293]Note from Munier, Palestine mission, Jerusalem, to ICRC Geneva, Jan. 30, 1948 (AICRC, G.59/I/G.C.).
[294]Note from Marti, Palestine mission, Jerusalem, to ICRC Geneva, Jan. 29, 1948 (AICRC, G.59/I/G.C.).
[295]Note from Marti, Palestine mission, 'Meeting with Mr. Leo Cohn (sic), Secretary of the Political Department of the Jewish Agency, Jerusalem,' to ICRC Geneva, Feb. 1, 1948 (AICRC, G.59/I/G.C.).

First, he said, Kohn deplored the Arabs' rejection of the partition plan, which was the source of the current confrontation. England had adopted an attitude of 'malevolent neutrality,'[296] leaving the Jews to defend themselves alone against the Arabs both inside and outside Mandatory Palestine. Resolution 181, by which the UN had approved the partition of Palestine, probably could not be put into effect. Of course, the UN had set up a United Nations Commission on Palestine to examine ways of implementing the partition plan; but from its first meeting the Commission had realized the difficulties involved, and, in view of the deteriorating situation in Palestine, it had decided to send six members of its secretariat to Palestine to find a local solution. The British, however, had opposed this rapid action, on the pretext that the members of the UN delegation would be in great danger from Arab hostility. The members of the UN Commission were not scheduled to arrive until May 1, 1948. Under these circumstances, the Commission could not be effective, since it would in fact have only two weeks before the British withdrawal to master the many intricacies of a complex administration.

The Jews feared for their future, and the Jewish Agency wanted the UN to send an international buffer force. This idea was under consideration, but Britain was unlikely to accept it. If Kohn's predictions proved accurate, outright war could be expected, and both sides were preparing for one, though with unequal means in manpower and arms. The Jews were few in number, Jewish immigration was subject to stringent controls, and their arms supply was strictly supervised, owing to a US embargo on arms shipments to the Near East. The Arabs, however, could circumvent the embargo by bringing in arms and men without restriction through Syria, Lebanon, and Transjordan, the British making no objection. There was little chance of a diplomatic settlement between Jews and Arabs. Only King Abdullah of Transjordan would be open to the idea, and his hands were tied; although his army comprised a majority of Transjordanians, it was financed and commanded by Britons,[297] led by Sir Glubb Pacha.

The humanitarian problem faced by the Jews could be described in one word: insecurity. Convoys of Jews, Kohn

[296]Ibid.
[297]Ibid.

explained, were attacked daily on the roads linking the Jewish sectors; those roads were lined by Arab villages, the source of the ambushes. The Jews were forced to defend themselves, but the British allowed them only an inadequate two guns per truck. In the Old City of Jerusalem, the Jewish Quarter was surrounded by Arabs, and its inhabitants were cut off from the New City in the west, where most of the approximately 100,000 Jewish residents of Jerusalem lived. The New City, in turn, was cut off from the western sector of Palestine, which had been assigned to the future Jewish state; the road linking Tel Aviv to Jerusalem, from the west, was almost entirely under Arab control. At present, the British army escorted the Jewish vehicles carrying supplies from Tel Aviv to the Jewish civilian population in Jerusalem, but what would happen after May 15, when the British left? Without an international buffer force, communications with Jerusalem might be completely cut off. Even farther away from the Jewish zones was the old Jewish cemetery on the Mount of Olives, north-east of Jerusalem. The funeral convoys were also exposed to Arab attacks.

If the war intensified, Kohn was inclined to believe the Jews would decide to apply the 1929 humanitarian conventions; he had no doubt the latter would be respected by the Jewish population. That said, the Jewish Agency had several requests. For one thing, it suggested that the ICRC set up a delegation in Jerusalem and make it accessible to both sides. This way, through the intermediary of the ICRC, Tel Aviv could hope to maintain contact with the Jewish population of Jerusalem. The Jewish Agency also wanted the ICRC to ask the Arab Higher Committee to make its combatants stop mutilating the dead and killing off wounded Jews. It asked, too, that Jewish medical personnel and ambulances be declared neutral in the spirit of the Geneva Convention, even though the Convention did not specify the red star of David that the Jewish relief society had used as its emblem since its inception in 1931. The Jewish Agency also expected the ICRC to persuade the Arab combatants to allow the funeral convoys traveling to the Mount of Olives to pass in safety, as well as the maintenance crews who worked in the cemetery, and who at present were regularly attacked. The Jewish Agency hoped the ICRC would help guarantee, by means yet to be studied, the provision of food, water, and electricity to Jewish sectors or neighborhoods surrounded by Arabs. Finally, Kohn asked the ICRC to make inquiries in Lebanon regarding the fate of five Palestinian Jews who had been sentenced on September 7, 1947, by a Lebanese military court and imprisoned in the Sables prison in Beirut.[298] The Jewish Agency hoped that the ICRC could assist them.

When the delegates expressed concern over the financing of the action, Kohn responded that the matter had already been taken up in Geneva between Eliezer Kaplan, director of the financial department of the Jewish Agency, and Max Wolf, who was, as noted previously, Ruegger's special advisor and a relative of the Warburg bankers. Kohn confirmed what Kaplan and Wolf had agreed, that Geneva could count on all the financial assistance desirable for a humanitarian operation in Mandatory Palestine.[299]

Having met with the authorities of the Palestinian Jewish community, on February 2, 1948, the ICRC delegates approached the local officials of the Arab Higher Committee, Hussein Khalidi and Emile Ghori. Khalidi and Ghori began by emphasizing the sovereignty of the Arab Higher Committee; the latter had not made any appeal to the ICRC, but it was happy to receive the ICRC representatives. However, the Arab Higher Committee had no requests to make. The neighboring Arab countries, according to Khalidi, had organized themselves at an inter-Arab conference on January 21, 1948, to provide the Arabs of Palestine with all the material and medical aid they might need. A center was to be established in Amman for that purpose. In Jerusalem, the Arab community had created a 'Higher First Aid Committee,' presided over by Khalidi himself and run by Dr. Tamous Canaan, president of the Arab Medical Association of Jerusalem, and Dr. Mahmud Taher Dejani, a well-known Palestinian doctor. Several Arab charitable organizations in Palestine were associated with this project. If, despite these arrangements, the ICRC still wanted

---

[298]On this subject see letter from Munier, Palestine mission, to Burnier, ICRC Beirut, Jan. 30, 1948 (CZA.S.25.207).

[299]Note from Marti, Palestine mission, 'Meeting with Mr. Leo Cohn (sic), Secretary of the Political Department of the Jewish Agency, Jerusalem,' to ICRC Geneva, Feb. 1, 1948 (AICRC, G.59/I/G.C.). I have found no trace in the ICRC archives of the talks between Kaplan and Wolf, a considerable part of the Committee's financial records for that period having been destroyed at a later date.

to help, it would be welcome, but the Arab Higher Committee was not requesting assistance.

Although it could not serve as a neutral intermediary in such an operation, the ICRC did propose assistance[300] – at least in principle, since the spheres, beneficiaries, and modalities of its action had not yet been defined. At that stage, it considered that the sole purpose of its presence in Mandatory Palestine was to seek the means of playing a role as a neutral intermediary, in the sense of Article VII of the International Red Cross Statutes.

The Arab Medical Association of Palestine, which served as the aid society of the Arab Higher Committee, subsequently offered the ICRC a warm, lavish reception, attended by officials of the British health service in Palestine. Marti, personally won over, was nevertheless uncomfortable, for he had a feeling that the Palestinian Arabs would perceive any aid extended to them as reflecting an emotional and political bias in favor of their cause. This was likely to make the ICRC's role of neutral, independent, and impartial intermediary very difficult.

Adapting the 'Red Cross Code'

The ICRC could scarcely hope to interpose itself between Jews and Arabs under these conditions. It was difficult to be a neutral intermediary between one party which presented needs and one which did not, since the factor of reciprocal interest was lacking.

The ICRC delegates therefore needed to adapt their usual procedures, their 'Red Cross code,' to use Marti's expression.[301] According to de Reynier, the only way of arousing an interest in, or even a demand for, assistance on the part of the Arabs would be to offer them at the outset the type of aid they would be willing to accept. But he knew that the Committee did not want to present itself as a simple relief agency.[302] It would have to find a way to create a reciprocal relationship between Jews and Arabs so that it could act as a neutral intermediary between the two. A solution was required for another problem, as well:

---

[300] Note from Marti, Palestine mission, 'Entretien avec le Dr H. F. Khalidi et M. Emile Ghori,' Jerusalem, Feb. 2, 1948 (AICRC, G.59/I/G.C.).

[301] Report by Marti, de Reynier, and Munier, Palestine mission, Jerusalem, Feb. 15, 1948 (AICRC, G.59/I/G.C.).

[302] According to de Reynier, Palestine mission, monthly report no. 1 (March), Jerusalem, to ICRC Geneva, March 31, 1948 (AICRC, G.59/I/G.C.).

How could the ICRC ask for a financial contribution from an Arab organization that asked for nothing? For the ICRC delegates, this question remained open.

At that stage in the negotiations, they were still listening to what the parties had to say, taking time to think it over, and continuing their evaluation. They toured the entire country, inspecting in particular the medical facilities of the regions they visited, as the British wished. From February 3–17, they inspected the medical facilities of Tel Aviv, Jaffa, Haifa, Acre, Safed, Tiberias, Taibeh, Afula, Nazareth, Nablus, and Bethlehem before returning to Jerusalem. They sent regular reports to the ICRC in Geneva, which began to worry that the mission was concentrating too heavily on health matters; the Committee reminded the delegates that the medical aspect was neither its only nor its main objective. Marti was asked to find out more about the prisoners in Palestine and explore the possibility of persuading the Jewish and Arab authorities to apply the 1929 Conventions.[303] The ICRC asked Marti to return to Geneva – possibly accompanied by his colleagues – as soon as these inquiries were completed, to make his report.[304]

The state of the conflict in mid-February, 1948

A report by High Commissioner Alan Cunningham, dated February 14, 1948[305] – just before the ICRC completed its study mission – summed up the situation in Palestine at the time, from the perspective of the Mandatory power: Some 1,000 to 2,000 Lebanese and Syrian Arab volunteers had crossed the Jordan River at Jisr Damiych. The Arab combatants in the Old City of Jerusalem who had surrounded the Jewish Quarter were mostly Syrians. On February 5, 1948, the Syrians had chaired a meeting in Damascus which was attended by, among others, Mufti Hadj Amin el-Husseini, Abdul Kader el-Husseini, and Hassan Salameh, the three war leaders of the Arab Higher Committee

---

[303]Telegram from President's office, ICRC Geneva, to Marti, YMCA Jerusalem, Feb. 12, 1948 (AICRC, G.59/I/G.C.).
[304]Ibid.
[305]Telegram from High Commissioner for Palestine, Jerusalem, to Secretary of State, Colonial Office, London, Feb. 14, 1948 (Cunningham Private Papers, III/1/94, St. Antony's College. Middle East Library, Oxford).

whom the British saw as the greatest threats to order in the country.

The Arab military leaders who met in Damascus decided to divide Palestine into four military zones: northern Palestine, including Samaria, where operations would be directed by Fawzi el-Kaukji; Jerusalem, which would be the responsibility of Abdul Kader el-Husseini (who was granted special powers for the purpose); the Lydda district, to be controlled by Hassan Salameh; and southern Palestine, which would be placed under Egyptian command. Jaffa was henceforth to be controlled by an Iraqi, Abdul Mahad Bey; and in Khan Yunis, Mahmud Labis recruited a corps of Egyptian volunteers from among the Muslim Brotherhood. A unified command was entrusted to General Ismail Sawfat. Following these military arrangements, Hassan Salameh and Abdul Kader el-Husseini entered Palestine through Transjordan, while the Mufti, accompanied by other members of the Arab Higher Committee, returned to Cairo.

In Samaria, the situation was fairly calm. The Syrian Arab Liberation Army exercised strict control over the Arab regions, and so far had avoided confrontations with the Jewish settlements. In the same area, the Haganah had abstained from acts of provocation. In Haifa, where there were frequent clashes between Jews and Arabs, tension was high. In Jerusalem, the Arabs had attempted to occupy the Jewish neighborhood of Yemin Moshe, which was defended by the Haganah. In the Old City, the Arabs had the Jews surrounded. The Mandatory power, goaded by international pressure, was advocating a truce to preserve Jerusalem and its holy places, but was balked by the refusal of the Arab Higher Committee.

Arabs and Jews were perfecting their organizational arrangements, and there was every indication that the conflict would continue to intensify. A more or less stable front had developed around Jaffa, where shooting could be heard day and night. In Galilee, the fighting centered on communication lines. In general, the Syrian Arab Liberation Army was aided by Arab Palestinian irregulars. The Haganah had stepped up its campaign of selective reprisals, without worrying about their consequences for noncombatants. The high commissioner saw the Stern group (Lehi) as a Communist threat to the country, likely to recruit new Russian immigrants,[306] despite Stern members' declarations that they would not tolerate Soviet imperialism any more than they did that of the United Kingdom.

The Jews were in a weak position. They had increasing difficulty in providing their urban populations with food and supplies. They had lost faith in the United Nations' ability to establish a Jewish state by diplomacy. The Jewish population in Palestine – according to Cunningham – believed that the Palestine question no longer interested the president of the United States, who was preoccupied by the upcoming presidential elections; it had been shifted to the defense department, which was more or less unaffected by electoral pressures, and had an interest in maintaining good relations with the Arab world. The Jews felt abandoned and alone; and the British continued to restrict Jewish immigration and to intern illegal immigrants in Cyprus.[307]

Devising a plan of action on the spot

Faced with this situation – of which they must have been aware, at least generally – the ICRC delegates devised a provisional plan of action, taking account of their talks with the local British, Jewish, and Arab authorities and discussing it with them before they submitted it to Geneva for examination and approval. The plan was based on a summary analysis, since the ICRC delegates had no idea of how the conflict would develop. They had observed that the Jews wanted a complete, practical solution in order to create their state, while the Arabs of Palestine, opposed to the partition of a country they considered as integrally theirs, seemed determined to fight to the last man to prevent the implementation of the partition plan.

Both sides were ready for ruthless combat, and were openly preparing for a large-scale war that would begin on May 15, as soon as the British forces pulled out. By February 15 there were already dozens of dead and wounded every day. The British army maintained some semblance of order, but usually declined

---

[306]On this particular British fear, see telegram from the High Commissioner for Palestine, Jerusalem, top secret 'Weekly Intelligence Appreciation,' to Secretary of State, London, Feb. 7, 1948 (Cunningham Private Papers, III/I/82, St. Antony's College. Middle East Library, Oxford).

[307]Telegram from High Commissioner for Palestine, Jerusalem, to Secretary of State, Colonial Office, London, Feb. 14, 1948 (Cunningham Private Papers, III/1/94, St. Antony's College. Middle East Library, Oxford).

to intervene. The battle lines kept shifting, and the Arab and Jewish zones were muddled. Everyone was either surrounded or surrounding, and every move meant crossing the territory of the other side, a problem that would have to be taken into account in organizing the ICRC delegation that would be put in charge of the Palestine action.

The two communities did not have the same needs. According to the ICRC delegates, the Arabs lacked material necessities, especially in the medical sphere. The Jews had different problems. They were not rich, of course, but their main problem was physical danger rather than poverty; they most required greater security. All of the civilian population faced the prospect of many small-scale battles over control of the communication routes, as well as the possible loss of facilities vital to the community: water, electricity, and other public services hitherto provided by the British.[308]

Starting from April 1, 1948, six months before the partition plan was due to take effect on October 1, 1948, the ICRC delegates proposed to set up a permanent delegation in Palestine composed of eight Swiss delegates assisted by ten Swiss nurses; the latter would replace the British 'matrons'[309] in the main government hospitals. The delegation's headquarters would be in Jerusalem, but in view of the fragmentation of Palestine and the instability of the battle lines, the ICRC would also establish offices in Tel Aviv, Jaffa, Gaza, Haifa, and Tiberias. Twenty-five locally recruited staff members would maintain the infrastructure and take care of some of the administrative tasks.[310]

As for what the future delegation was to do, the ICRC envoys had kept in mind the wish expressed by the Committee on February 12, 1948, that the delegation's focus would be on persuading the parties to the conflict to respect the 1929 Conventions and on promoting the ICRC's role of neutral intermediary. They proposed that the future delegation's first objective should be to ensure that the Conventions' principles were applied to all the

---

[308]Report from Marti, de Reynier, and Munier, Palestine mission, Jerusalem, Feb. 15, 1948 (AICRC, G.59/I/G.C.).

[309]Ibid. The English word was used in the delegates' report.

[310]Report by Marti, de Reynier, and Munier, Palestine mission, Jerusalem, Feb. 15, 1948 (AICRC, G.59/I/G.C.). See also telegram from High Commissioner for Palestine, Jerusalem, to Secretary of State, Colonial Office, London, Feb. 17, 1948 – copy to UK Delegation Washington (Cunningham Private Papers, III/I/103, St. Antony's College. Middle East Library, Oxford).

victims of the Palestinian conflict, regardless of their membership in one or the other of the two camps, Arab or Jewish, but according to categories of existing law or law in the making: The delegation would help the wounded and the sick, prisoners and noncombatant civilians, without distinction as to race, nationality, or religion.

On the practical level, the ICRC would have to do the following:

- try to protect the existing institutions dedicated to humanitarian goals for the benefit of the general public, by designating them with a red cross;
- try to obtain free access to hospitals and cemeteries for medical or funeral convoys displaying the red cross, crescent, or Magen David (star of David);
- generate, receive, coordinate and allocate aid equitably between the Arabs and the Jews according to their respective needs, and control its distribution, although making use of local facilities and manpower where possible;
- create safety zones outside the combat zones where civilians could seek refuge from the hostilities, and organize assistance for those civilians.[311]

The issue of the men held in the Sables prison in Beirut was to be dealt with separately by Georges Burnier, the ICRC's representative in Lebanon. There were apparently no prisoners in Mandatory Palestine. On February 15, 1948, the date that the delegates put the final touches on their plan of action, the parties to the conflict did not appear to be taking any prisoners. The ICRC, who saw its main purpose as visiting prisoners of war, would have to adapt to this situation.

The delegates and nurses sent to Palestine would have to develop personal contacts with all the groups and communities in the areas where they would be conducting their activities; they would need to establish a network of humanitarian solidarity. And since the countries of the Arab League were equally

---

[311]Ibid. See also the plan of action, rewritten for publication, as presented in CICR, 'Le Comité international de la Croix-Rouge en Palestine (1er décembre 1947–1er mai 1948),' *RICR* (May 1948): 332–333. This plan had a purpose of its own, as will be seen in Chapter 4.

THE ICRC ACHIEVES ITS AIM

committed to the Palestinian issue, the ICRC delegation would maintain steady communication with them.[312]

The cost of the operation was estimated at one million Swiss francs, for a period extending up to the following October 1. Since the ICRC did not have even a fraction of this sum at its disposal, it intended to ask each of the parties concerned to assume responsibility for one-third of the budget. To this end, the ICRC first approached Britain, which agreed, after referring the matter to the United Nations in regard to the months following its withdrawal.[313] The Colonial Office implied, however, that its financial participation would be conditional on the orientation of the Committee's activities[314]: It wanted the delegation to confine itself to health care and to give the Arabs priority. The Jewish Agency agreed to make the contribution requested. Kohn opined that the ICRC could expect the same from the Arabs, who, according to him, had the means but had developed an inferiority complex which the British had fostered.[315] Since the Arabs had not requested aid, however, the ICRC delegates preferred to consult Geneva before discussing the matter with them.

Marti returned to Geneva on February 18, 1948, to deliver his report, while his two colleagues visited several hundred civilian internees and German members of the Order of Templars in the villages and camps of Wilhema and Waldheim, whom the British wished to evacuate with their possessions, possibly to Australia, since their active support for the anti-Zionist cause had aroused the hostility of the Jews. Munier subsequently returned to Cairo, and Jacques de Reynier, destined to become the head of the ICRC delegation in Mandatory Palestine, remained in Jerusalem.

---

[312]Report by Marti, de Reynier, and Munier, Palestine mission, Jerusalem, Feb. 15, 1948 (AICRC, G.59/I/G.C.). See also CICR, 'Le Comité international de la Croix-Rouge en Palestine (1er décembre 1947–1er mai 1948),' *RICR* (May 1948): 332–333.

[313]According to telegram from High Commissioner for Palestine, Jerusalem, to Secretary of State, Colonial Office, London, Feb. 17, 1948, copy to UK Delegation Washington (Cunningham Private Papers, III/I/103, St. Antony's College. Middle East Library, Oxford).

[314]Letter from Bondeli, ICRC Geneva, to ICRC delegation, London, Feb. 27, 1947 (AICRC, G.59/I/G.C.).

[315]Note from Marti, mission in Palestine, 'Entretien avec M. Léo Cohn (sic), Secrétaire du Département politique de l'Agence juive, Jérusalem,' Feb. 1, 1948, to ICRC Geneva (AICRC, G.59/I/G.C.).

Fitting the operation to a strategy

In Geneva, on February 28, 1948, the ICRC began debating general policy for its future operations in Palestine, on the basis of the joint report by Marti, Munier, and de Reynier. In three weeks the Special Commission to Study Ways and Means of Reinforcing the Efficacy of the Work of the ICRC would meet in Paris for the last time before the Stockholm Conference. During this period the Committee was preparing to show the Commission that the ICRC's effectiveness would be reinforced by the consolidation of international law and by the mention of the ICRC in future conventions – not by changes in its composition or in the structure of the International Red Cross. In terms of the development of humanitarian law, the draft article providing for the application of conventional principles to non-international conflicts such as civil wars was of prime importance, as has already been emphasized.[316]

This was the context in which the ICRC established the conditions and guidelines of its future activities in Palestine. Its main rule was not to embark upon any activity without first having obtained the warring parties' respective commitments to honor the essential principles of the 1929 Conventions.[317] This condition was perhaps a product of the ICRC's experience in World War II. In that war, the USSR had not acceded to the Prisoners of War Convention, nor allowed the ICRC to do anything for the 'Fascist' prisoners it held. Consequently, the ICRC had not been able to operate the 'lever of reciprocity'[318] on behalf of the Soviet prisoners of war who were in the hands of enemies of the USSR. This is what the ICRC explained to the Communists when they reproached it for failing to protect Soviet prisoners in German hands. The ICRC had already received an oral assurance that the Jewish side would do everything necessary to ensure the conventions were applied, but it had not received a similar promise from the Arab side.[319]

The ICRC therefore decided to launch an appeal to the parties

---

[316] See Chapter 1, pp. 34–5, and Chapter 2, pp. 66–8.
[317] ICRC, procès-verbal, Bureau meeting of Feb. 28, 1948 (AICRC, no file number).
[318] Frédéric Siordet, *Inter Arma Caritas*, p. 90.
[319] Letter from de Bondeli, ICRC Geneva, to ICRC London, Feb. 27, 1947 (AICRC, G.59/I/G.C.).

to the conflict in Mandatory Palestine, asking them to respect the essential principles of the conventions – principles the ICRC would have to clarify, since they were still poorly defined at that point in the evolution of the law. Once it had persuaded the parties to adhere to the principles of the *'Geneva Conventions'* (author's emphasis), the ICRC could remind the Jews and the Arabs of their undertaking to treat wounded and ill, prisoners, and civilians properly without requirement of reciprocity, and mediate between the Jews and the Arabs for all these categories of victims. This would also allow it to decide what it would do for each side; for example, it could emphasize protection for the Jews on one hand, and concentrate on material assistance for the Arabs on the other hand. The principle of reciprocity would be respected in relation to the ICRC, which after obtaining an advantage for the victims of one of the communities would be able to ask for an equivalent, if not analogous, gesture on behalf of the other. As Jacques Chenevière, a Committee member, pointed out, in Palestine any relief operations carried out would not serve as a 'doorway to protection'[320] – that is, a way of reaching prisoners and gaining entry to prison camps, as they had in Yugoslavia and Poland during the war; there, the ICRC's relief operations had given it access to camps of German prisoners, and in this way it had been able to protect them. In Mandatory Palestine it would have to create the link between material aid and the protection of war victims. Making its relief action conditional on a commitment by the parties to the conflict to respect the principles of the conventions would, it was hoped, allow the ICRC to connect the two branches of its activities: assistance and protection.[321]

Finally, before embarking on its official operation in Mandatory Palestine, the ICRC wanted to make doubly sure that the Arabs would participate in the cost of the enterprise, in order to strike a balance between all the parties and not lay itself open to accusations of bias. This accorded with its more general ambition to universalize its financing. The ICRC therefore decided to send Marti and Munier off immediately to raise funds in the countries of the Arab League, as well as Iran and Turkey. They would also

[320]ICRC, procès-verbal, Bureau meeting of March 4, 1948 (AICRC, no file number).
[321]Ibid.

take the opportunity to explain the significance of the Stockholm Conference to the leaders of the countries they visited and encourage them to participate.[322]

The conditions the ICRC posed before beginning its activities in Mandatory Palestine were well-defined from then on. The ICRC would negotiate with the belligerents for their agreement to respect the essential principles of the 1929 Conventions. This would give it the means of stimulating reciprocal interests between them, on the basis of which it would begin to exercise its role of neutral intermediary. Once this role was well-accepted, it would develop a program to supply material relief to those who most needed it, the Arabs. Finally, it would make every effort to obtain a financial contribution from all the parties concerned. This would be a step towards universalizing its sources of funds, to consolidate its sought-after independence from Switzerland.

All these arrangements arose out of the discussions between Marti and the Committee members, and reflected a mutual understanding between the team in the field and Geneva; they also make a counterpoint for the Committee members' preoccupation with the upcoming Stockholm Conference. If they were carried out, they would make the ICRC's enterprise in Mandatory Palestine a kind of model.

The ICRC archives do not yield up any concrete plans for specific operations to be conducted for the benefit of this or that sector of the Palestinian population affected by the war. For wounded Jews and Arabs, for the Arab civilians who had been streaming out of the area since December, 1947 – and whom the three visiting delegates must have seen on the roads – for the inhabitants of the Arab-ringed Jewish Quarter in the Old City of Jerusalem, for other categories of war victims – the ICRC did not recommend anything specifically adapted to their needs. In Geneva the concern was to reaffirm the ICRC's role of neutral intermediary as such. It was the ICRC delegates in the field who would decide on a day-to-day basis how to apply Geneva's general guidelines to the situations that arose and the suffering they confronted.

In a press release dated March 5, 1948, the ICRC publicly

---

[322] AICRC, G.59/I/G.C.

announced its delegates' financial prospecting mission in the Near East and recalled the foundation and the point of departure of its action in Palestine: The organization was responding to a spontaneous appeal from the British government. It had sent delegates to the country to offer 'to all concerned the customary services of the Committee as a neutral intermediary, having in mind especially the protection and care of wounded, sick, and prisoners.'[323] Obviously, the ICRC had no intention of keeping a low profile; it wanted to publicize its activities and explain their purpose.

Reaffirming threatened functions

Having been informed by Geneva that the Committee wanted its traditional neutral intermediary activities developed as quickly as possible in Palestine, de Reynier, who had remained in Jerusalem, paid a visit on March 11 to Sir Henry Guerney, adjutant to the British high commissioner, Sir Alan Cunningham, at the King David Hotel in Jerusalem. Cunningham happened to be present as well. This time de Reynier imposed the ICRC's views, referring explicitly to Article VII of the International Red Cross Statutes. He then went down into the basement of the hotel, where the members of the UN Special Commission on Palestine were hidden away. Although they had not been scheduled to arrive until May 1, they had actually been in the city since the beginning of March, in the greatest secrecy; fearing for their safety, they dared not leave the building.

De Reynier explained the Committee's intentions to the head of the UN mission, Pablo Azcarate; he needed the UN's approval for the operations the ICRC would undertake after the British left. Azcarate promised to refer the matter to his superiors, but in the meantime, like the British, he emphasized the primordial necessity of a medical and sanitary operation. De Reynier reiterated that the ICRC did not want to assume responsibility for the medical needs of the Arab population in Palestine. It did not exclude the medical aspect from its future activities, and should the UN request it, the delegation would examine the health problems that arose, on a case-by-case basis. What the ICRC

---

[323]ICRC, 'Mission of the International Red Cross Committee in Palestine,' press release no. 359b, Geneva, March 5, 1948 (Press Release Collection, ICRC Library).

most wanted to do in Mandatory Palestine, however, was to insure that the conventions were respected and to humanize the war in accordance with ICRC traditions, 'to help as much as possible on a moral basis if not a legal one.'[324] This indicated that the ICRC might not adhere to the letter of the conventions, but rather would allow itself to act according to its interpretation of their principles – thereby setting itself up as a moral authority.

The question was, however, whether the UN would accept the ICRC's mission as a neutral intermediary, and whether it too might be prepared to make a financial contribution to further that mission – perhaps by subsidizing the operation of the public health services. The UN's response arrived on March 31: The UN Commission agreed to permit a delegation 'of the International Red Cross' (sic) to function in Palestine after May 15, 1948.[325]

Back in Geneva, however, the Committee was concerned by the contacts its delegate in Jerusalem had established with the UN Commission. The Arabs, hostile to the United Nations, were likely to misunderstand relations between an ICRC delegate and members of the UN Commission, even if such relations in no way compromised the ICRC's independence. This could make the Committee's mission difficult. As Geneva wrote to de Reynier, 'the very nature of this mission in Palestine obliges you not to "tag along" after anyone, and to maintain a complete freedom of movement that cannot be questioned by either of the parties, since the latter can only trust you by reason of the apolitical nature of your activities.'[326]

Securing the legal grounds for intervention

On March 12, 1948, the day after de Reynier's visits to Sir Henry Guerney and the members of the UN Commission, the Committee proceeded to the next stage of its negotiations: securing from the belligerents a commitment to respect the humanitarian conventions, which would provide the delegation with legal grounds for intervention. The ICRC launched a public appeal, entitled

[324]Note from de Reynier, 'Entretien avec la Commission de l'ONU,' Jerusalem, to ICRC Geneva, March 11, 1948 (AICRC, G.59/I/G.C.). [Translation: M.G.]

[325]This consent was sent to de Reynier by telegram on March 31, 1948, according to a note from de Reynier, Jerusalem, to ICRC Geneva, April 8, 1948 (AICRC, G.3/82, G.49/I/G.C.).

[326]Note from de Bondeli, ICRC Geneva, to de Reynier, ICRC Jerusalem, March 25, 1948 (AICRC, G.59/I/G.C.). [Translation: M.G.]

'Application in Palestine of the *Principles* of the *Geneva Conventions*, Appeal by the ICRC in Geneva' (author's emphasis).[327] There was a reason that only the principles, rather than the 1929 Conventions themselves, were cited: The revised and new draft conventions as they stood on March 12, 1948, provided that in a civil war or any other conflict arising within the territory of a contracting party, the parties to the conflict would be asked to respect the *principles* of the conventions, on condition of reciprocity. In formulating its appeal to the parties at war in Palestine, the ICRC did not lose sight of the fact that this text could constitute a precedent for the promotion of an article extending the field of application of future conventions to situations of civil war.

At the same time, the ICRC could not ignore the possibility of an international conflict – a possibility suggested, in particular, by the entry into Palestine of the Syrian Arab Liberation Army. Such a conflict could lead to open warfare if two new states, Jewish and Arab, were to emerge; but the ICRC could not afford either to appear alarmist, or to assume the partition plan would take effect. It therefore took certain oratory precautions: 'Although the incidents now taking place do not constitute a conflict between two Powers,'[328] the ICRC called upon the parties, 'unless they decide meanwhile to abandon the use of force – to act in obedience to the traditional rules of international law, and to apply, as from today, the principles embodied in the two Conventions signed at Geneva on July 27, 1929.'[329]

What were the principles that the ICRC had in mind? At that stage in the evolution of humanitarian law, the principles the ICRC cited had not yet been extracted from the conventions and formulated as general rules, but the ICRC was seeking to do this in the revised or new draft conventions it was to present at the Stockholm Conference. In particular it intended to facilitate by this means the interpretation of the article – if it was accepted at the next diplomatic conference – providing for the application of these principles in non-international conflicts. In this context, the appeal of March 12, 1948, was an opportunity for the ICRC to enunciate the principles mentioned in the title of the appeal.

Thus, according to the March 12 appeal, the wounded and ill

---

[327]'Application in Palestine of the Principles of the Geneva Conventions, Appeal by the ICRC in Geneva,' Geneva, March 12, 1948 (AICRC, CP 312).
[328]Ibid.
[329]Ibid.

should 'be treated without discrimination in a spirit of humanity and receive the care which their condition demands. The vehicles for the transport of sick and wounded, the medical establishments (both fixed and mobile), as well as the members of the medical personnel and the medical stores shall be respected and protected in all circumstances.'[330] This wording is almost identical to that proposed by the ICRC in the draft revision of the Geneva Convention that it planned to present in Stockholm. In the revised Geneva Convention, protection would no longer be limited to the wounded and sick 'in armed forces in the field,' and 'without distinction of nationality,' but would cover all the wounded and ill in time of war, who would be protected and cared for 'in all circumstances.'[331] On the local level, this principle corresponded to Kohn's request that the Arabs respect medical convoys and personnel.

The second principle demanded 'respect shown to the dead, to their bodies and to the funeral arrangements for their burial.'[332] This provision also reflected the spirit of the draft revision of the Geneva Convention, which stipulated that the belligerents would take the necessary measures to seek out the dead and prevent them from being despoiled,[333] but the fact that the ICRC spelled it out indicates that the organization was concerned by what the Jewish Agency had said about the mutilation of the dead by Arab combatants and the attacks against Jewish convoys on their way to the cemetery on the Mount of Olives.

Next, the ICRC introduced the principle of civilian immunity, which it planned to emphasize in future conventions.[334] It affirmed the right to 'security for all persons who are non-comba-

---

[330]Ibid.

[331]'Revision of the Geneva Convention of July 27, 1929, for the Relief of the Wounded and Sick in Armies in the Field,' Chapter II, 'Wounded and Sick,' Art. 10, in ICRC, XVIIth International Conference of the Red Cross, Stockholm, August 1948, *Draft Revised or New Conventions for the Protection of War Victims, established by the International Committee of the Red Cross with the assistance of government experts, national Red Cross societies and other humanitarian associations* (Geneva: ICRC, May 1948), p. 9.

[332]'Appeal by the ICRC in Geneva,' March 12, 1948 (AICRC, CP 312 G).

[333]'Revision of the Geneva Convention of July 27, 1929, for the Relief of the Wounded and Sick in Armies in the Field,' Chapter II, Art. 12, in ICRC, XVIIth International Conference of the Red Cross, Stockholm, *Draft Revised or New Conventions*, p. 11.

[334]'Convention for the Protection of Civilian Persons in Time of War,' Part II: 'General Protection of Populations against Certain Consequences of War,' Art. 11, in ibid., p. 158.

THE ICRC ACHIEVES ITS AIM

tant, especially women, children and the aged,'[335] thus preparing the public mentally for the future establishment in Palestine of safety zones for the protection of civilian populations.

Finally, the ICRC came back to a principle already enshrined in the existing conventions, and extended it to include all combatants, regular or otherwise, nationals or not, since it was to be applied in the context of civil wars: the 'right of every combatant falling into the hands of the adverse party to be treated as a prisoner of war.'[336] The revised draft of the Prisoners of War Convention also tended in this direction, but did not go as far, since it listed the categories of combatants that could be considered as prisoners of war if captured – namely, the combatants belonging to organized forces and the civilian populations of occupied territories who fought openly, a definition that implicitly excluded 'franc-tireurs' or irregulars.[337]

The appeal of March 12, 1948 was conceived within the perspective of future law, not only existing law. Its application could therefore be expected to enrich the ICRC's tradition and, by creating a precedent, contribute to the advancement of international humanitarian law. It was in fact consistent with the drafts the ICRC was to submit to the Stockholm Conference, to which the ICRC in Geneva was adding the final touches in March, 1948.

The appeal was prepared and issued a few days before the Special Commission met for the last time before the Stockholm Conference. The Commission met in Paris on March 18 to decide which proposals concerning the revision of the IRC Statutes it wanted to recommend. At the same time, the ICRC began to lobby openly in favor of reinforcing its legal grounds for intervention instead of changing the structure of the International Red Cross. The March 12 appeal thus provided a good opportunity to reaffirm the argument that without legal grounds for intervention the ICRC could not do its best – its usual response to the criticisms regarding its weak efforts on behalf of the victims of Hitler's persecution. The same idea was reiterated at the end

---

[335]'Appeal by the ICRC in Geneva,' March 12, 1948.
[336]Ibid.
[337]'Revision of the Convention Concluded at Geneva on July 29, 1929, Relative to the Treatment of Prisoners of War,' Part I: 'General Provisions.' Art. 3, in ICRC, XVIIth International Conference of the Red Cross, Stockholm, *Draft Revised or New Conventions*, pp. 52–53.

of the appeal, where the ICRC stressed that the undertaking of the parties to the Palestinian conflict to respect the spirit of the conventions was 'imperative for the proper carrying out, in obedience to the principles which [the ICRC] is called upon to defend, of any humanitarian scheme in behalf of those who are suffering through the present distressing events.'[338]

At Geneva's request, de Reynier had the appeal disseminated in Palestine, in English, Hebrew, and Arabic, by all possible media: newspapers, radio, press conferences. At the same time, the Committee sent the text of its communiqué to those press agencies with offices in Geneva. Obviously, it was not intended solely for the parties locally engaged in the conflict. Given the international community's interest in Mandatory Palestine, the ICRC may have hoped that its message would be widely transmitted, enhancing understanding of the spirit of its work.

Arab reluctance: Jewish ICRC delegates?

In Jerusalem, de Reynier followed up the March 12 appeal with negotiations with the Jewish Agency and the Arab Higher Committee. The Jewish Agency made no difficulties. The Va'ad Le'umi had been prepared since February 15, 1948, to agree to a Committee request to respect the principles of humanitarian law.[339]

It remained only to convince the Arab Higher Committee. Recently, however, the representatives of the Arab Higher Committee had been maintaining a hostile distance from de Reynier.[340] During the same period, Marti and Munier, who had begun their tour of the Near East a week previously, met with very tepid courtesy in the countries they visited: Syria, Transjordan, and Iraq. What was going on? De Reynier heard by word of mouth that the Arabs believed his fellow delegates to be Jews: Marti, because of the mission he had carried out in aid of the Jewish refugees of the *Exodus 47*, and Munier, because he had assisted the Jewish exiles in Asmara and, later, in Kenya. The president

---

[338]'Appeal by the ICRC in Geneva,' March 12, 1948.
[339]'Projet de réponse du Va'ad Le'umi à un appel éventuel du CI sur l'application des Conventions,' annex to report by Marti, de Reynier, and Munier, Palestine mission, Jerusalem, Feb. 15, 1948 (AICRC, G.59/I/G.C.).
[340]Note from de Reynier, Palestine mission, Jerusalem, to ICRC Geneva, Delegations Division, March 10, 1948 (AICRC, G.59/I/G.C.).

THE ICRC ACHIEVES ITS AIM

of the Syrian Red Crescent sent a telegram to the ICRC in Geneva asking it to 'please take into consideration the non-presence of Jews among the special envoys.'[341] Hussein Khalidi, through whom de Reynier was trying to secure the Arab Higher Committee's promise to respect the conventions, complained that the ICRC was undertaking nothing in Palestine, but was nevertheless trying to collect money from the Arabs.[342]

De Reynier hastened to allay the Arabs' suspicions. He showed the consuls of the Arab countries in Jerusalem the letter of introduction that Azzam Pacha had given the ICRC envoys in January, 1848, when they visited Cairo. He wrote to Geneva: 'I went around to these consuls ..., casually showed the letter and explained our work, mentioning the *Exodus 47* but also the fact that Dr. Marti spent the entire war in Germany on behalf of the Allies, which proves his religion, since he is still alive.'[343] De Reynier went on to suggest that the passports of the delegates sent to Palestine should indicate that they were Christians.[344] Marti and Munier, for their part, asked Geneva to provide all the delegates and nurses sent to the Near East with a certificate of 'Arianism' (sic).[345] The Committee did not react to its delegates' shocking suggestions.

The ICRC's entire operation in Mandatory Palestine was at stake. In every Arab or Moslem country they visited, the ICRC delegates delivered a memorandum, dated March 14, 1948, in which they announced the ICRC's intention to act in Palestine, described the 1929 Conventions, asserted that the Jewish Agency and the Arab Higher Committee had promised to respect them – which at that point was apparently stretching the truth in the case of the Arab Higher Committee – and appealed for financial contributions from the Arab countries concerned by the fate of the victims of the Palestinian conflict.[346]

---

[341]Telegram from Dr. Kadry, President of Syrian Red Crescent, to ICRC Geneva, March 10, 1948 (AICRC, G.59/I/G.C.). [Translation: M.G.]

[342]Note from de Reynier, Palestine mission, Jerusalem, to ICRC Geneva, April 1948 (AICRC, G.59/I/G.C.).

[343]Note from de Reynier, Palestine mission, Jerusalem, to ICRC Geneva, Delegations Division, March 10, 1948, (AICRC, G.59/I/G.C.). [Translation: M.G.]

[344]Ibid.

[345]Note from Marti and Munier, mission to Arab countries, Baghdad, to ICRC Geneva, March 23, 1948 (AICRC, G.59/I/G.C.).

[346]ICRC, memorandum, March 14, 1948 (AICRC, G.59/I/G.C.).

As soon as the ICRC envoys heard they were thought to be Jews, they denied it orally. The Committee backed them up. On April 2, the ICRC wrote to the minister of foreign affairs in Damascus that Marti and Munier were 'both Swiss citizens and Christians.'[347] Unlike de Reynier, Marti, and Munier, it did not adopt the Nazi racial definition as the criterion for its delegates' non-Jewishness. In its letter to the Syrian Red Crescent, however, it used more ambiguous terms: The delegates Marti and Munier were 'both authentically Christians' and 'neither [was] of Israelite ancestry.'[348] The ICRC wrote to the president of the Iraqi Red Crescent that, as Munier and Marti had probably been able to confirm in person, neither of its special envoys was 'of the Israelite religion, not even partially: Dr. Marti, in particular, was head of our delegation in Berlin throughout the war, and it is obvious that he could not have filled that post if he had not been a Christian.'[349] As the ICRC explained to its correspondents, it offered these clarifications to demonstrate that it considered itself duty-bound to observe constant objectivity and the strictest neutrality in choosing the delegates it sent abroad.[350]

The ICRC's conditions are met

The belligerents undertake to respect the conventions

The ICRC achieved its goal: On March 30, in response to the appeal of March 12, the representatives of the Arab Higher Committee in Palestine, their fears allayed by the ICRC, orally agreed to make a formal commitment in the near future to respect the basic principles of the conventions. De Reynier informed the press immediately, without waiting for the written undertaking.[351] On April 3, 1948, Khalidi finally signed a document stating: 'The Higher Arab Committee, representing the Arab people of Palestine, having perused the said appeal, and in con-

[347]Letter from Gloor, Vice-President, ICRC Geneva, to Jamil Mardam Bey, Minister of Foreign Affairs, Damascus, April 2, 1948 (AICRC, G.59/I/G.C.).
[348]Letter from Gloor, Vice-President, ICRC Geneva, to Central Committee of the Syrian Red Crescent, Damascus, April 2, 1948 (AICRC, G.59/I/G.C.).
[349]Letter from Gloor, Vice-President, ICRC Geneva, to Syied Arshad el-Omari, President of the Red Crescent of Iraq, Baghdad, April 2, 1948 (AICRC, G.59/I/G.C.). [Translation: M.G.]
[350]Ibid.
[351]Reuter dispatch, Jerusalem, 'Convention Croix-Rouge en Palestine' (ICRC translation), March 30, 1948 (AICRC, G.59/I/G.C.).

THE ICRC ACHIEVES ITS AIM

formity with Arab and Moslem tradition and customs in respect of humanitarian issues, agree and will do everything humanely possible to abide by the minimum conditions enumerated in the ... appeal.'[352] This letter, however, emanating as it did from a local authority, was not enough for the ICRC. The Mufti had not yet given his consent. He was in Damascus, and the ICRC delegate in Egypt, Albert de Cocatrix, did his best to contact him. On April 7, 1948, the ICRC in Cairo learned from the Arab League that the Mufti would accept, but on condition of reciprocity.[353]

The Jewish Agency, for its part, had, on April 4, 1948, given its 'formal assurance that the competent Jewish authorities in Palestine will, during the present conflict, respect the Geneva Conventions of 1929, both in regard to military personnel and to the civilian population,'[354] but with this reservation: It would protect civilian populations only in so far as 'the said conventions apply to civilian populations.' The 1929 Conventions did not apply to civilian populations – as the Jewish authorities could not help being aware – but it was the goal towards which the ICRC, encouraged by the government experts consulted in 1947, was orienting its new and revised draft conventions.[355]

On April 9, 1948, the Mufti spoke. Acknowledging receipt of the ICRC's appeal on March 30, 1948 (the date that de Reynier informed the press of the Arab Higher Committee's agreement to undertake in writing to respect the conventions), he declared that the 'principles contained in this appeal are already applied by the Arabs in the present struggle for the defense of their Homeland and their liberty,' and that 'consequently, the Arab Higher Committee for Palestine takes the opportunity to express

---

[352] Letter from Khalidi, AHC Jerusalem, to ICRC in Palestine, April 3, 1948 (AICRC, G.59/I/G.C.). See also CICR, 'Le Comité international de la Croix-Rouge en Palestine (décembre 1947–1er mai 1948),' *RICR* 353 (May 1948): 335.

[353] Letter from Azzam Pacha, League of Arab States, Cairo, to ICRC Cairo, April 7, 1948 (AICRC, G.59/I/G.C.).

[354] Letter from Golda Myerson and Itzhak Ben Zevie (sic), Tel Aviv, to ICRC in Palestine, Jerusalem, April 4, 1948 (AICRC, G.59/I/G.C.). See also CICR, 'Le Comité international de la Croix-Rouge en Palestine,' *RICR* 353 (May 1948): 335.

[355] 'Revision of the Geneva Convention of July 27, 1929, for the Relief of the Wounded and Sick in Armies in the Field,' Chapter III: 'Medical Units and Establishments,' Art. 18, p. 15; 'Convention for the Protection of Civilian Persons in Time of War,' Part II: 'General Protection of Populations against Certain Consequences of War,' Art. 12, p. 158; and Annex A: 'Draft Agreement Relating to Hospital and Safety Zones and Localities,' pp. 214–218; all in ICRC, XVIIth International Conference of the Red Cross, Stockholm, *Draft Revised or New Conventions*.

its formal agreement with the four clauses formulated in'[356] the ICRC's appeal.

The ICRC had not waited for the Mufti's letter to decide that it could officially begin its operation on behalf of the victims of the Palestine conflict. On April 8, 1948, it wrote to Marti, then making his tour through the Near East, that 'now that the two parties to the conflict have accepted the primordial condition posed by the ICRC, namely to respect the spirit of the Red Cross conventions, our plan of action can be put into effect.'[357] The ICRC published the pledges of both the Jewish Agency and the Arab Higher Committee, but in the case of the latter, it preferred to show the text signed by Khalidi rather than the one signed by the Mufti.[358]

It should be noted, too, that the ICRC did not approach el-Kaukji, the head of the Arab Liberation Army, who was leading the offensive in northern Palestine. We have no indication as to whether this was a conscious decision on the ICRC's part. The Mandatory power may have preferred to remain ignorant of that foreign Arab army's presence on mandated territory – the question remains open. Whatever the reason, the ICRC did not seek out el-Kaukji until May 9, 1948, when it discreetly made contact with him in Jenin.[359]

The legal grounds for intervention that the ICRC had secured by obtaining the consent of the parties in the Palestine-EY conflict were modeled on the provisions the ICRC hoped to insert in the future Geneva Conventions, if and when those conventions were extended to conditions of civil war. In this respect, the appeal of March 12, 1948 constituted a precedent.

From civil war to international war: a stormy transition

On May 14, 1948, however, the nature of the conflict changed, and the ICRC was obliged to adapt its legal basis for intervention

---

[356]Letter from Chairman of the Arab Higher Committee for Palestine, Cairo, to ICRC Cairo, April 9, 1948 (AICRC, G.59/I/G.C.). [M.G. translation from ICRC translation of original Arabic.]

[357]Note from Dunand, ICRC Geneva, to Marti, care of ICRC delegation in Cairo, April 8, 1948 (AICRC, G.59/I/G.C.). [Translation: M.G.]

[358]CIRC, 'Le Comité international de la Croix-Rouge en Palestine (décembre 1947 au 1er mai 1948),' *RICR* 353 (May 1948): 329.

[359]Report from Jean Courvoisier, ICRC Nablus, to ICRC Geneva, May 14, 1948 (AICRC, G.59/I/G.C.).

THE ICRC ACHIEVES ITS AIM

to the new situation. When the state of Israel declared independence on May 14, 1948, five Arab armies from the neighboring countries – Lebanon, Syria, Iraq, Transjordan, and Egypt – attacked. The ICRC was no longer dealing with a civil war, but an international one, which implied the integral application of the 1929 Conventions, insofar as the belligerents had acceded to them. Egypt and Iraq were signatories of the two conventions that were most important to the ICRC in the Palestine-EY conflict, namely the Geneva Convention for the Amelioration of the Condition of the Wounded and Sick in Armed Forces in the Field, and the Prisoners of War Convention. Lebanon and Syria had acceded to the first one, but not to the second. Transjordan had not acceded to either.[360] Israel, which had just come into being as a sovereign state, had not yet had the time to accede formally to the conventions, and consequently was not officially bound by them. The Arab Higher Committee, in turn, was bound only by its declaration of the preceding April. The situation was complex and the ICRC could not simply remind the belligerents of their conventional obligations. To complicate matters still further, the Arab countries did not recognize Israel as a state.

On May 24, 1948, the ICRC addressed a public appeal to all the belligerents,[361] urging them to respect the provisions of the 1929 Conventions and offering its services as 'a neutral intermediary acting according to the traditions of the Red Cross and the Red Crescent...'[362] It went on to mention the relevant articles of the Prisoners of War Convention, concerning the Central Tracing Agency for prisoners of war and, by extension, for civilian internees, although the latter were not yet protected by a convention. This appeal is a good example of the way that the ICRC, looking ahead to future conventions, saw them in relation to existing conventions. To quote Max Huber, who after World War II was no longer interested in upholding the legalist view but

---

[360] According to letter from de Bondeli, ICRC Geneva, to Hadi Hakki, Syria Legation, Bern, April 15, 1948 (AICRC, G.59/I/G.C.). A clarification should be made regarding Transjordan. On March 15, 1932, Transjordan – by a royal edict published in the official *Gazette* 345 (May 1932), and conforming to Article 19, Paragraph 2, of the Organic Law – announced its wish to accede to the 1929 Conventions. That accession was not made according to the normal procedure, however, in that the Swiss government was not notified of it.

[361] Ruegger, President of the ICRC, untitled memorandum, May 24, 1948 (AICRC, G.59/I/G.C.).

[362] Ibid. [Translation: M.G.]

wanted the ICRC to assume a role of moral authority, what 'matters in the Convention is its humanitarian substance, which must be maintained outside or above the law.'[363]

Of those who were sent the May 24 memorandum, the Arab League was the first to react. Azzam Pacha declared that the Arab combatants were already respecting and would continue to respect the conventions, but this intention might go by the board if the Zionists, who were all terrorists, did not behave humanely. He was referring to the massacre of some 200 innocent civilians which had been perpetrated by the Irgun in the Arab village of Deir Yassin on April 9, 1948.[364] The specter of a war of reprisals appeared on the horizon, worrying the ICRC.

To avoid the risk of offending the Arab countries, the ICRC had addressed its May 24 appeal personally to Moshe Shertok, the minister of foreign affairs of the provisional government of Israel, rather than to the Israeli government as such.[365] Shertok replied on May 27, declaring that his 'government has the intention of observing very strictly all provisions of the Geneva Convention for the protection of prisoners of war and civilian detainees who fall into its hands.'[366] He hoped that the ICRC would appreciate this official response, considering that the memorandum had been addressed to him personally.[367]

Israel's undertaking to respect the 1929 Conventions aroused the fury of the Arab countries. All of them referred to the massacre of Deir Yassin to bolster their calls to struggle against the 'Zionists' – a term they gave a pejorative significance – whom they characterized without exception as 'bandits' and 'terrorists.' Phalangist Lebanon[368] was the first to express the Arab rage, followed by Iraq.[369] Their words betraying the weakness of their

---

[363]ICRC procès-verbal, Bureau meeting of April 11, 1946 (AICRC, no file number). [Translation: M.G.]

[364]Telegram from Azzam Pacha, Secretary of the Arab League, Cairo, to ICRC Geneva, May 26, 1948 (AICRC, G.59/I/G.C.). See pp. 128–33 for the Deir Yassin massacre

[365]Telegram from Ruegger, President of the ICRC, to Moshe Shertok, Minister of Foreign Affairs, Tel Aviv, May 24, 1948 (AICRC, G.59/I/G.C.).

[366]Telegram from Shertok, Minister of Foreign Affairs, Provisional Government of the State of Israel, to Ruegger, President of the ICRC, Geneva, May 27, 1948 (AICRC, G.59/I/G.C. and ISA/MEA/1987.7). [Translation: M.G.]

[367]Ibid.

[368]Radiogram from Hamid Frangié, Minister of Foreign Affairs, Beirut, to ICRC Geneva, May 29, 1948 (AICRC, G.59/I/G.C.).

[369]According to telegram from ICRC Cairo to ICRC Geneva, June 2, 1948, citing the Iraqi communication (AICRC, G.59/I/G.C.).

knowledge about the International Red Cross and the 1929 Conventions, these countries threatened to quit the International Red Cross if the ICRC allowed a state which they considered illegitimate to adhere to the 1929 Conventions, and asserted that the other Arab states would follow suit.

The ICRC's relations with the Arab world were liable to deteriorate seriously if the organization did not find a way to extricate itself from the controversy. Under no circumstances could it afford any involvement with the Arab opposition against Israel, since that would make its role of neutral intermediary impossible. Moreover, the US and the USSR had recognized the Jewish state. The ICRC had to reach an understanding somehow with the Arab states, and to that end it chose to explain to them certain facts about the organization.

The first point was that although the ICRC helped draft conventions, it played no further role once the time came to ratify them. It was the Swiss Confederation – which, it should be noted, had not yet recognized Israel – which was the depository for the 1929 Conventions and which collected the states' instruments of accession. The ICRC had no control over which states acceded,[370] but, in principle, accession to the conventions facilitated the ICRC's task by providing a legal basis for ICRC intervention.

The second point was that a state's accession to the humanitarian conventions did not in itself make that state a member of the International Red Cross, but it was one of the conditions necessary for a state's national society to be accepted by that organization. Accordingly, if the state of Israel formally acceded to the 1929 Conventions, the question of recognizing the Israeli National Society as a member of the International Red Cross could arise. The Israeli society would also have to give up the red star of David in favor of the red cross.

The ICRC would have to reassure the Arab states about its intentions regarding the possible recognition of the Israeli relief society if the latter agreed – unlikely though that was – to adopt the red cross as its emblem. The ICRC decided that if the Arab countries raised the question, it would reply that on principle it did not recognize new National Societies while hostilities were in progress. In deciding on this course, it drew on its experi-

---

[370]Letter from Gallopin, ICRC Geneva, to Ruegger, President of the ICRC, Jerusalem, May 31, 1948 (AICRC, G.59/I/G.C.).

ence in World War II.[371] This way, it would be able to explain to the Arab countries that in its eyes the Magen David Adom (the Hebrew for 'red shield of David'[372]) did not constitute a Red Cross society, but was a charitable society like any other, with which it maintained de facto relations.

Between June 2–11, 1948, the ICRC wrote letters explaining these points to the governments of Lebanon, Iraq, and other countries hostile to Israel. It dispatched several envoys to the diplomatic representatives of these countries in Switzerland in order to supplement the letters with oral clarifications where necessary. These efforts to set the record straight did have some effect, for the Arab countries ultimately accepted the ICRC's aid to the Arab Palestinians in Israel or in the areas controlled by the Jews. But there were to be constant gaps between the Arab states' declarations of principle, which affirmed their intention of respecting the conventions, and their armies' actual behavior towards the Jews.

The ICRC's explanations did not give it much more latitude in its relations with Israel, either; in its local public communications, it continued to address the 'Jewish' civil and military authorities when it meant Israel and its army. After May 14, 1948, the date the state of Israel came into being, de Reynier had the delegation's official paper printed with the letterhead 'Delegation of the International Committee of the Red Cross for Palestine.' In 1948 the ICRC did not speak of the 'Arab-Israeli' conflict, as the Jews did, or of the 'Arab-Jewish' conflict, as the Arabs did. For as long as the war lasted, the ICRC used a third term, the 'Palestine' conflict, after the former Mandatory Palestine. These measures, intended to be neutral and to soothe Arab sensibilities, irritated the Israelis.

First official act: at Deir Yassin

De Reynier performed the first official act of the ICRC delegation in Mandatory Palestine, without consulting Geneva, on April 11, 1948 – just after the agreement by the Jewish Agency and the Arab Higher Committee to respect the essential principles of

---

[371]In-house note from Pictet, 'Doctrine à fixer quant à des Croix-Rouge demeurant dans une situation anormale,' cited in ICRC, procès-verbal, Bureau meeting of Aug. 29, 1946 (AICRC, no file number).

[372]For the origin of this term, see Chapter 4, p. 146.

THE ICRC ACHIEVES ITS AIM

the Geneva Conventions. De Reynier, still on his own in Palestine, was called by representatives of the Arab Higher Committee to the little Arab village of Deir Yassin, the population of which had been savagely massacred by the IZL on April 9, 1948. The village was located about five kilometers from Jerusalem, in the direction of Jaffa. De Reynier arrived on the scene accompanied by a member of the IZL and a Magen David Adom medical team. The commander of the troops occupying the village told de Reynier that just before the attack, the women and children had been warned and called upon to surrender. His story, as reported by de Reynier, was that some 150 people – mostly women and children, but also a number of wounded men – had responded to the call and given themselves up to the British army. The IZL had apparently deemed those who remained to be combatants, and attacked the village. De Reynier's informant estimated the total death count at about 200 people.

De Reynier explained the purpose of his mission. The ICRC did not want to set itself up as a judge or arbiter. De Reynier had come only to 'return the wounded and dead to the Arab zone.'[373] However, since the bodies had been carried out of the village, de Reynier was not able to see them. Passing through the ruined village, he discovered in the rubble a little girl of about ten who was still alive, and he immediately put her into the care of the medical team accompanying him. Back in Jerusalem at midday, de Reynier mediated between the Arabs and the Jews. After a long discussion with the representatives of the Arab Higher Committee, de Reynier contacted an IZL official (whose name is unrecorded), and gave him the following instructions in the name of the ICRC:

- The dead were to be buried where they were.
- The IZL was to provide a list of the dead, together with their identity cards, so that the ICRC could inform the Arab authorities and possibly the families of the victims.
- The wounded survivors were to be delivered to him at a place agreed upon, where an Arab ambulance would await them.

De Reynier formulated these requirements in the spirit of the

---

[373]Report from de Reynier, ICRC Jerusalem, to ICRC Geneva, April 13, 1948 (AICRC. G.3/82). [Translation: M.G.]

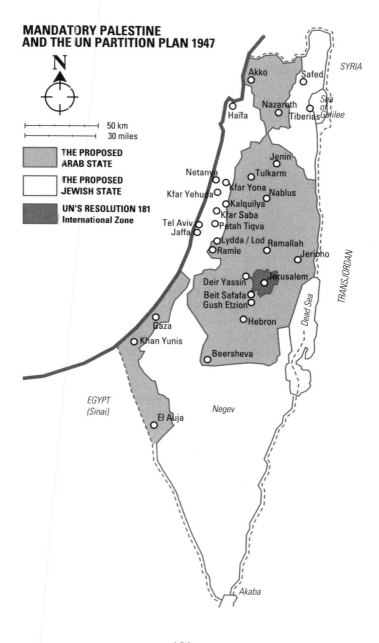

THE ICRC ACHIEVES ITS AIM

role of neutral intermediary and moral authority that the ICRC had allocated to itself.

At about 5:00 p.m., an old woman, seriously wounded, was brought to the appointed place. There was apparently no other survivor of the massacre, besides the little girl mentioned above.

Following these events, de Reynier went to the Jewish Agency to protest the atrocities. He mentioned the Jewish Agency's pledge to respect the 1929 Conventions, and declared that this crime violated them in both letter and spirit. The Jewish Agency expressed indignation and regret, but replied that the massacre had been perpetrated by the IZL, whose actions it could not control – a fact it hastened to confirm publicly. In a communiqué dated April 11, it condemned the massacre, which, committed by dissident organizations, was contrary to the spirit of the Jewish community of Palestine – pointing out first, however, that although this was no excuse, no one had ever spoken up against the murders and mutilations committed in Palestine by Arabs against Jews.[374]

To judge by de Reynier's report to the Committee,[375] and contrary to what has often been claimed since, the ICRC delegate did not denounce this collective crime. He told Arabic radio that at his instigation, two ambulances, a truck, three doctors, and a few Jewish medical workers had been completely given over to the relief action.[376] The Arabic radio station in Jerusalem broadcast a statement by the Arab Higher Committee, which in apportioning the blame for the massacre relied on an oral report that de Reynier had made to it. The ICRC representative in Palestine himself considered that he could not condemn the atrocities in the name of the ICRC, because the latter was not mandated to serve as a judge,[377] but as a neutral intermediary.

Arab reprisals against Jews were not long in coming. In

---

[374] The exact wording of the Jewish Agency's statement can be found in the Israel State Archives: 'Statement Regarding Deir Yassin,' April 11, 1948 (ISA/MEA/2106.2). For a press source, see, for example, Eric Downton, '200 Died in Terrorist Massacre of Arabs, Reprisal Attack on Jewish Settlement Opens,' *Daily Telegraph* (April 12, 1948): 1 and 4.

[375] Report from de Reynier, ICRC Jerusalem, to ICRC Geneva, April 13, 1948 (AICRC, G.3/82).

[376] See, for example, Downton, '200 Died in Terrorist Massacre of Arabs,' pp. 1 and 4.

[377] Ibid.

northern Palestine, the Arab Liberation Army attacked Kibbutz Mishmar Ha'emek. The Arab League appealed to the Arabs in Palestine not to carry out reprisals against Jewish villages. The 1929 Conventions prohibited reprisals, and the ICRC conveyed its appreciation of the Arab League's gesture through the intermediary of the Egyptian government.[378]

Deploying forces

The ICRC sent its first delegates and nurses to Palestine between April 14–29, 1948, all of them armed with documents attesting to their Christian affiliation. One of them reportedly had an 'Aryan' certificate furnished by a lecturer at the University of Geneva, though the teacher had supposedly asked him not to use it unless his life depended on it, since the Jewish race did not exist.[379]

Jean Courvoisier moved into the Nablus Triangle, headquarters of the Syrian Arab Liberation Army commanded by el-Kaukji. Maximilian de Meuron was based in Haifa, a Jewish port city where the ICRC had been planning since April, 1948, to send material aid for the Jewish sector in Palestine when the time came. Robert Gouy established an office in Tel Aviv and moved into the Cliff Hotel in Jaffa. Courvoisier, De Meuron, and Gouy had all been demobilized from the Paris delegation, which had cut back its activities after carrying out the last repatriations – the liberation of German prisoners of war held by the French. These delegates, like their colleagues in the Paris delegation, were aware of the ICRC's difficulties and concerned for its future.[380]

The same was true of Pierre Gaillard, who held a post in the ICRC Delegations Division and had the task of traveling back and forth between Palestine and Geneva. In this way he provided a link between the field, where personal initiative predominated, and the ICRC in Geneva, which was anxious that the operation

---

[378]Letter from Martin Bodmer, Vice-President of ICRC, to Abdul Karim Bey Sawfat, Envoy Extraordinary and Minister Plenipotentiary of His Majesty the King of Egypt, Legation of Egypt, Bern, April 23, 1948 (AICRC, G.59/I/G.C.).

[379]As reported by Pierre Gaillard in a conversation with the author in the summer of 1981. Since the ICRC did not give me access to the personal files of the ICRC delegates, I must cite this information with some reservations.

[380]Melchior Borsinger, report of Paris mission, Geneva, Sept. 27, 1947 (AICRC, G.8/51).

THE ICRC ACHIEVES ITS AIM

be carried out in its spirit, whatever the circumstances. None of these first delegates to Mandatory Palestine was a doctor, in accordance with the wishes of de Reynier, who at the beginning of April, 1948, had remarked that the delegation had more use for 'a civilian delegate familiar with ICRC work than [for] a good doctor who is not,' and that the ICRC would save 'more people with properly applied conventions than with doctors ...'[381]

Nonetheless, in May, 1948, the ICRC was obliged to send in more doctors: Raoul Pflimlin and Pierre Fasel, on their first mission, and Otto Lehner, an old hand at the ICRC, who had been a delegate for the organization in the Nazi protectorate of Bohemia-Moravia (Czechoslovakia under Hitler's occupation). The ICRC also had nurses in various government hospitals of Palestine, who worked in obscurity under the authority of the local delegate. They did not make systematic written reports on their work, since their role, though necessary, was considered of secondary importance in the ICRC's scale of priorities.

The ICRC delegation's headquarters in Palestine were in Jerusalem at the YMCA hostel, opposite the King David Hotel, just where the Jewish New City of Jerusalem was closest to the Arab Old City and overlooking it. The two areas were separated by a no man's land down below. The ICRC delegation's headquarters were thus accessible to both parties from the moment the official operation began, but they were also potentially in the line of fire.

---

[381] Note from de Reynier, ICRC Jerusalem, to ICRC Geneva, April 5, 1948 (ICRC, G.59/I/G.C.). [Translation: M.G.]

Chapter Four

THE RED CROSS IN PALESTINE–ERETZ-YISRAEL: FUNCTION, SIGNIFICANCE, AND USAGE

The flag

The first thing the British expected the ICRC to do, in January, 1948, was to take steps to insure the continued operation of the Palestine government health system after the Mandate ended, when the United Nations relieved the Mandatory power for the transition period that would precede the implementation of the partition plan. The Palestine government health facilities provided most of the medical services available to the Arab Palestinians, whereas the Jewish Agency had created its own health-care system. The British considered that failing to provide for the continued smooth operation of their hospitals after they left Palestine would amount to abandoning the Arab population in the sphere of public health.

The ICRC did not feel, however, that it could assume direct responsibility for the hospitals and other health services, and even if it could, at that moment, it would still be unwilling. It did not wish to care for war victims itself, but rather to fulfill its role of neutral intermediary, thereby reaffirming the wartime task entrusted to it by Article VII of the International Red Cross Statutes. Moreover, it did not want to undertake anything that, a priori, would constitute a derogation of the principle of impartiality as the ICRC interpreted it: intervening on behalf of the victims of both camps. At the beginning of 1948, however, the Arab Palestinians in particular required the services of hospitals that were secure enough so that the medical personnel would agree to remain in them. The Jewish Palestinians, on the other hand, required protection of their facilities and ambulances against Arab attacks.

The solution – obligatory, from the ICRC's standpoint – that would permit the reconciliation of all these goals was to persuade the parties to the conflict to recognize the immunity of health-care facilities and any other stationary or mobile medical equipment or supplies, in accordance with the principle laid down in the Geneva Convention.[382] As mentioned earlier, at the beginning of April, 1948, both parties had agreed to observe the basic principles of the conventions, including the right of the wounded and sick to be collected and cared for in all circumstances. Safeguarding the hospitals was therefore the responsibility of the belligerents.

The red cross: a label and a symbol

This recourse to international humanitarian law implied that health-care facilities benefiting from immunity should be indicated by a distinctive sign, which, under the Geneva Convention, could be a red cross, a red crescent, or else a red lion and sun.[383] In this case, the red cross (or the equivalent symbol) served as a label with a protective function: The military authorities on both sides were to use it to mark visibly, whenever it seemed useful, the members of the medical corps, the buildings, and the material that the Geneva Convention ordered the belligerents to protect and respect,[384] so that the adversary could see and spare them. The Geneva Convention did not forbid the caregiving personnel to bear arms in their own defense, nor to provide establishments indicated by the protective emblem with a police force responsible for the security of the hospitals or the medical convoys.[385] However, it would clearly be a serious violation of the principles of the Geneva Convention to hide arms or troops in the establishments or ambulances marked with the red cross (or equivalent emblem), thus making them into camouflaged combat bases. The

---

[382]'Geneva Convention of July 27, 1929, for the Amelioration of the Condition of the Wounded and Sick in Armed Forces in the Field,' Chapter II: 'Medical Formations and Establishments,' Art. 6, in ICRC/LRCS, *Handbook*, p. 60.

[383]Ibid., Chapter VI: 'The Distinctive Emblem' Art. 19, in ICRC/LRCS, *Handbook*, p. 64.

[384]Ibid., Art. 22, in ICRC/LRCS, *Handbook*, p. 65.

[385]Ibid., Chapter II: 'Medical Formations and Establishments,' Art. 8, in ICRC/LRCS, *Handbook*, p. 61.

red cross could not be used to designate material or personnel serving any categories of war victims except wounded and sick army personnel The convention also provided that in wartime the red cross could be called 'Geneva Cross.'[386]

Finally, only the army medical services were entitled to use the red cross for protection; the personnel of duly recognized and authorized voluntary aid societies could use it on condition that they placed themselves under the military authority.[387] No other entity was permitted to do this,[388] not even the National Red Cross Societies or the International Committee of the Red Cross.

The International Committee described itself as 'of the Red Cross' because the emblem had a symbolic value for it; there was, however, no direct relation with the distinctive, protective function of the red cross as defined by the Geneva Convention. For the ICRC, the red cross symbolized the principles underlying the International Red Cross and of which it was the guardian, the ideals and the spirit of the work it had originated. It had made its flag from the red cross emblem registered in the Geneva Convention. The emblem evoked Switzerland, since it was formed by reversing the colors of the federal flag; and it evoked Geneva, the birthplace of the Geneva Convention. Geneva was also the headquarters (contested by some) of the ICRC.

For a long time the ICRC had arrogated to itself the right to use its flag for its own protection as well, a use that had no basis in the Geneva Convention. Nor did the ICRC limit that use to the wounded and sick; for example, ICRC delegates provided themselves with armbands bearing the red cross emblem when they visited prisoner-of-war camps. The sides of the ICRC ships that had plied the seas during World War II to deliver Red Cross parcels to prisoners of war had been marked with large red crosses so the belligerents could let them pass in safety if possible.[389] The ICRC had done this for practical reasons, but the

---

[386]Ibid., Chapter VI: 'The Distinctive Emblem,' Art. 24, in ICRC/LRCS, *Handbook*, p. 65.

[387]Ibid., Art. 20, in ICRC/LRCS, *Handbook*, p. 64.

[388]Ibid., Chapter VIII: 'Suppression of Abuses and Infractions,' Art. 28 a), in ICRC/LRCS, *Handbook*, pp. 66–67.

[389]ICRC delegation to Stockholm, preparatory meetings, July 20, 1948 (AICRC, CR 25).

ICRC's members and workers also had an emotional attachment to the organization's emblem. The Red Cross emblem, which doubled as the ICRC's flag, symbolized their ideal, and they relayed it from one person to the next.

The National Red Cross Societies and their personnel were no less attached to the flag with the red cross on the white background; they, too, considered it as their own. They took the same liberties as the ICRC in using it, despite the risk. In fact, being closely tied to their respective governments and their particular political and cultural contexts, they were more likely than the ICRC to forget the conventions and the principles that inspired them, to deny them or to interpret them in a way that betrayed the original ideal of the work. During World War II, for example, German Red Cross members used a red cross to mask disgraceful acts such as the pseudo-medical experiments conducted by Nazi doctors in the concentration camps.

That, of course, was a recent, extreme case; there were others, much less serious, but ideologically disturbing in view of the problems with unity and harmony that the International Red Cross faced at the beginning of the Cold War. For instance, major National Societies like the American and Australian Red Crosses carried out 'military welfare' activities – namely, aid benefiting the able-bodied soldiers of their armies, which was contrary to the spirit of the Geneva Convention.[390]

Rallying under one flag

In a divided International Red Cross, in which the members drifted from the straight and narrow in interpreting the spirit of the work and the conventions, the ICRC had the feeling that the Red Cross was in 'peril'[391] and needed defending, which meant defending its symbol, its flag. In that effort, constant confusion reigned between two possible usages of the red cross on the white background: the label, or the sign of the red cross; and the symbol, or the emblem of the Red Cross, and of the ICRC.

Thus, in the draft revision of the Geneva Convention of 1929

---

[390]ICRC, procès-verbal, Bureau meeting of Jan. 27, 1948 (AICRC, no file number).
[391]Ibid.

for the Amelioration of the Condition of the Wounded and Sick, which it was to present at Stockholm, the ICRC proposed, with the approval of the government experts it had consulted, that 'the organisms of the International Red Cross and their duly recognized personnel' should be 'authorized to use the sign of the red cross on a white ground at any time,'[392] on condition that they used it only to indicate activities involving the wounded and sick.[393] This provision, introduced as much for the protective function of the emblem as for its symbolic value, might link the Red Cross societies and their League more closely to the spirit of the work as expressed in the Geneva Convention, and prevent them from drifting off course. The ICRC may have had this in mind when it proposed including the provision in future conventions.

For itself, the ICRC added a clause intended to protect its role of neutral intermediary and its right of initiative against a revision, by unenlightened minds, of the International Red Cross Statutes – meaning the proposed internationalization of the Committee's membership or the ICRC's subordination to the Standing Commission of the International Conference of the Red Cross. The ICRC suggested that the revised Geneva Convention should include an article stipulating that 'the provisions of the present Convention do not constitute an obstacle to the humanitarian activities which the International Committee of the Red Cross may undertake for the protection of wounded and sick, of members of the medical personnel and of chaplains, and for their relief, subject to the consent of the Parties to the conflict who may be concerned.'[394] If this article were adopted, it would allow the ICRC to base its activities as a neutral intermediary on the Geneva Convention, in the framework of which the red cross emblem had been instituted. By attaining a place in the Geneva Convention, an instrument which could not be dissociated from

---

[392]'Revision of the Geneva Convention of July 27, 1929, for the Relief of the Wounded and Sick in Armies in the Field,' Chapter VII: 'The Distinctive Emblem,' Art. 36, in XVIIth International Conference of the Red Cross, Stockholm, August 1948, *Draft Revised or New Conventions for the Protection of War Victims*, pp. 25–26.

[393]Ibid.

[394]'Revision of the Geneva Convention of July 27, 1929, for the Relief of the Wounded and Sick in Armies in the Field,' Chapter I: 'General Provisions,' Art. 7, in XVIIth International Conference of the Red Cross, Stockholm, August 1948, *Draft Revised or New Conventions for the Protection of War Victims*, p. 8.

the work of the Red Cross in general, the ICRC would anchor itself firmly at the core of that work.[395]

The fight against the inflation in emblems

Under the threat of schism in the International Red Cross, an idea that the ICRC had been defending for many years re-emerged with a vengeance. The ICRC wanted the governments that adopted the revised Geneva Convention to renounce the emblems equivalent to the red cross, namely the red crescent and the red lion and sun, leaving the red cross as the sole emblem. The variety of signs in fact emphasized the particular characteristics of those signs, be they religious, national, or political, whereas a single emblem would be easier to present as the neutral conveyor of a simple, universal message. The ICRC wanted that single emblem to be the red cross, to which it was so closely tied.

Concentrating on this objective, the ICRC was defending a rather unrealistic point of view, namely that the red cross had no religious or political significance. It was, claimed the Committee, a neutral sign, devised merely to distinguish both the persons who devoted themselves to the care of the wounded, and the fixed and mobile equipment that they used. Every soldier was supposed to be instructed to spare equipment marked with a red cross on a white background. If a number of different signs existed, said the ICRC, it would be more difficult to insure that the combatants recognized and respected them. The ICRC also pointed out that the red cross was the symbol of a single ideal. Multiplying the symbols implied a danger of impairing the unity of the ideal; each country might imbue 'its' symbol with its own interpretation of the Red Cross principles and ideals.

The question of reinstating the red cross as the sole protective emblem in the revised Geneva Convention had been discussed at the Preliminary Conference of National Red Cross Societies in

---

[395] It should be noted that up until then, only the Prisoners of War Convention – which was not a 'Geneva Convention' proper, but rather a convention concluded *at* Geneva which did not mention the red cross emblem – recognized a right of humanitarian action, and even that only with respect to prisoners of war.

Geneva in 1946.[396] At the time, the representative from Egypt had expressed the view that Moslem sensibilities would make the Arab countries unwilling to accept the cross. This led the ICRC to assume – in the absence of the Alliance of Red Cross and Red Crescent Societies of the USSR, which was boycotting the conference – that if the Moslems of the Arab countries were apt to react negatively, the same might be true of those in the Moslem republics of the USSR. The ICRC was eager to appease the USSR, and in particular its Alliance of Red Cross and Red Crescent Societies, which, about ten days before the conference, at the session of the Board of Governors of the League of Red Cross Societies held in Oxford, had proposed simply to do away with the ICRC altogether and replace it with the League. Since 1946, then, the ICRC had not dared to suggest suppressing the red crescent, for fear of unleashing reactions that would increase the risk of schism in the International Red Cross.

The Committee had therefore chosen to compromise, encouraged by National Society and government experts. At the Stockholm Conference it would propose maintaining the red crescent, but it would recommend that every effort be made to avoid accepting any new emblem – such as the red star of David – in future conventions.[397] This would not prevent it from continuing, over the long term, to militate in favor of returning to a single emblem, the red cross – as it had been doing since the beginning of the century.[398] But there was to be an intermediate phase in that struggle, during which the ICRC would oppose adding to the emblems valid since 1906 in the 1948 revision of the Geneva Convention.

The ICRC's use of the red cross

These issues had implications for the ICRC's activities in Palestine, as a review of some of those activities indicates. The ICRC's

[396]ICRC, *Report on the Work of the Preliminary Conference of National Red Cross Societies for the Study of the Conventions and of Various Problems Relative to the Red Cross* (Geneva: ICRC, 1947), pp. 43–44. See also Chapter 1, p. 24.

[397]Letter from Claude Pilloud, ICRC Geneva, to H.W. Dunning, LRCS Geneva, March 10, 1948 (AICRC, CR 195).

[398]On the ICRC's efforts to maintain the unity of the Red Cross symbol, see François Bugnion, *The Emblem of the Red Cross, A Brief History* (Geneva: ICRC, 1977), 85 pp.

first project, of course, was to keep the health services of the Palestine government running.

At the beginning of March, 1948, the hospitals that most concerned the government of Palestine were those of Jerusalem, Bethlehem, Haifa, Nablus, Jaffa, Beersheva, Gaza, Tel Aviv, and Safed. When they withdrew, the British planned to hand as many of their health-care facilities as possible over to the Jewish and Arab municipal authorities. Thus, for example, the government hospitals of Tel Aviv and Bnei Brak were to be turned over to the Va'ad Le'umi, and those of Nablus, Jaffa, Beersheva, and Gaza to the local Arab authorities.[399]

The most urgent problem was Jerusalem and Bethlehem, for which United Nations Resolution 181 prescribed an international regime, as yet undefined. As long as the future sovereignty of the Holy City and its environs remained undecided, Britain could not hand the government hospitals of Jerusalem and Bethlehem over to one or the other of the parties, Arabs or Jews, without derogating from the political neutrality it claimed it wanted to observe. It was also unthinkable to transfer responsibility for the hospitals to the UN Special Commission on Palestine, since this would be unacceptable to the Arabs[400]; in any case, in March, 1948, the UN Commission was inoperative, since its members were hiding in the cellars of the King David Hotel. The government of Palestine therefore looked upon the ICRC as an unhoped-for alternative, probably thinking along the lines of what Lord and Lady Mountbatten had told Ruegger in December, 1947, in New Delhi.[401]

There were two buildings in particular in Jerusalem and Bethlehem, respectively, that the British wanted to hand over quickly to a third party – in the event, the ICRC: the big government hospital of Jerusalem in the Russian Compound, which treated mostly Arabs, and the Bethlehem hospital for the mentally ill, which cared for both Jews and Arabs.

The ICRC was faced with the problem of reconciling the British request to take responsibility for the government hospitals with

---

[399]Telegram from Cunningham, High Commissioner for Palestine, Jerusalem, to UK Delegation New York, March 15, 1948, copy to Secretary of State, Colonial Office, London (Cunningham Private Papers, III/2, St. Antony's College. Middle East Library, Oxford).

[400]Ibid.

[401]See Chapter 1, p. 39.

its usual role of neutral intermediary, the utility of which it wanted to reaffirm. The mental asylum in Bethlehem is a good example of how it did this. In mid-March, 1948, the ICRC and the government of Palestine drew up a sort of standard contract to provide for that hospital and the other government hospitals. The terms of the transaction, for which the British had obtained the approval in principle of the UN Commission on Palestine,[402] were as follows:

- The government of Palestine would turn the Bethlehem hospital over to the ICRC, in trust. The ICRC accepted this, but would put its seal on the hospital: the Red Cross emblem. The emblem would serve two functions: It would indicate that the hospital enjoyed immunity under the Geneva Convention, and it would show that it had been handed over to the ICRC.
- Once the ICRC had taken possession of the hospital, it would assume the position of a temporary guardian, an intermediary between the Mandatory power and the international authority, as yet undefined, that would succeed the British in Jerusalem and Bethlehem when they withdrew.
- While waiting for this hypothetical legal and international authority which was to take responsibility for the Jerusalem-Bethlehem sector, the ICRC would entrust the administrative, financial, and medical management of the Bethlehem hospital to the Arab Medical Association of Palestine.
- Since the hospital would be marked with the emblem of the Red Cross – which was shared by the ICRC – the Arab Medical Association undertook to use the sign in conformity with the essential principles of the Geneva Convention and to accept any suggestion of a humanitarian nature that the ICRC might make to it.
- The Mandatory power would finance the hospital for a period not to exceed two months after the end of the Mandate. The money would be paid to the ICRC in Geneva.

This contract was signed by the government of Palestine, the Arab Medical Association, and the ICRC delegate in Palestine. The agreement regarding the Bethlehem mental hospital, signed

---

[402]Letter from Azcarate, United Nations Commission for Palestine, to ICRC Jerusalem, March 25, 1948, cited in note from de Reynier, ICRC Jerusalem, to ICRC Geneva, April 8, 1948 (AICRC, G.59/I/G.C.).

April 28, 1948, took effect on May 1, 1948.[403] The ICRC was to use it as a model for various transactions with other authorities who owned hospitals in Palestine and wanted to protect their facilities. Wherever possible, the ICRC entrusted the management of the buildings the Palestine government turned over to it to the Arab Medical Association or charitable organizations serving the Arabs. At the end of April, de Reynier transferred the government hospital in the Russian Compound to the Arab Medical Association, and, to compensate, he handed the English Mission Hospital of Jerusalem over to the Jewish Agency's relief society, the Magen David Adom.[404]

By means of contracts like the one described above, the ICRC achieved a number of objectives:

- It met Britain's expectations without abdicating its own principles. In fact, it insured that the hospitals of the Palestine government continued to function after the Mandate ended, and it increased the number of beds available for Arab Palestinians, yet without playing a purely medical role.
- It performed the function of a neutral intermediary – under an inventive interpretation – between Great Britain and the United Nations or any other hypothetical authority that might exercise lawful power over Jerusalem or in Palestine after the departure of the Mandatory power.
- It undertook a humanitarian initiative for the category of victims protected by the Geneva Convention and made use of the red cross, which accorded well with the new provisions it proposed to include in the revised Geneva Convention.
- It obliged the beneficiaries of the contracts to obey the rules of the Geneva Convention, which was a way of setting itself up as a moral authority in respect to that convention, of promoting the convention's essential principles, and of indicating its own link with it.

---

[403] Agreement between Director of Medical Services, Government of Palestine (signature illegible), the ICRC, signed by de Reynier, and the Palestine Arab Medical Association (signature illegible), Jerusalem, April 28, 1948 (AICRC, G.20 and G.59/I/G.C.).

[404] De Reynier, ICRC Jerusalem, to ICRC Geneva, April 25, 1948 (AICRC, G.59/I/G.C.).

An emblem signifying moral authority

Despite these achievements, the ICRC had created a rather unorthodox fusion between the sign of the red cross, designated by the Geneva Convention as a distinguishing mark to protect medical facilities from warfare, and the emblem of the ICRC, identical in appearance, which symbolized that institution's ideal. In the ICRC's hospital contracts with the government of Palestine, the ICRC emblem annulled and replaced the sign of the red cross that the belligerents, who had undertaken to respect the Geneva Convention, were to post on medical equipment to indicate its immunity so the adversary could spare it. This initiative, arbitrary in terms of humanitarian law, was doubtless motivated at that time by the ICRC's desire to promote the red cross over the red crescent and the red star of David.

The initiative was facilitated by the fact that at the time no military authority of a country that had signed the Geneva Convention – and that therefore might use the red cross for protection – seemed likely to take over from the British when they left Palestine. The Jews used the red star of David, and the Arabs the red crescent – if not the cross and crescent together, as Transjordan did. There was little hope that the Arabs would respect the red star of David and the Jews would respect the red crescent.

By giving its own emblem a protective function, the ICRC was thus filling a predictable gap, and possibly protecting the wounded from the hostilities. At the same time it was indicating its link with the Geneva Convention and placing itself above the convention, as a moral authority, since it obliged those who used its emblem to obey the essential rules of that convention.

This way of proceeding concealed a danger, however: If the sight of the red cross did not elicit respect from the combatants – to speak plainly, if the combatants were to shoot at the people, buildings, and material designated with the emblem – not only the targets themselves would be injured, but the ICRC as well, since the red cross was its own flag.

The news that the ICRC was taking charge of certain government hospitals was soon making the rounds in Palestine. Numerous private bodies, British or foreign, many of them linked to the countries that had voted for the partition plan, appealed to the ICRC to protect from the effects of the war not only their

PLATES

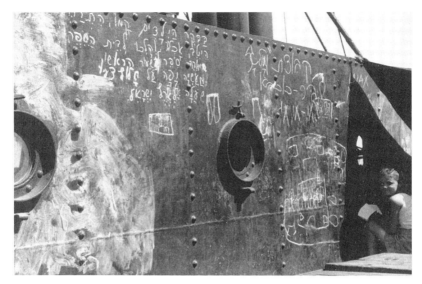

1. 'All day long, you can see the schools studying on the decks, writing with chalk on the black parts of the ships.' Picture Marti. (See p. 84.)

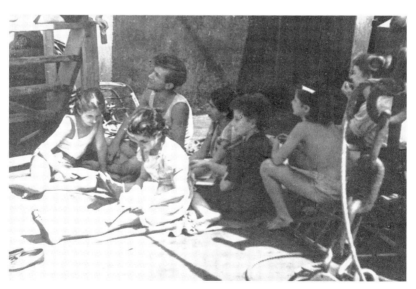

2. School on the *Runnymede Park*. Picture and caption ICRC. (See p. 84.)

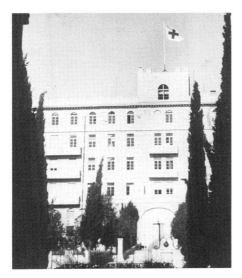

3. The King David Hotel under the Red Cross flag. Picture ICRC. Caption D.D.J. (See p. 172.)

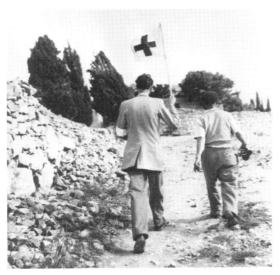

4. 'Jerusalem, May 10, 1948 – 48 hours' armistice. M. Jean Courvoisier, ICRC's delegate, crosses the firing line in order to fetch back the bodies of Arabs fallen in the ruins of Katamon, a district of Jerusalem.' Picture and caption ICRC. (See p. 200.)

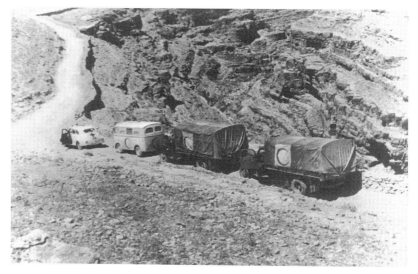

5. The positioning of the red cross and the red crescent for a joint repatriation convoy. Picture ICRC. Caption D.D.J. (See p. 196.)

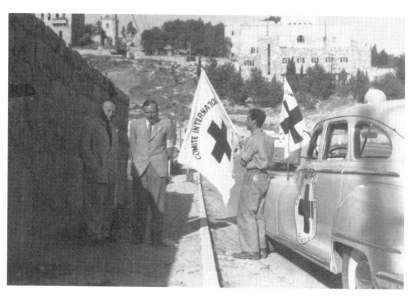

6. President Ruegger, accompanied by Wolf, attending to the evacuation of the inhabitants of the Jewish Quarter. Picture de Reynier. Caption D.D.J. (See pp. 209-11.)

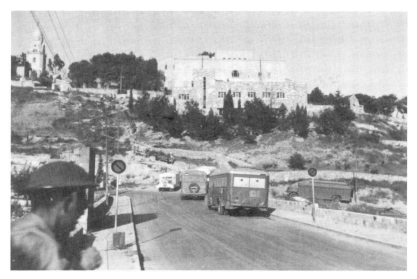

7. Evacuation of the inhabitants of the Jewish Quarter of the Old City. Picture de Reynier. Caption D.D.J. (See p. 210.)

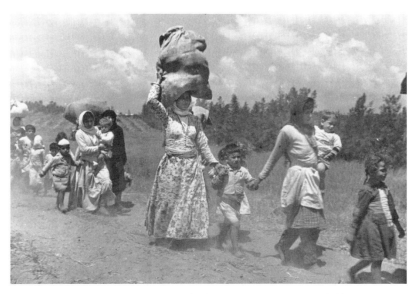

8. Kfar Yona, June 18, 1948: "At their demand 1,100 women and children are transferred from Natanya to the Nablus Triangle." Picture D.D.J. Caption ICRC (See p. 216.)

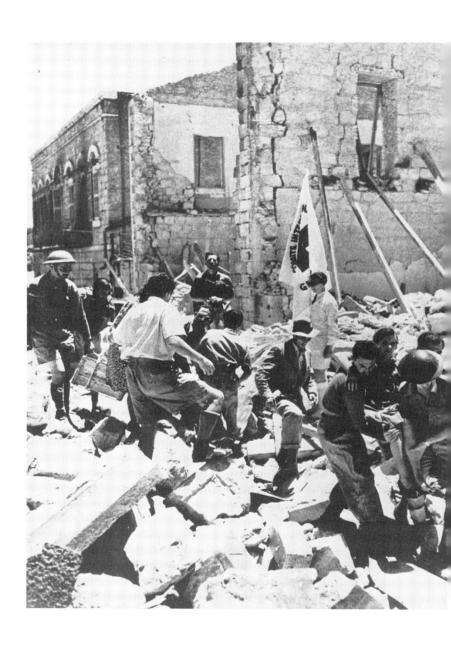

9. The ICRC's delegates preparing an exchange of civilians. Picture ICRC. Caption D.D.J. (See p. 212.)

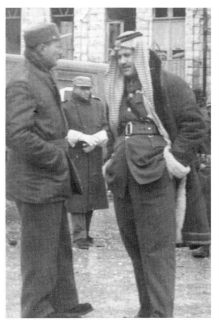 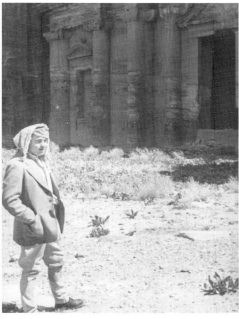

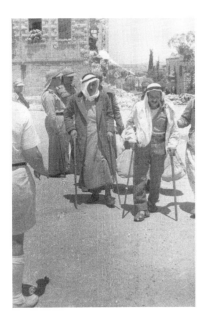

10. (above left) Moshe Dayan and Abdullah Tel meet for the repatriation of wounded Arab prisoners. Picture Munier. Caption D.D.J. (See p. 217.)

11. (above right) Munier wearing the keffiyeh in Petra. Picture Munier. Caption D.D.J. (See p. 228.)

12. (left) 'Repatriation of Arab POWs. Two wounded.' Picture and caption Munier. (See p. 217.)

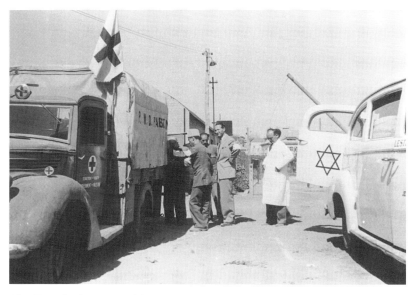

13. 'Transferring some of the Arab old people and wounded from Tel Aviv to Jaffa. Summer 1948.' Picture H. Pinn. Caption ICRC. (See p. 214.)

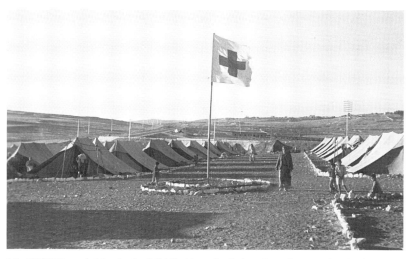

14. 'ICRC's activities in the Middle East. Assisting the refugees of Palestine, June 1949, Ramallah – Nebi Jacoubs refugee camp.' Picture ICRC. Caption D.D.J. (See p. 259.)

medical facilities, but also the buildings housing their charitable, missionary, educational, and social enterprises. Without any legal basis for doing so, de Reynier allowed them to post the emblem of the Red Cross, on condition that the buildings that bore it were at least partially used to provide free medical care for the sick and wounded.

Accordingly, the sisters of the Bethany convent transformed part of their Arab girls' school into an infirmary, the American Colony Hotel set up a dispensary, and so on. Often the establishments furnished with the ICRC emblem remained in their owners' hands, but in some cases the ICRC handed them over to the Arab Medical Association. Very rarely, private hospitals were transferred to Jews. Soon an impressive number of medical establishments in Mandatory Palestine – especially in Jerusalem but also in Jaffa – displayed the Red Cross emblem.

On May 14, 1948, when the conflict entered its international phase, the ICRC called all the belligerents' attention to the immunity of the hospitals, and asked them to spare the buildings and equipment marked with the Red Cross emblem. De Reynier gave the Jewish and Arab military authorities a list of the hospitals the ICRC had placed under its protection. He was ready to add to the list if the parties to the conflict submitted written requests to that effect.[405] The belligerents, apparently not very familiar with the conventions, accepted the moral authority that the ICRC had attributed to itself and which was symbolized by the Red Cross emblem, as used in Palestine.

Acceptance of the red cross by the local communities

The Moslems

For the Arab Moslems in Palestine, using a red cross instead of a red crescent posed a cultural and religious problem. In the Koran, the crescent represents the cycle of the moon, the basis for the Moslem calendar of prayer and pilgrimage. Whereas the cross evoked for them the idea of Western and Christian domination, the crescent stood for the primacy of Islam. The Moslems recognized themselves in the crescent emblem, and tended to reject the cross. However, since in the Palestine conflict

---

[405]De Reynier, memorandum to the civil and military authorities in Palestine, Jerusalem, May 14, 1948 (AICRC, G.59/I/G.C.).

they considered things Christian as neutral elements,[406] they were frequently willing to use the red cross. They had few facilities of their own, and if they could obtain additional ones as long as they displayed the sign of the Red Cross on them, they did not object. In fact, it appears from the ensemble of de Reynier's reports that the great organization of inter-Arab aid that was supposed to be set up to help the Palestinian Arabs – according to what Khalidi had told the ICRC delegates in February, 1948 – had never materialized, even though, encouraged by the ICRC, sporadic assistance from Arab countries arrived in various forms and in an apparently unconcerted manner.

The Jews

For the Jews, the cross was no more acceptable than it was for the Moslems. They held by the star of David, representing the divine shield, symbol of the protection that the One God accorded to His people.[407] The star of David was par excellence the symbol of the life and culture of the Jewish people. It had decorated their synagogues for centuries, distinguishing them from Christian churches. A yellow star of David was used to identify Jews during the Nazi persecutions. A blue star of David was part of the Zionist flag, and, since May 14, 1948, of the national flag of Israel. For religious Jews the sign of the cross was unacceptable, since in their eyes it could not be separated from its Christian significance. It was likely, in fact, to wound the sensibilities of the entire Jewish people, which for centuries had suffered from Christian persecution and which, in Europe, had recently been subjected to the most horrifying treatment – treatment against which the Catholic Church had taken no firm stand.

The leaders of the young state of Israel, for their part, hoped that future humanitarian conventions would recognize the red star of David in the same way and for the same distinguishing and protective functions as the red cross, the red crescent, and the red lion and sun. It was therefore in their interest to promote

---

[406]See Chapter 3, p. 98.

[407]'The Lord is my rock, and my fortress, and my deliverer; the God of my rock; in Him will I trust: He is my *shield* ['*magen*'], and the horn of my salvation, my high tower, and my refuge, my savior; Thou savest me from violence.' 2 *Samuel*, 22:2–3.

its use. This annoyed the ICRC which, having decided to combat the multiplication of protective signs in the upcoming revision of the Geneva Convention, wanted the Jews to use the cross.

Nonetheless, not all the Jews of Palestine were opposed to using the red cross, if doing so would actually save their buildings. Kohn, for example, came up with the idea spontaneously in March, 1948,[408] as a pragmatic approach to protecting the Hadassah university hospital and the Hebrew University of Jerusalem. These institutions were located on Mount Scopus and completely enclosed by an Arab population zone in East Jerusalem. In March, 1948, they were targets for numerous attacks by the irregulars of Abdul Kader el-Husseini, a noted Higher Committee war leader in the region. On March 30, 1948, Kohn asked de Reynier to provide these precious buildings with the Red Cross emblem.

De Reynier could have responded in the letter of the Geneva Convention and explained to the head of the political department of the Jewish Agency that the decision to mark buildings and medical material with the red cross was, under humanitarian law, the prerogative of the military authorities of the contracting parties, referring him to the relevant articles in the 1929 Geneva Convention. He could have encouraged him, in this way, to study the convention and absorb its spirit. However, if he allowed the Jewish Agency to use the red cross emblem autonomously, he would in effect be repudiating the convictions that were leading him, with the approval of the ICRC in Geneva, to undertake the Jerusalem and Bethlehem hospital initiative in concert with the British. De Reynier wanted the ICRC to confer its emblem for protective purposes and with strings attached: The users had to undertake to use the buildings displaying the red cross in conformity with the provisions and spirit of the Geneva Convention, as well as any suggestion that the ICRC might make. Consequently, the ICRC representative was willing to bestow the Red Cross emblem on the Mount Scopus buildings only under the following conditions:

– The Hebrew University would have to devote part of its facilities to the care of the sick and wounded.

---

[408]Note from Leo Kohn to David Ben-Gurion, Jerusalem, March 30, 1948 (ISA/MEA/2106.2).

- Access to the buildings of the Hadassah Hospital and the Hebrew University would be prohibited to everyone except hospital personnel – which meant the patients could not be visited by their relatives.[409]
- Buildings marked with the Red Cross emblem would have to renounce all armed protection.[410]

The first condition was consistent with the Geneva Convention; the second was arbitrary, but allowed de Reynier to assure the Arabs that the Mount Scopus buildings would not be infiltrated by soldiers; and the third seemed to be contrary to the Geneva Convention, which stipulated that an armed guard was not cause for denying a medical establishment immunity under the convention.[411]

Since at the time the legal frame of reference for such matters was undergoing revision and was therefore in a shaky state, de Reynier allowed himself to deviate from the letter of the Geneva Convention. He set the ICRC up as a moral authority, above the law, and dictated his own law to those who recognized that authority, symbolized by the Red Cross emblem.

Kohn, who apparently had not read the convention carefully, accepted the ICRC's authority regarding the use of the emblem; he did not perceive the distinction that should have been made between, on one hand, the red cross, a sign that belligerent signatories of the Geneva Convention had the duty to post on their medical facilities and equipment so that the enemy could spare them; and, on the other, the Red Cross emblem, the sign of the ICRC in Palestine, which had a primarily symbolic impact.

For reasons of security, however – not because de Reynier's

---

[409]Ibid.

[410]Note from de Reynier, ICRC Jerusalem, to ICRC Geneva, April 25, 1948 (AICRC, G.59/I/G.C.).

[411]'The following conditions are not considered to be of such a nature as to deprive a medical formation or establishment of the protection guaranteed by article 6: — (1) that the personnel of the formation or establishment is armed, and that they use the arms in their own defence or in that of the sick and wounded in charge; (2) that in the absence of armed orderlies the formation or establishment is protected by a piquet or by sentries; (3) that small arms and ammunition taken from the wounded and sick, which have not yet been transferred to the proper service, are found in the formation or establishment...' 'Geneva Convention of July 27, 1929, for the Amelioration of the Condition of the Wounded and Sick in Armed Forces in the Field,' Chapter II: 'Medical Formations and Establishments,' Art. 8, in ICRC/LRCS, *Handbook*, p. 61.

conditions were inconsistent with the Geneva Convention – the Jewish Agency rejected the restrictions, particularly the prohibition on an armed guard. It examined all sorts of other ways to protect the buildings on Mount Scopus. Finally, at the beginning of July, 1948, as a last resort Israel and the Arab Legion agreed to make Mount Scopus, which also comprised the Augusta Victoria Arab hospice and the Arab village of Issawiya, a demilitarized zone under the control of the United Nations.[412]

On May 17, 1948, Kohn, in the name of the Jewish Agency, wrote to the ICRC asking it to take under its protection 20 hospitals in Jerusalem, which he listed.[413] He then added a rider to his request by telephone: He wanted to juxtapose the red star of David and the red cross. Kohn's proposal may have been inspired by an initiative of Transjordan, which had juxtaposed the crescent and the cross.

De Reynier was reluctant to grant the Israeli request. He was probably afraid of creating a precedent that would hinder the ICRC's efforts to combat the increase in protective signs; but in this particular case, he may also have wished to avoid putting the ICRC emblem into overly close contact with the Jewish symbol, for fear the ICRC would lose credibility in the Arab world – which, it will be recalled, had recently suspected the organization of employing Jewish delegates. Whatever the reason, de Reynier rejected the idea of a double emblem, and misled Kohn into thinking that the aid societies of the belligerent countries were responsible for supervising the use of the sign, when the Geneva Convention – which he mentioned – clearly stipulated that this was the exclusive responsibility of the mili-

---

[412]'Agreement reached between the Arab and Jewish military commanders in the Jerusalem area for the demilitarisation of Mount Scopus Area commencing on Wednesday, the 7th July, 1948' (ISA/MEA/1986.8). This decision was made after the ICRC had proposed to make the area a safety zone to shelter civilians threatened by the war.

[413]Letter from Kohn, JA, Jerusalem, to ICRC Jerusalem, May 17, 1948 (CZA.S.25.8943). The hospitals were as follows: Hadassah First Aid Hospital, Hassolel St.; Shaare Zedek, Jaffa Rd.; Bikur Holim, Chancellor St.; Misgav Ladach, Old City; Dr. Ticho's Eye Clinic, Rabbi Kook St.; Dr. Feldman's Clinic, Romema; Mekor Haim, transferred to Abyssinian St.; General Workers' Sick Fund Clinic, Ben Yehuda St.; National Workers' Clinic, Ben Hillel St.; Ezrat Nashim, Romema; Dr. Shadowsky's Maternity Home, Bezalel St.; Wizo Baby Home, Bezalel St.; Old People's Home, Romema; Institute for the Blind, Montefiore St.; Strauss Health Center, Chancellor St.; School for Crippled Children, Ben Yehuda St.; Schneller Hospital, Geula Rd.; Beit Tseirot Misrachi, Rachi St.; St. Joseph's Hospital, Street of the Prophets.

tary authority. This fallacious postulate dictated the conclusion that Israel did not have an aid society that met the requirements to join the International Red Cross. In short, since Israel had not yet officially acceded to the Geneva Conventions and its aid society would not adopt the red cross as its emblem, the ICRC could not recognize the Magen David Adom as a member of the International Red Cross. De Reynier thus set the ICRC up as the substitute for an 'Israeli Red Cross' that did not exist, by way of asserting that only the ICRC had the power to use the Red Cross emblem.[414] De Reynier's letter ended with a number of unfeasible proposals – which I will not describe here – that were of a nature to discourage the Israelis from persisting in their request.

There were additional letters in the same vein from the head of the ICRC delegation 'in Palestine,' which, lacking any definite, reasonable frame of reference, kept his Jewish correspondents in a state of confusion. Kohn finally resorted to reading the 1929 Geneva Convention himself, and presumably discovered that the ICRC did not have the right to use the red cross, nor to decree the uses that could be made of it. He read that hospitals were supposed to enjoy absolute immunity as long as they provided care for sick and wounded soldiers, and that it was the military authorities which had the legal responsibility of affixing the red cross to medical buildings and material.[415] On May 21 he planned to iron out the matter with de Reynier, but decided against it, for unknown reasons.[416] It seems likely, however, that the head of the ICRC delegation had lost credibility with Kohn, who was in charge of Israel's political contacts with the ICRC. Kohn and the Israeli military leaders had learned a lesson from the affair: When, on May 21, Egypt bombed a Tel Aviv infirmary marked with the red star of David,[417] the Israelis, taking matters into their own hands, asked de Reynier to inform the Egyptians that

---

[414]Letter from de Reynier, ICRC Jerusalem, to Leo Kohn, Jewish Agency, Jerusalem, May 20, 1948 (ISA/MEA/2406.4).
[415]Letter Kohn, JA, Jerusalem, to de Reynier, ICRC Jerusalem, May 21, 1948. Draft, not sent (ISA/MEA/2406.6).
[416]Ibid.
[417]Telegram from Gouy, ICRC Tel Aviv, to ICRC Geneva, May 21, 1948 (AICRC, G.59/I/G.C.). On June 2 Israel bombed the Egyptian Red Crescent hospital in Ramle, apparently in retaliation.

from then on all the hospitals in Tel Aviv and the surrounding areas would be marked with the red cross.[418]

On May 30, 1948, de Reynier took the initiative again regarding the use of the red cross, announcing publicly to all the military and civilian authorities, Jewish and Arab, that the ICRC would be willing to offer the protection of its emblem to the hospitals of both the Magen David Adom and the Red Crescent societies, under the same conditions it had posed when it turned the government hospitals in Jerusalem and Bethlehem over to the Arab Medical Association, and the English Mission Hospital over to the Magen David Adom aid society.[419] It was the right moment to prove the usefulness of the red cross: With this single emblem, the belligerents would, in theory, no longer be able to distinguish between their own protected facilities and those of the enemy. This may have been one of de Reynier's motives in making the offer. With a single sign, the buildings would be safer than with a variety of signs each of which emphasized national and religious characteristics, and with them the user's link to the enemy.

But Kohn had realized that he did not need the ICRC's authorization to use the red cross. On June 8, 1948, he informed de Reynier that the Jewish hospitals of Jerusalem that he had listed on May 17 – except for two which had been put out of commission by the war – would display no sign other than the red cross.[420] Moreover, he would not make any contract with the ICRC for these hospitals.

On June 11, 1948, the first truce between the Arabs and the Israelis took effect. It had been negotiated for a limited period by Bernadotte, who on May 21 had accepted the post of United Nations mediator for Palestine. The ICRC delegates, expecting a renewal of hostilities at the end of the truce, took advantage of it to post the Red Cross emblem on medical establishments that

[418]Telegram from Gouy, ICRC Tel Aviv, to ICRC Geneva, May 21, 1948 (AICRC, G.59/I/G.C.).

[419]De Reynier, 'Memorandum aux autorités civiles et militaires en Palestine: Proposition de mise sous drapeau Croix-Rouge des hôpitaux du Croissant Rouge et du Bouclier Rouge à Jérusalem,' Jerusalem, May 30, 1948 (AICRC, G.59/I/G.C.).

[420]Letter from Kohn, JA Jerusalem, to de Reynier, Jerusalem, June 8, 1948 (CZA.S.25.8943). The two hospitals taken off the list were the Hadassah First Aid Clinic on Hassolel St., and the Misgav Ladach Hospital in the middle of the Jewish Quarter of Jerusalem, which had fallen into the hands of the Arab Legion on May 28 and was no longer controlled by Israel.

wanted it, thus carrying the ICRC standard to many parts of a territory up to then divided into two camps and two communities: the state of Israel, which, established by UN resolution on a limited section of Palestine, considered itself to be in a defensive position; and the Arabs, who saw Palestine as an indivisible Arab entity, invaded by the Zionists, whose state was illegitimate. The ICRC hoped that when hostilities resumed, the hospitals displaying the red cross would be respected.

De Reynier, who had tried to insure that this emblem would appear on the greatest possible number of establishments in Palestine, did not let his desire to promote the Red Cross prevent him from doing anything to protect the buildings that still displayed the red star of David. He wrote to the ICRC that one of his greatest successes had been to secure the Arabs' pledge to respect buildings showing the red star of David. He did not give details on those negotiations, however, nor on the people with whom he had conducted them,[421] and in practice, the red star of David was not respected by Arab combatants.

The fate of hospitals displaying the ICRC emblem

The evolution of the conflict and the partition of Jerusalem between Israel and Transjordan raised questions regarding the fate of the government hospitals which were under ICRC contract and displayed its emblem. It should be remembered that the Mandatory power had entrusted them provisionally to the ICRC, while waiting for a future legitimate authority to succeed it in Palestine – the United Nations in Jerusalem's case.

Each case was different. Usually, the ICRC delegates tried to negotiate matters so that the Arabs of Palestine could continue to use the establishments. This did not, in general, pose any major problems with Transjordan, as long as it controlled Arab Palestine, the Old City of Jerusalem, and its eastern sector.

The case of the government hospital in the Russian Compound in Jerusalem, however, revealed the bias of the ICRC delegation head, who for a long time resisted handing it over to the Israelis. On July 25, 1948, during a second truce between the Arabs and the Israelis – established for an indeterminate period in the hope that it would lead to a peace accord – the medical service of the

[421]Note from de Reynier, ICRC Jerusalem, to ICRC Geneva, May 17, 1948 (AICRC, G.59/I/G.C.).

Israeli army, which had occupied the first floor of the hospital by force, proposed that the hospital continue to operate and that the first floor be reserved for Israeli sick and wounded. If the ICRC requested its return, the Israeli medical service undertook, with reasonable advance notice, to restore it in perfect condition. The ICRC could inspect the premises at any moment to verify that they were in good condition, and, in addition, it would be given every means of assuring itself that the medical personnel were acting in conformity with Red Cross practices.[422]

The Israeli proposal corresponded with the provisions of the Geneva Convention, which stated that if a hospital fell into the hands of the enemy, it should not be prevented from performing its usual function of caring for the sick and wounded, whatever their nationality.[423] De Reynier consulted the Arab administrator of the hospital, Dr. Bichara, who desired an immediate evacuation of the wounded and the Arab medical staff. This was his right, recognized by the Geneva Convention, which stipulated that in such situations the wounded could be kept as prisoners of war, but the belligerents would be 'free to prescribe, for the benefit of wounded or sick prisoners, such arrangements as they may think fit beyond the limits of the existing obligations,'[424] and the medical personnel was to be repatriated 'as soon as ... military considerations permit'[425] – which, of course, was the case in the middle of a truce.

However, de Reynier dissuaded the Arab Medical Association from abandoning the hospital. 'We would like,' he wrote to Geneva, 'to avoid being accused of having made the Arabs abandon a hospital in order to give it to the Jews, but also [to avoid] perhaps being reproached for not having managed to insure the protection of a hospital which is, after all, located in the first line of fire.'[426] The affair was finally concluded at the end of October,

---

[422]Letter from Walter Eytan, Provisional Government of the State of Israel, Ministry of Foreign Affairs, to de Reynier, Head of the ICRC Delegation in Palestine (sic), Oct. 28, 1948 (ISA/MEA/2406.4).

[423]'Geneva Convention of July 27, 1929, for the Amelioration of the Condition of the Wounded and Sick in Armed Forces in the Field,' Chapter IV: 'Buildings and Material,' Art. 15, in ICRC/LRCS, *Handbook*, p. 63.

[424]Ibid., Chapter I: 'Wounded and Sick,' Art. 2, in ICRC/LRCS, *Handbook*, p. 59.
[425]Ibid., Chapter III: 'Personnel,' Art. 12, in ICRC/LRCS, *Handbook*, p. 62.

[426]De Reynier, report of meeting with Glubb Pacha, Abdullah Tel, Musa Husseini, Dr. Husseini (Augusta Victoria Hospice), Dr. Canaan, President of the Arab Medical Association, de Reynier, and Gaillard, Jerusalem, Aug. 3, 1948 (AICRC, G.59/I/G.C.). [Translation: M.G.]

1948, when Walter Eytan, director-general of the Division of International Organizations in the Israeli Ministry of Foreign Affairs, himself decided the fate of the government hospital in the Russian Compound. Citing the relevant articles of the Geneva Convention, he decreed that the medical personnel was to be evacuated to behind Arab lines; the hospital would continue to be used for its original purpose, caring for the sick and wounded; Israel would not appropriate any supplies or equipment belonging to Britain, but reserved the right to use them 'so long as no final arrangements have been made between the Government of the United Kingdom and the Governments succeeding to the mandatory regime in Palestine.'[427] Eytan concluded with a sentence that revealed his perception of the ICRC policy concerning the hospitals: 'the means of hospitalization for the Jewish population of Jerusalem are – contrary to what may be generally thought – insufficient, and this new hospital with its equipment would help remedy, to a certain degree, the consequences of the siege and the war in the city of Jerusalem.'[428] Thus, in its hospital policy, the ICRC, following its own rules, was competing with the provisions of the Geneva Convention as implemented by Eytan, Israel's representative.

Apparently, however, Israel was anxious not to exacerbate the tension between it and the ICRC. Katznelson, the minister of health, whom the ICRC delegates admired for his understanding attitude, signed a contract with the organization on the model of the one covering the mental hospital in Bethlehem. The ICRC agreed to take 'under its protection' the government hospital of Jerusalem, including its annexes, and to hang the Red Cross flag on all its buildings. In return, the health minister of the Israeli government would take responsibility for insuring that the hospital was run in accordance with the Geneva Conventions and any suggestions the ICRC might make.[429]

---

[427]Letter from Walter Eytan, Provisional Government of the State of Israel, Ministry of Foreign Affairs, to de Reynier, Head of the ICRC Delegation in Palestine (sic), Oct. 28, 1948 (ISA/MEA/2406.4). [Translation: M.G.]

[428]Ibid.

[429]Agreement, signed for Ministry of Health, Provisional Government of Israel, by A. Katznelson; signed for International Committee of the Red Cross Geneva, by J. de Reynier (AICRC, G.59/I/G.C.).

In Jerusalem: the flag in the service of politics

Safety zones around British buildings

While working on his hospital initiative, de Reynier was developing another project as well, which he linked, like the other one, to the use of the ICRC emblem: protecting civilian populations from the effects of combat, in 'safety zones' that would enjoy an immunity similar to that of hospitals. Indeed, back in March, 1948, when the ICRC and the British had agreed that the ICRC would undertake to place the Palestine government hospitals under the Red Cross emblem to indicate that they were protected, de Reynier had considered extending this provision to important buildings used by the British administration in Jerusalem: Government House in the south-east of Jerusalem and the King David Hotel, located across from the YMCA hostel where de Reynier had set up his office, which overlooked the Arab-controlled Old City.[430]

When they began their retreat, the British feared that their positions would be immediately taken over by the Jews, bringing Arab censure down on their heads. They would obviously be very happy if the ICRC did the same as it had for the hospitals and placed the Red Cross emblem on British administrative buildings in order to protect them until they were turned over to the UN authority that would succeed the Mandatory power in Jerusalem.

The ICRC, for its part, wanted to create 'safety zones' in Palestine for civilian populations, which could be established more or less around the buildings that the British were leaving. This idea was very important to the ICRC in respect to certain political events taking place in Switzerland – which will be described further on – as well as within the perspective of the draft conventions it was to present at the Stockholm Conference.

Their convergent interests led the British government and de Reynier to plan, in March, 1948,[431] the creation of safety zones

---

[430]During the last weeks of the British Mandate, some of these buildings and their surroundings had been converted into entrenched camps, militarily protected against the attacks of Jewish extremists; they had also served as strategic and preventive buffer zones between Jewish and Arab sectors in Jerusalem who were apt to clash with each other. The British called them 'Security Zones A and B.' The Jews dubbed them 'Bevingrad.'

[431]De Reynier, ICRC mission in Palestine, to ICRC Geneva, March 24, 1948 (AICRC, CR 201).

for civilian protection around the government buildings – primarily the King David Hotel and Government House – that the Mandatory power wanted to preserve intact, in the hope of eventually handing them over to the United Nations.[432] Later, if the experiment was a success, the ICRC could create more and more zones of this type, thereby contributing to the progressive demilitarization of Jerusalem and facilitating its transition to an international regime. The location of zone no. 1 would also tend to protect the Old City, especially the large Arab quarter of Jerusalem, against a possible Jewish advance. The plan was thus partly political. It was also humanitarian indirectly, since it would result in saving human lives. De Reynier therefore believed that it could be put into effect.[433]

Here it may be useful to define the concept of safety zones and its legal basis, and to discuss what they represented for the ICRC. Between the two world wars, an association called 'Lieux de Genève' (Places of Geneva) had proposed the creation of places of refuge to shelter civilian victims of war, especially from aerial bombardments. The idea had been studied by numerous entities, including the ICRC, which competed to come up with the appropriate juridical concept. The details are irrelevant, but the important point is that in October, 1938, mandated by the XVIth International Conference of the Red Cross in London, the ICRC organized a meeting of government experts who approved a plan to create hospital localities and zones. The central idea was to offer belligerents the possibility of designating, *before* hostilities began, localities or zones that would take in wounded soldiers and that, as a result, would benefit by analogy with hospitals from the immunity offered by the Geneva Convention. That immunity would be indicated by a red cross. The secondary effect of these zones would be to protect the civilians living in them.[434] The ICRC tried to persuade the experts' meeting in 1938

---

[432]On this subject, see 'Les zones de sécurité constituées en Palestine sous le drapeau du Comité international de la Croix-Rouge. Les bâtiments des zones de sécurité,' *RICR* 354 (May 1948): 411–412.
[433]Note from de Reynier, ICRC Jerusalem, to ICRC Geneva, April 25, 1948 (AICRC, CR 201).
[434]The text of this draft is cited without a title in CICR, *Rapport du Comité international de la Croix-Rouge sur le projet de convention pour la création de localités et zones sanitaires en temps de guerre, adopté par la Commission d'experts réunie à Genève les 21 et 22 octobre 1938* (Geneva: CICR, 1939), p. 9.

to approve a draft creating safety zones to shelter civilians. It was partly successful: The experts declared that the idea should be examined. From the beginning of World War II, and undoubtedly with the intention of creating a precedent, the ICRC suggested that the belligerents agree to organize such zones[435] to protect the civilian population from the effects of the war, particularly indiscriminate bombing. Plans for concentrating the civilian population in 'safety zones' in Germany and France were considered up to the end of the war, but the ICRC's efforts in this direction were unsuccessful.

Creating a legal precedent and serving Switzerland

Following the advent of the American atomic bomb and the general massacre of the civilian population of Hiroshima and Nagasaki in the summer of 1945, and in the context of the very beginning of the Cold War, the idea of safety zones made a strong comeback. On June 24, 1946, Emil Anderegg, national councilor for the Canton of Saint Gall in Switzerland, in association with other political figures, called on the Swiss people to appeal for the establishment of a diplomatic convention stipulating that entire countries could be 'neutralized' and thereafter offer a refuge to civilian populations under the sign of the red cross.[436] What he was basically suggesting was to transform entire countries into 'safety zones.' Anderegg was obviously thinking of Switzerland. This worried Petitpierre, the head of the Federal Political Department; if Switzerland supported the project, the international community could accuse it of giving in to war paranoia and taking measures to guarantee its own security under cover of a generous proposition.[437] Petitpierre felt the best solution would be to encourage the ICRC's efforts in revising and drafting conventions,[438] with an eye to persuading the states to accept the possibility of creating hospital localities or zones for the protection of sick and wounded soldiers and, by extension,

---

[435]CIRC, 'Mémorandum sur les localités sanitaires et sur les localités et zones de sécurité', Sept. 9, 1939 (M. 832. AICRC, CR 225).

[436]'Appel au peuple suisse,' signed by Albert Steffen and Emil Anderegg, cosigned by 41 Swiss federal parliamentarians and 7 senators, Saint Gall, June 24, 1946 (AICRC, CR 201).

[437]'Réponse de M. le Conseiller fédéral Max Petitpierre au postulat Anderegg du 24 juin 1946,' Conseil national, Dec. 17, 1946. (AICRC, CR 201).

[438]Ibid.

civilians – and, while they were about it, safety zones to shelter civilian populations.

At the April, 1947, Conference of Government Experts, the idea of hospital localities and zones to protect the wounded and sick was approved and written into the draft revision of the Geneva Convention: The immunity enjoyed by hospitals was to be extended to zones that would be defined or localities that would be chosen by means of an accord between the states concerned, *before* the fighting began. These localities and zones would be designated, like hospital buildings, by a red cross on a white background. The ICRC was thus able to include this proposal in the draft conventions it would present in Stockholm. The experts, however, were less amenable to the ICRC's suggestion of extending the application of future conventions to the general civilian population, and to the idea of permitting the establishment of safety zones and localities intended specifically for civilian use. The ICRC was given a mandate to examine the question further[439]; consequently, it had an interest in creating precedents, if possible, by its actions.

On January 12, 1948, when the ICRC delegates were getting ready for their study mission in Palestine, Anderegg reaffirmed his proposal.[440] Not long afterwards, the ICRC instructed Marti and de Reynier to examine the possibility of creating safety zones in Palestine. Indeed, the plan of action that the ICRC delegates devised on February 15, 1948, provided, in theory, for the institution of safety zones in Palestine to shelter civilian populations,[441] although the delegates' daily reports give no indication that any systematic evaluation of the needs of those populations was made.[442] Another document specifies that de Reynier went to Palestine 'in view of constituting safety zones there.'[443] He went there, it should be noted, on January 20, 1948, or not long

---

[439]ICRC, *Report on the Work of the Conference of Government Experts*, p. 300.

[440]According to letter from de Haller, Federal Council's Delegate for Mutual International Aid, Bern, to Ruegger, Minister of Switzerland, London, Feb. 10, 1948 (IZG, Zurich, Fonds Ruegger).

[441]See Chapter 2, p. 110.

[442]Report by Marti, de Reynier, and Munier, Palestine mission, Jerusalem, Feb. 15, 1948 (AICRC, G.59/I/G.C.).

[443]Joint meeting League—ICRC at headquarters of the League of Red Cross Societies, May 11, 1948, at 15:00, procès-verbal no. 9, point IV (AICRC, CRI 1). [Translation: M.G.]

after Anderegg decided to renew his proposal. The ICRC thus intended to create safety zones in Palestine for two reasons: to neutralize Anderegg's proposals, and to create a legal precedent. These plans had, for Switzerland and for the ICRC, a value that was not directly related to the needs of the civilian populations threatened by the fighting in Mandatory Palestine.

On April 21, 1948, after long negotiations, de Reynier announced to the press a plan for establishing safety zones in Jerusalem.[444] The following zones were to be transformed into places of refuge for noncombatant civilians, for which purpose they would enjoy an immunity comparable to that of hospitals:

- Zone no. I, comprising the building and grounds of the King David Hotel, the YMCA hostel with all its annexes, the Terra Sancta school and an adjacent children's home. The zone thus demarcated would accommodate some 2,000 people.
- Zone no. II, as compact as the first, which would encompass Government House and the surrounding grounds, the Jewish agricultural school for girls, and the Arab governmental college, extending up to the Allenby barracks. This zone could accommodate 2,000 to 5,000 people.
- Zone no. III, for which de Reynier had not yet received all the necessary guarantees, depended in particular on the consent of the Jews and was to encompass the Italian school and a former Italian hospital that had been turned into a British barracks, up as far as Abyssinian Street.

De Reynier announced that the three zones together would offer a total accommodation capacity of 15,000 people. The zones would be designated by the Red Cross emblem.

The head of the ICRC delegation had little to guide him, caught as he was at a key moment in the development of ICRC tradition, between the 1929 Conventions and the future treaties. He was obliged to administer the institution of the safety zones both heedfully and audaciously, considering only the good of the victims. It was a tremendous responsibility, demanding outstanding human qualities.

When de Reynier established the safety zones in Jerusalem, he

---

[444]Palestine Post Staff, 'Geneva Areas for Jerusalem,' *Palestine Post* [Jerusalem], (April 22, 1948): 1.

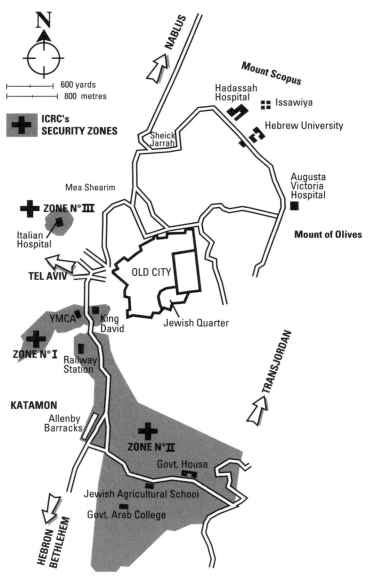

Since no graphic depiction of the safety zones in Jerusalem could be found in the ICRC archives, this map was drawn on the evidence of written documents, and is consequently approximate.

considered their implications for Swiss politics, but he did not know the details of the revised and new draft conventions that ought to have guided the conception and implementation of the zones.[445] He knew only that these drafts extended conventional immunity to individual civilians and civilian populations in their entirety, and that they offered protection from the effects of armed conflict to those civilians in the safety zones.[446] The gap widened rapidly between the way de Reynier conceived of the safety zones in Jerusalem and the relevant provisions in the legal texts that the ICRC had prepared in Geneva to submit at the Stockholm Conference.[447] The different outlooks can be summed up as follows:

- In Jerusalem, if the conflict intensified, the safety zones were potentially in the front lines and contained important administrative buildings, such as the King David Hotel and Government House; according to the ICRC drafts, however, the zones should have been well back behind the lines and devoid of any buildings that might have a strategic value.[448]
- In Jerusalem, the zones were designated by the Red Cross emblem; but the ICRC drafts stipulated that the zones reserved for the civilian population would be indicated by oblique red

---

[445] In-house note from Pilloud, Legal Division, to Marti, Medical Division, May 10, 1948 (AICRC, G.59/I/G.C.).

[446] See, for example, de Reynier, 'Procès-verbal de l'entrevue de la délégation du CICR en Palestine et du corps consulaire de Jérusalem du 1er mai 1948,' Jerusalem, May 1, 1948 (AICRC, G.59/I/G.C.).

[447] 'Revision of the Geneva Convention of July 27, 1929, for the Relief of the Wounded and Sick in Armies in the Field,' Chapter III: 'Medical Units and Establishments,' Art. 18, in XVIIth International Conference of the Red Cross, Stockholm, August 1948, *Draft Revised or New Conventions for the Protection of War Victims*, p. 15; 'Convention for the Protection of Civilian Persons in Time of War,' Part II: 'General Protection of Populations against Certain Consequences of War,' Art. 12, in XVIIth International Conference of the Red Cross, Stockholm, August 1948, *Draft Revised or New Conventions*, p. 15; and XVIIth International Conference of the Red Cross, Stockholm, August 1948, *Draft Revised or New Conventions*, Annex A: 'Draft Agreement Relating to Hospital and Safety Zones and Localities,' pp. 214–218. These documents are revised versions of the documents resulting from the consultation with experts in October, 1938, on the issue of hospital and safety zones and localities.

[448] 'Draft Agreement Relating to Hospital and Safety Zones and Localities,' Art. 4 c): 'They shall be far removed and free from all military objectives, or large industrial or administrative establishments'; Art. 4 d): 'They shall not be situated in areas which, according to every probability, may become important for the conduct of the war.' In XVIIth International Conference of the Red Cross, Stockholm, August 1948, *Draft Revised or New Conventions*, p. 215.

bands on a white ground, the red cross to be used only for the wounded and sick.[449]
- In Jerusalem, the safety zones were set up during an emergency situation; the ICRC drafts, however, following the recommendations of the 1938 studies, stipulated that the belligerents should agree in advance on the establishment of the zones, and that the protecting powers or the ICRC should lend their good offices to that end.[450]

Given these differences, de Reynier's establishment of safety zones in Jerusalem did not constitute a precedent that the ICRC could invoke in the strict sense at the Stockholm Conference. Nonetheless, if de Reynier's experiment succeeded, it would not only save lives, but it would also win the ICRC enormous prestige.[451]

With this in mind, de Reynier first sought to arrange the means of feeding thousands of hypothetical refugees – for if they escaped the bullets only to die of hunger, the ICRC's credibility would suffer, he warned.[452] The ICRC obtained funds from the American Red Cross, taking the opportunity to give that organization a detailed report of its other activities in Palestine, emphasizing its role as a neutral, independent intermediary.[453] Geneva also sent a circular letter out to the National Societies, calling on them to join in its efforts.[454]

The inauguration of the safety zones created considerable publicity for the ICRC in United Nations circles, as was confirmed by

---

[449]'Draft Agreement Relating to Hospital and Safety Zones and Localities,' Art. 6, in XVIIth International Conference of the Red Cross, Stockholm, August 1948, *Draft Revised or New Conventions*, p. 216.

[450]'Revision of the Geneva Convention of July 27, 1929, for the Relief of the Wounded and Sick in Armies in the Field,' Chapter III: 'Medical Units and Establishments,' Art. 18, in XVIIth International Conference of the Red Cross, Stockholm, August 1948, *Draft Revised or New Conventions*, p. 15. 'Convention for the Protection of Civilian Persons in Wartime,' Part II: 'General Protection of Populations against Certain Consequences of War,' Art. 12, in XVIIth International Conference of the Red Cross, Stockholm, August 1948, *Draft Revised or New Conventions*, p. 158.

[451]Note from de Reynier, ICRC Jerusalem, to ICRC Geneva, April 19, 1948 (AICRC, G.59/I/G.C.).

[452]Ibid.

[453]Letter from Gloor, Vice-Chairman, ICRC Geneva, to James Nicholson, Vice-Chairman, American Red Cross, May 4, 1948 (AICRC, G.59/I/G.C.).

[454]CICR, 'Zones de sécurité en Palestine,' May 4, 1948 (AICRC, CP 316).

Margarita Straehler,[455] ICRC delegate to the UN at Lake Success[456] since March, 1948 and one of the rare ICRC workers who spoke Russian.[457]

A neutral Jerusalem under the Red Cross emblem?

At the end of April, the Americans and the British combined and intensified their efforts to safeguard Jerusalem, particularly the holy places. The US prepared a proposal for the Security Council which would immediately place Jerusalem under provisional trusteeship, in accordance with Chapter XII of the United Nations Charter. The idea of a cease-fire in Jerusalem was being studied, but its chances of success were still uncertain. While waiting for final arrangements concerning the security and the future of the Holy City, the British proposed that an independent, neutral individual be placed temporarily at the head of the Jerusalem municipality while the city was still under British authority. This commissioner, whose function would be to intermediate between the Jewish and Arab communities of Jerusalem, should be from a neutral country so that he would be acceptable to both parties; by the same token, he could not be appointed by the United Nations, since the Arabs rejected its authority, but would have to be named by the government of Palestine.

Moshe Shertok, consulted as the representative of the Jewish Agency, expressed no views on the matter, but said he would have to refer the matter to Tel Aviv. Jamal el-Husseini, the representative of the Arab Higher Committee at Lake Success, where the UN debates on Palestine's future were taking place, declared himself in favor of the idea from the outset, and suggested de Reynier for the post.[458] On May 1, Alexandre Parodi, the French representative to the United Nations, also proposed the appoint-

---

[455]Note from Straehler, ICRC Delegation to the United Nations, New York, to ICRC Geneva, May 13, 1948 (AICRC, G.59/I/G.C.).

[456]East of New York City, Lake Success was at the time the headquarters of the United Nations. Those headquarters were moved to Manhattan in 1951.

[457]Straehler had served as an interpreter to Marcel Junod, an ICRC delegate who, during World War II, had tried to establish contacts with official representatives of the USSR in Ankara.

[458]Report from Secretary of State, New York, signed P.T.O., to High Commissioner for Palestine, Jerusalem, May 1, 1948 (Cunningham Private Papers, III/5/13, St. Antony's College. Middle East Library, Oxford).

THE IMPERILED RED CROSS

ment of de Reynier. The press highlighted this information.[459] The idea was never adopted, however, mainly because in the meantime the head of the ICRC delegation had been working secretly on a much more ambitious project, which a press leak was soon to reveal – all too soon, from the Committee's point of view[460]: a plan to make all of Jerusalem a single hospital and safety locality under the Red Cross flag.[461]

A letter from Kahany indicates that the ICRC was not the originator of this ambitious idea. According to Kahany, it was suggested by a certain S. Adler-Rudel, a veteran Zionist who dealt with questions coming within the purview of the Intergovernmental Committee on Rufugees, during a visit he reportedly made to the ICRC in the spring of 1948. Adler-Rudel knew Wolf, the ICRC president's special assistant. According to Kahany, 'it was Adler-Rudel and Wolf – each one for a different reason but both with the best intentions – who conceived this plan for placing the whole of Jerusalem under the protection of the Red Cross.'[462] Convinced in his turn, Ruegger apparently gave his delegation head the task of implementing the plan.[463]

If this was indeed the case, however, the Jewish Agency was unaware of it at the beginning of May, 1948. It saw the plan as a de Reynier initiative that was contrary to its own interests and favorable to the wishes of the English and the Arabs, 'who tried hard to replace any interference of the UN in Jerusalem by some 'humanitarian' arrangement, under the auspices of a non-political and neutral 'international' body like the ICRC.'[464] Britain, for its part, considered that de Reynier had exceeded the ICRC

[459]Jesse Zel Lurie, Palestine Post Correspondent [Lake Success, Sat., May 1], 'Superman for Jerusalem,' *Palestine Post* (May 2, 1948): 1.
[460]Telegram from Straehler, ICRC New York, to ICRC Geneva, May 5, 1948 (AICRC, G.8/47a).
[461]According to a private letter from de Reynier, ICRC Jerusalem, to Gloor, Vice-President of the ICRC, April 23, 1948, mentioned in a message from de Reynier, ICRC Jerusalem, to Munier, ICRC Cairo, May 4, 1948 (AICRC, G.59/I/G.C.). See also Jesse Zel Lurie, Palestine Post Correspondent, 'Red Cross Wants Its Flag over All Jerusalem Area,' *Palestine Post* (May 4, 1948): 1.
[462]Letter from Kahany, Provisional Government of Israel, no place given, to Walter Eytan, Ministry of Foreign Affairs, Tel Aviv, July 29, 1948 (ISA/MEA/547.1).
[463]Ibid.
[464]Ibid.

mandate in embarking on a political operation.[465] Fletcher Cooke, the British delegate to Lake Success, was delighted with the plan, but a little worried.[466]

On May 6, 1948, de Reynier sent the Committee in Geneva the details of his plan, which he had worked out in cooperation with his colleagues. First, the request for the neutralization of Jerusalem would have to come, in writing, from the Arab and Jewish authorities. Jerusalem would be demilitarized, a status that would be indicated by the emblem of the Red Cross. At the moment the neutralization took effect, the Arab and Jewish positions would be frozen. The administration of the city would be assumed by the authorities already exercising the power locally. The perimeter of the neutral zone would be the perimeter of the city at the moment of its neutralization. The ICRC would provision the city by means of the Tel Aviv-Jerusalem road, under the protection of the Red Cross emblem.[467]

On May 8, 1948, Geneva sent de Reynier its approval in principle, but expressed reservations regarding the mode of implementing the plan: De Reynier could not ask the authorities concerned to send the ICRC a written request, as he had done in connection with the hospitals, for the ICRC could not assume a direct responsibility that might later put it in a position where it had to arbitrate. De Reynier should settle for facilitating the conclusion of an agreement between the parties. He should not take on the task of provisioning the town.[468] The ICRC would do nothing more than monitor the parties' fulfillment of their undertakings and report to those concerned.[469]

Wishing to see the project implemented in the spirit of the new

[465] According to note from Straehler, ICRC New York, Lake Success, to ICRC Geneva, May 13, 1948 (AICRC, G.59/I/G.C.).
[466] Telegram from Straehler, ICRC New York, to ICRC Geneva, May 5, 1948 (AICRC, G.8/47a).
[467] Telegram from de Reynier, ICRC Jerusalem, to ICRC Geneva, May 6, 1948 (AICRC, G.59/I/G.C.).
[468] This would be essentially to the advantage of the Jews living in West Jerusalem, it might appear biased, and consequently it was apt to be frowned upon by the Arab Higher Committee. When Article 8 of the first truce provided that the ICRC was to provision the city of Jerusalem, the ICRC refused to do so, on Courvoisier's advice, for fear of arousing hostility among the Arabs of Palestine. On this subject see AICRC, Dossier 'Mission Courvoisier' (G.3/82), as well as Chapter 5, p. 227.
[469] Intercroixrouge telegram, Geneva to ICRC Jerusalem, via Amman, May 8, 1948 (AICRC, G.59/I/G.C.).

articles of law that it would present in Stockholm, the Committee gave the relevant extracts from those articles to Marti,[470] whom it sent to Jerusalem in great haste to help de Reynier stay on the right track. But Marti arrived too late. De Reynier and his colleagues had already presented their plan to members of all the parties involved: the Jewish Agency in Tel Aviv and Jerusalem, the Arab Higher Committee in Jerusalem and Damascus, el-Kaukji in Jenin, King Abdullah of Transjordan, and Azzam Pacha, the secretary-general of the Arab League in Amman.[471] Their plan was in part the result of these consultations. The Jewish Agency's delegates did not report its reaction to the principle, but it seems to have been deeply opposed. It could not, of course, afford to give the impression that it opposed the pacification of Jerusalem; so it merely raised the difficult question of supplying the approximately 100,000 Jewish inhabitants of Jerusalem.[472] The ICRC therefore thought of taking charge of the matter itself.

The different Arab parties reacted favorably on the whole to de Reynier's plan. King Abdullah, in particular, who saw himself reigning over a decentralized Palestinian state in which the Jews would have an autonomous status, said that he would be satisfied with this measure[473] to protect the holy places that would eventually be within his own kingdom. The Arab Higher Committee imposed a condition: It demanded that the Jews evacuate the Arab neighborhood of Katamon in West Jerusalem, which the Haganah[474] had attacked on April 30 as part of an offensive to establish a densely populated Jewish zone inside the New City.

[470]Pilloud, note to Marti and appended extracts of the Stockholm drafts, Geneva, May 10, 1948 (AICRC, G.3/82).

[471]For a review and the procès-verbaux of all the meetings, see note from Reynier, 'Jerusalem, zone neutre de sécurité sous pavillon ICRC,' Jerusalem, June 9, 1948 (AICRC, CR 201. For el-Kaukji, see Jean Courvoisier, report, Nablus, to ICRC Geneva, May 14, 1948 (AICRC, G.549/I/G.C.) – which cannot be found in the collection of procès-verbaux mentioned above. The ICRC seems to have considered el-Kaukji to be of secondary importance.

[472]Gaillard, procès-verbal of May 2, 1948, meeting with Leo Kohn in Jerusalem, May 12, 1948. Appended to note from Reynier, 'Jérusalem, zone neutre de sécurité sous pavillon CICR,' Jerusalem, June 9, 1948 (AICRC, CR 201).

[473]Gaillard, 'Procès-verbal d'entretien entre S. M. le Roi Abdullah, Tujunji et Krikorian, Gaillard et de Reynier, à Amman le 6 mai 1948 au Palais Royal,' Jerusalem, June 9, 1948. Annexed to note from de Reynier, ibid.

[474]The Haganah was a voluntary Jewish self-defense organization established in Palestine during the Mandate. It gave rise to the Israel Defense Force (IDF), which replaced it.

Since the Arabs controlled the water pumps that supplied the city with water, the Arab Higher Committee threatened to cut off the water supply in retaliation against the Jewish population of Jerusalem if its demand was not met.[475] The UN Commission, in the person of its chief, Pablo Azcarate, promised not to put any obstacles in the way of the ICRC plan. Finally, the British also supported the project initially, and tried to impose a truce in Katamon.

On May 12, 1948, at Lake Success, Andrei Gromyko surprised everyone by telling the Security Council essentially that implementing the plan was actually a way of promoting Anglo-Arab interests, under cover of the Red Cross. The USSR saw no objection to the ICRC carrying out humanitarian projects in Palestine, on condition that it did not exceed its traditional role.[476] Gromyko's warning served the interests of the Jewish Agency, which could not express opposition to the ICRC's plan, unfavorable though that plan was to it, without creating the impression that it was hindering the efforts to pacify Jerusalem.[477]

In the diplomatic corps in Switzerland, it was felt that Gromyko's contention had merit,[478] and should give the ICRC pause. The ICRC, however, had formed the impression from its international contacts that many states that could be considered to favor the internationalization of Jerusalem were pinning great hopes on the ICRC. Accordingly, fully aware of the political implications of its decision, it resolved to undertake the project of making Jerusalem a neutral city under the Red Cross flag.[479]

---

[475]Gaillard, 'Rapport d'entretien entre Dejani, Husseini (du Caire), un représentant des autorités militaires arabes de Jérusalem, de Reynier et Gaillard (sic) à l'hôpital Beit Safafa,' Jerusalem, May 2, 1948. Place not mentioned, procès–verbal not dated. Also Munier report on his mission to Damascus and his talks with the Mufti and Isaac Darwich Bey on May 7 and 8, 1948, Amman, May 8, 1948. Appended to note from de Reynier, ibid.
[476]UNO, Security Council, *Official Records*, Third Year, 291st Meeting, Lake Success, 12 May 1948. See also note from Straehler, ICRC Delegation to the United Nations, New York, to ICRC Geneva, May 13, 1948 (AICRC, G.59/I/G.C.).
[477]When the United Nations decided to place Jerusalem under an international regime, the Jewish Agency agreed. But as it began to realize that the United Nations would not be capable of implementing such a regime, the Jewish Agency gradually changed its policy.
[478]De Haller, 'Commentaire sur la lettre du Ministre Bruggmann en date du 21 mai,' Bern, June 4, 1948 (ADPF.2001 [E] 5).
[479]ICRC, procès-verbal, Bureau meeting of May 13, 1948 (AICRC, no file number).

The ICRC was thus prepared to play a political card in the negotiations regarding the future status of Jerusalem.[480] Nevertheless, in order to 'depoliticize' the operation and to bring it into its own purview, the ICRC deemed that it would absolutely have to be carried out in the spirit of the 'Draft Agreement Relating to Hospital and Safety Zones and Localities' and other provisions relative to the creation of safety zones and localities that the ICRC would present at Stockholm,[481] drafts whose political and legal importance I have already emphasized. Marti, armed with the relevant excerpts from those documents, arrived in Jerusalem on May 13, 1948. He gave the papers to de Reynier, and relayed the Committee's instructions to him. Unfortunately for the ICRC, though, negotiations were already too far advanced to make the changes in de Reynier's plan that Geneva thought necessary.

Until May 17, 1948, the ICRC delegates focused all their efforts on achieving the neutralization of Jerusalem. But the plan failed, for reasons that are unclear from the evidence of the ICRC archives. De Reynier's explanations were numerous, contradictory, unclear, more emotional than analytical; and he gave way to an emotional conclusion: 'Our plan was not signed. The Arabs were willing but the Jews kept promising, kept arguing over tiny details, and never signed. ... The Jews' absolute bad faith was the real reason for the failure of this final attempt to save the city.'[482] In Geneva, the Committee did not pay any attention to this remark. What mattered to it was that the project had been shelved.

---

[480]In this spirit, Ruegger wrote on Aug. 13, 1948, to Anderegg that 'the Committee is also ready, at a moment when no other authority is dealing with the problem, to consider assisting in the neutralization of the whole of Jerusalem – despite the fact that the problems posed by the implementation of this program are, practically speaking, enormous and imply very great good will on the part of all.' See Ruegger's personal letter to Anderegg, National Councilor, Aug. 13, 1948 (AICRC, CR 201). [Translation: M.G.]

[481]Letter from Gallopin, ICRC Geneva, to de Reynier, ICRC Geneva, May 14, 1948 (AICRC, CR 201).

[482]Note from de Reynier, ICRC Jerusalem, to ICRC Geneva, May 16, 1948 (AICRC, G.59/I/G.C.). [Translation: M.G.]

Settling for safety zones

For the time being, the ICRC had no alternative but to fall back on the safety zones scheme, which it had not ceased to promote for an instant. Nor were the zones empty; when he had begun to publicize the idea, de Reynier had been obliged to accept some unusual refugees: many consuls who had begun to seek shelter after some of them, envoys of countries that had voted in favor of partition, had been attacked. De Reynier resisted the pressure of the consular corps for as long as possible, since the presence of these political figures in the safety zones could damage the ICRC's neutral image. He finally had to give in, however, though not without imposing preliminary conditions: The consuls had to be unarmed, they could not exercise any professional function within the zones, and they would be considered ordinary civilians of foreign nationality.[483]

On May 13, 1948, de Reynier informed the civil and military authorities in Mandatory Palestine, without asking for their approval, that 'as of now the following buildings benefit from the protection of the Red Cross in the capacity of safety zones'[484]: the Franciscan school of Terra Sancta, the YMCA hostel, the King David Hotel, Government House, the Arab college, the Jewish agricultural school, and the adjacent territory extending up to the Allenby barracks, including the grounds surrounding these buildings. If he had adhered strictly to the draft conventions that would be presented in Stockholm, de Reynier would have had to settle for offering the belligerents the ICRC's good offices to help them come to an agreement on the establishment of the zones. But Marti had only just arrived in Palestine with the relevant drafts, and de Reynier may not have had the time yet to consult them. At best, he could have seen them on the same day that he presented his proposal to the authorities concerned. Nonetheless, de Reynier took other liberties. For one thing, contrary to what had been decided at the beginning of the negotiations, he no longer guaranteed that the refugees would be

---

[483]Correspondence and notes relative to the talks with the consular corps in Jerusalem, April-May 1948 (AICRC, G.59/I/G.C.). See also de Reynier, monthly report no. 2, April, Jerusalem, May 1, 1948 (AICRC, G.59/I/G.C.).

[484]ICRC delegation in Palestine, 'Aux autorités civiles et militaires en Palestine, concerne: zones de sécurité,' Jerusalem, May 13, 1948 (CZA.S.25.8943 and ISA/MEA/2406.4).

provisioned; they would find only temporary shelter in these buildings.[485]

There was a conspicuous gap between de Reynier's perspective and that of the Committee in Geneva, but the Committee did not seem to be aware of it. De Reynier's main concern, judging by his May 13, 1948, communications to the parties to the conflict, seemed to be protecting the buildings that the British wished to preserve from possible control by the Jews – the same buildings and grounds that he had turned into safety zones. Geneva's focus was on the creation of safety zones along the lines stipulated in the drafts for Stockholm, in order to create a precedent. Given this outlook, Geneva could not, in particular, afford to promote the zones unilaterally, without the consent of the belligerents, and therefore in its official publications laid emphasis on the fact that both parties had accepted the establishment of safety zones as conceived by de Reynier.

According to the *Revue internationale de la Croix-Rouge*, de Reynier received, on May 9 and 17, 1948, respectively, the written undertakings of the Arab Higher Committee and the Jewish Agency to honor the zones established by the ICRC.[486] The ICRC's source for these dates was de Reynier's reports, yet the ICRC archives do not appear to contain any communication from an official of the Arab Higher Committee or any other Arab authority agreeing to respect the ICRC safety zones. Munier had met with the Mufti on May 7, 1948, in Damascus, in the course of the negotiations for the 'neutralization' of Jerusalem. It is possible that on that date or shortly afterwards Hadj Amin el-Husseini gave Munier an oral consent to the establishment of the safety zones; there is no evidence either to confirm or to exclude this possibility, but it would have been to his advantage to agree, since the location of the King David zone in particular represented a potential strategic asset for the Jews.

As for Israel, I did not find the written consent of May 17, 1948, in the ICRC archives.[487] The Israel State Archives, however,

[485]Ibid.
[486]'Les zones de sécurité constituées en Palestine sous le drapeau du Comité international de la Croix-Rouge,' *RICR* 354 (June 1948): 409–413.
[487]De Reynier asked the ICRC for a copy of it at the end of January 1949, but the ICRC could not find it. See note from de Reynier, Beirut, Jan. 20, 1949, concerning 'lettre des autorités juives du 17 mai 1948 acceptant les zones de sécurité' (AICRC, G.59/I/G.C.).

THE RED CROSS IN PALESTINE–ERETZ-YISRAEL

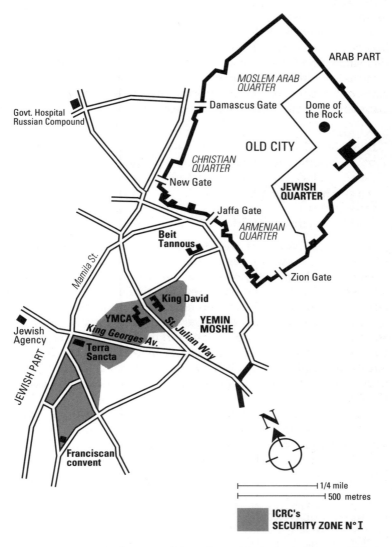

Since no graphic depiction of the safety zones in Jerusalem could be found in the ICRC archives, this map was drawn on the evidence of written documents, and is consequently approximate.

contain a copy of a letter from the Jewish Agency to the ICRC, dated May 17, which is not in the ICRC archives. It is addressed to de Reynier, from Kohn. In it Kohn acknowledges receiving de Reynier's May 13, 1948, announcement that the British buildings had been placed under the protection of the Red Cross flag and that safety zones had been established around them. He was not opposed to the institution of such zones, but made a request concerning zone no. 1, comprising the YMCA and the King David Hotel with their adjoining grounds:

> As regards the determination of the zones, we consider that they should not include any main road so that there may be no interference with the zone arrangement through the passing along such roads of military personnel. For this reason we suggest that zone I, ... should be broken into three zones so that St Julian's Way and King George Avenue should be left out of the zone.[488]

St. Julian's Way[489] passed between the King David and the YMCA, in the middle of zone I, and governed access to the Jewish neighborhood of Yemin Moshe in West Jerusalem. A Haganah unit which was then stationed next to Beit Tannous, not far from Jaffa Gate and the Old City, intended to try to join another unit located at Yemin Moshe and to attempt from there to go to the assistance of the civilian population in the Jewish Quarter, which was surrounded by the Arab armies in the Old City. To carry out this operation successfully, a unit of the Israeli army would have to pass through St. Julian's Way – which explains Kohn's request.[490]

Under the draft conventions, Kohn's request could have been granted. They stipulated that military convoys could, if necessary, cross the zones without stopping. De Reynier, who by now must have been able to acquaint himself with the details of the drafts Marti had brought him on May 13, could therefore have

---

[488]Letter from Kohn, JA (no place given), to de Reynier, ICRC Jerusalem, May 17, 1948 (ISA/MEA/2406.4).

[489]The Israelis later changed the name of St. Julian's Way to 'Rehov David Hamelech' (King David Street).

[490]According to telephone interview by author (Geneva) with Netanel Lorch (Jerusalem), May 3, 1993. On the operation as a whole, see, for example, Avi Shlaim, *The Politics of Partition, King Abdullah, the Zionists and Palestine, 1921–1951*, revised ed. (1st ed. 1988 under the title *Collusion Across the Jordan*) (Oxford: Oxford University Press, 1990), 465 pp., p. 180.

responded to Kohn's request accordingly. But he did not: 'We agree to consider King George as outside of zone I, but it is impossible to do the same for St. Julian's Way because the King David and the YMCA form a solid block that cannot be divided.'[491] In the end, since the Israeli army could not take another route, a few trucks from the unit that had been ordered to join the forces at Yemin Moshe simply raced the few hundred meters of St. Julian's Way, for lack of any other solution.[492]

On May 19, 1948, shortly after the international hostilities began and when the Arab Legion was on the point of entering Jerusalem, the Committee in Geneva officially announced the existence of the safety zones to the Arab League countries and Israel. Geneva claimed – sincerely, it appears – that they had been established with the consent of the Arab and Jewish parties, and asked the belligerent armies to respect them.[493] The Arab countries agreed, and Shertok, the minister of foreign affairs of the provisional government of Israel, responded on May 25 as follows:

> we had already informed the ICRC delegates in Jerusalem that we would scrupulously respect any safety zone established by the Red Cross. We merely asked that our liaison officers in Jerusalem, Messieurs Kohn and Eytan, be informed whenever such a zone is instituted. We take it as understood that no safety zone will be used as any kind of base for attack with any weapon. . . .[494]

This message, dated May 25, 1948, is the only written Israeli agreement to the establishment of safety zones that I was able to find.

Adopting the same logic as de Reynier, who on May 13 had presented the safety zone scheme as a way of neutralizing, first, buildings with major strategic or administrative value, and, next,

---

[491]Letter from de Reynier, ICRC Jerusalem, to Kohn, JA Jerusalem, May 20, 1948 (ISA/MEA/2406.4). [Translation: M.G.].

[492]Author's telephone interview with Netanel Lorch, Jerusalem, May 3, 1993. Information confirmed in dossier 'Mission de Reynier' (AICRC, G.3/82).

[493]ICRC, 'The Conflict in Palestine: An Appeal of the International Committee of the Red Cross to the Forces Engaged,' press release no. 363b, Geneva, May 21, 1948 (Press Release Collection, ICRC Library).

[494]Radiogram from Shertok, Tel Aviv, to Ruegger, ICRC Geneva, May 25, 1948 (AICRC, G.59/I/G.C.). [Translation: M.G.].

the lands surrounding them, Kohn asked that a safety zone be set up for the Jewish population in the middle of the Jewish Quarter in the Old City, which was surrounded by the Arabs. This safety zone would be organized around the Misgav Ladach Hospital, which the Jewish military authorities had provided with a red cross in accordance with the Geneva Convention.[495] Kohn assured de Reynier that the Jewish Agency would be willing to recognize a similar zone established by the Arabs, on the basis of reciprocal respect.[496]

The extension of the Misgav Ladach Hospital's immunity to the land surrounding it for the protection of civilians threatened by the fighting was consistent with the drafts that would be presented in Stockholm, but could also have prevented the Arab military forces from conquering the Jewish Quarter of the Old City. The situation was analogous to that of the existing safety zones, which de Reynier had established around buildings that the British wanted to keep out of the hands of the Jews. Yet to the request regarding the Misgav Ladach Hospital, de Reynier responded that the ICRC had not 'received up until now the signed consent of the two parties concerning this hospital.'[497] As for the authorities of the Arab Legion, whom he had apparently contacted immediately, he declared that they had told him 'that they did not wish to make a decision to change the status of that hospital in the middle of the battle.'[498]

The draft laws concerning the establishment of hospital and safety zones provided that the latter would be established by

[495]Kohn had understood from de Reynier's memorandum of May 13 that buildings of all types could be marked with the red cross and declared 'safety zones.' He therefore asked that safety zones under Red Cross protection be instituted in the following buildings: Jerusalem Girls' College, Ussishkin Street; Strauss Medical Health Center, Chancellor Street; Spitzer School, David Street; Bukarian Quarter; Tachkemoni School, Kerem Quarter; Menorah Club, Ben Yehuda Street; Etz Haim Rabbinical College, Mahane Yeduda Quarter; Teachers' Training College, Bet Hakerem. Letter from Kohn, JA Jerusalem, to ICRC Jerusalem, May 19, 1948 (ISA/MEA/2406.4). De Reynier answered on May 20: 'Although we perfectly understand the motives for your request, we must nonetheless make it clear here that it is not possible to create new safety zones by unilateral decision and without first having obtained the consent of the interested parties.' Letter from de Reynier, ICRC Jerusalem, to Kohn, JA, Jerusalem, May 20, 1948 (ISA/MEA/2406.4). [Translation: M.G.]

[496]Letter from Kohn, JA, no place given, to de Reynier, ICRC Jerusalem, May 17, 1948 (ISA/MEA/2406.4).

[497]Letter from de Reynier, ICRC Jerusalem, to Kohn, JA, Jerusalem, May 20, 1948 (ISA/MEA/2406.4). [Translation: M.G.]

[498]Ibid.

accord between the belligerents[499]; thus, regarding the proposal to make the Misgav Ladach Hospital a safety zone, de Reynier was using the frame of reference that Marti had given him, namely the draft conventions that were to be presented in Stockholm. But this was not the reference point he had used in establishing the other safety zones; in that instance, he had announced their creation unilaterally.

Kohn did not understand de Reynier's attitude. Since the Misgav Ladach Hospital already displayed the red cross, why couldn't the grounds around it be turned into a safety zone, as de Reynier had done with the grounds around the King David, Government House, and other buildings? Looking for legal arguments, Kohn consulted the 1929 Geneva Convention, which contained no provision for hospital and safety zones. There he read that the neutralization of a hospital was not subject to the previous consent of an adversary.[500] He understood still less why a difference should be made for a safety zone established as an extension of the hospital concept when he recalled that on May 13 de Reynier had unilaterally announced the creation of safety zones around British buildings, without asking in advance for the belligerents' consent. On May 21, incensed, Kohn drafted an impulsive letter of protest to de Reynier, pointing out that hospitals were supposed to enjoy unconditional immunity in times of war, according to the Geneva Convention. In the end, however, he decided not to send it.[501]

Certain delegates' partiality and anti-Jewish attitudes

This affair reflected a drift away from Red Cross principles: De Reynier was showing evidence of bias. He was inconsistent, changing rules that he himself had established – something the Israelis could not understand at the time, but which later, when taking stock before the Diplomatic Conference of 1949, they would consider to have been the main reason for the failure of the ICRC safety zones. They would regret that the zones had not

---

[499]'Art. 12 (Projets civils)', annexed to note from Pilloud to Marti, ICRC Geneva, bound for Palestine, May 10, 1948 (AICRC, G.59/I/G.C.).
[500]Letter from Kohn, JA, Jerusalem, to de Reynier, ICRC Jerusalem, May 21, 1948. Draft, not sent (ISA/MEA/2406.6).
[501]Ibid.

been conceived and negotiated in the spirit of the draft conventions that were to be presented in Stockholm.[502]

At the moment, however, in May, 1948, tension continued to mount between the ICRC's Israeli contacts in Jerusalem and the head of the ICRC delegation 'in Palestine.' The bad relations between de Reynier – and other ICRC delegates as well – and the Israeli authorities in Jerusalem did not bode well for the success of an operation that, in the letter and spirit of the international humanitarian conventions and the Red Cross Statutes, depended on the good faith of the belligerents – the ICRC being expected to play, at most, a modest role as neutral intermediary between the parties to the conflict.

Since May 24, 1948, following the Arab Legion's entry into Jerusalem, Jews and Arabs had been fighting in the middle of safety zone no. III, around the Italian hospital, this zone having become highly strategic. It contained no refugees. Since it had not been established by agreement between the belligerents, the ICRC annulled it unilaterally on May 27.[503] At that time, the Jewish Quarter in the Old City, surrounded by the Arab Legion, was on the point of surrendering. On May 28, 1948, Kohn wrote to the ICRC: 'the whole idea of the safety zones is of little significance at a time when the Arab Legion is shelling indiscriminately the Jewish Quarter of Jerusalem and no safety zone can offer any protection. In fact, nothing could be more dangerous at the present time for women and children than to congregate in the gardens and courtyards of the safety zones as proposed by you.'[504] Indeed, the ICRC safety zones were not likely to offer shelter to Jews, and their locations were such as to hinder Israeli military operations.

While the safety zones were in effect, several incidents brought Israelis and ICRC delegates into conflict, reducing still further

---

[502]According to Hochman to Golan, 'Ezorei bitahon ve ezorei beit holim beyerushalaim,' [Safety and hospital zones in Jerusalem], Jerusalem, April 17, 1949 (ISA/MEA/1987.4).
[503]ICRC, memorandum to civil and military authorities in Palestine, Jerusalem, May 30, 1948 (AICRC, G.59/I/G.C.). See also 'Les zones de sécurité constituées en Palestine sous le drapeau du Comité international de la Croix-Rouge,' RICR 354 (June 1948): 410.
[504]Letter from Kohn, JA Jerusalem, to de Reynier, ICRC Jerusalem, May 28, 1948 (CZA.S.25.8943).

THE RED CROSS IN PALESTINE–ERETZ-YISRAEL

the trust that had existed between the authorities of the Jewish community and the ICRC delegation in Palestine at the very beginning of the ICRC's operations. Zone no. I, for example, sheltered a very small number of refugees,[505] among whom were Arabs of military age.[506] Both it and safety zone no. II, around Government House, employed only Arabs. On June 2, 1948, the Stern group complained that three of its fighters had been shot at from the grounds of the YMCA, as they passed not far from there, near the American consulate. The group issued a warning to the ICRC: If by noon on June 3 all the armed Arabs and Arab workers in the establishments protected by the ICRC in Jerusalem – except for sick and wounded – were not removed from the premises, the Stern group would no longer consider the ICRC a neutral organization.[507] In a less imperative manner, the Israeli provisional government asked that the Arabs of combat age be evacuated, and that the ICRC dismiss half of the Arab employees and replace them with Jewish workers for balance.

Another bone of contention between the Israeli authorities and the ICRC was that two drivers working for the ICRC delegation in Jerusalem turned out to be spying on Israel. One of them was denounced by de Reynier himself.[508] The other one, a German, was arrested by the IZL and handed over to the Jewish military authorities. Pflimlin, one of the ICRC delegates stationed in the zone, demanded the driver's return, declaring that working in Israel made anyone more anti-Semitic than before[509] – which naturally angered the officer to whom he was speaking.[510]

[505] According to a report by Juliane Beauverd, a social worker for the ICRC in Palestine who had stayed in safety zone no. I before being transferred on July 22 to Courvoisier's office in Nablus, the safety zone sheltered approximately 85 refugees in the YMCA, half of them children, 50 in the Franciscan convent of Terra Sancta, and none in the King David Hotel. J. Beauverd, ICRC Ramallah, to Lucie Odier, ICRC Geneva, Sept. 5, 1948 (AICRC, G.59/I/G.C.).

[506] Sikum taskir b'inyan pgisha mar Tchizik im mar de Reynier ve mar Gouy mehatslav ha'adom be'yom 22.6.1948 [summary of memorandum regarding meeting of Mr. Tchizik with Mr. de Reynier and Mr. Gouy from the Red Cross on June 22, 1948] (ISA/MEA/2406.1).

[507] Note from Fighters for the Freedom of Israel, Jerusalem, to ICRC Jerusalem, June 2, 1948 (JISA/MEA/2406.6).

[508] According to letter from Gaulan, Liaison Officer, Jerusalem, to Pflimlin, ICRC, July 18, 1948 (ISA/MEA/2406.6).

[509] Gaulan, 'doch katzar mesiha im Pflimlin, bacoah hatslav ha'adom habenle'-umi be-yerushalaim me'yom 16.7.48 [short report of conversation with Pflimlin, in the International Red Cross force in Jerusalem on June 16, 1948], Jerusalem, June 17, 1948 (ISA/MEA/1896.8).

[510] Ibid.

The Israeli authorities decided to express their indignation to the Committee in Geneva. Kahany, now the Israeli provisional government's representative to the United Nations and the ICRC in Geneva, went to see Wolf and Marti at ICRC headquarters to protest both Pflimlin's remark and de Reynier's biased attitude. In the Israelis' view, de Reynier had neglected the traditional tasks of the ICRC in order to embark on political activities that were harmful to Israel – particularly his attempt to place Jerusalem under the Red Cross flag[511] at a time when Israel had the upper hand in the Jewish, western part of Jerusalem. Wolf and Marti promised that Pflimlin would soon be dismissed[512] and reassured Kahany as to de Reynier's friendly feelings for the Israelis. Following these talks, Kahany tried to calm the authorities in Tel Aviv, particularly with respect to de Reynier: 'As far as I can judge,' he wrote to Eytan at the Israeli Ministry of Foreign Affairs,

> de Reynier is the type of a soldier (he is an officer of the Swiss Army) and he has neither diplomatic qualities nor is he able to understand the psychology of our people. But what you said of him in your letter, namely that 'his failure consists in neglecting the established routine work of the Red Cross and his embarkation on political activities, such as making proposals for placing the whole of Jerusalem under the protection of the Red Cross' is certainly erroneous. These proposals have not germinated in de Reynier's 'goyish'[513] brain.[514]

It was then that Kahany explained that the idea of safety zones had originated with Adler-Rudel, who, passing through Geneva, had given it to Wolf; he in turn had mentioned it to Ruegger.[515] However, Kahany, in Geneva, was far removed from

---

[511] According to letter from Kahany, Provisional Government of Israel, no place given, to Eytan, Ministry of Foreign Affairs, Tel Aviv, July 29, 1948 (ISA/MEA/537.1).

[512] This promise was not kept; Pflimlin was transferred to safety zone no. II and later to Gaza.

[513] In Hebrew, the word *goy* means 'people,' and the Jewish people is a 'goy' like any other. Nonetheless, in common parlance many Jews use the word 'goy' to designate non-Jews – a usage which apparently originated in the Jewish villages (*shtetls*) of Eastern Europe.

[514] Letter from Kahany, Provisional Government of Israel, place not given, to Eytan, Ministry of Foreign Affairs, Tel Aviv, July 29, 1948 (ISA/MEA/537.1.)

[515] See p. 164.

the realities of the conflict taking place between Arabs and Israelis in Jerusalem, and from the causes for resentment that de Reynier had given Israel, notably owing to his obstinate determination to maintain and administer the safety zones according to rules that favored the British and the Arabs.

Bernadotte in Palestine

While the ICRC's safety zones were beginning to pose problems in Jerusalem, endangering the Red Cross's image, Count Bernadotte, who had just accepted the post of United Nations mediator for Palestine, was setting out for Jerusalem himself. Shortly before, he had told the press that he was not very optimistic as to the outcome of the negotiations he was charged to conduct.

From the ICRC's point of view, Bernadotte's mission was ambiguous. Bernadotte had not in fact given up his functions as president of the Swedish Red Cross and chairman of the Standing Commission of the International Conference of the Red Cross when he accepted his mediating role; to Bernadotte's mind, the Red Cross's mission should not be limited to humanizing the war, but should also consist in preventing it. By this token, political missions could be conducted under the banner of the Red Cross. Bernadotte's view was similar to that of the Red Cross societies of the Communist countries, but was received with a marked lack of enthusiasm by the ICRC, which sought to retain a neutral, independent image. At a time when the promotion of peace was one of the main themes of Communist propaganda, the ICRC preferred to keep a low profile on the issue, pacifism being too political and too controversial. As Max Huber wrote cautiously in 1948: 'Certainly, the men and women who work for the Red Cross should also join in the supreme task of establishing permanent peace, but even whilst pursuing this exalted aim, they must remember that the work of the Red Cross organizations must be safeguarded against the possibility, however remote, that war may again break out.'[516]

Moreover, the ICRC feared that if his political peace mission should fail, Bernadotte would choose to turn to humanitarian actions, with the support of the National Societies. He might

---

[516]ICRC, XVIIth International Red Cross Conference, Stockholm, August 1948, *Report of the International Committee of the Red Cross on Its Activities during the Second World War*, Vol. I, p. 22.

thus 'checkmate' the ICRC in the Israeli-Arab war. To ward off these risks, Ruegger decided at the end of May, 1948, to go to Jerusalem himself, hoping to arrive before the mediator. The ICRC president wished to find common ground with Bernadotte. He would try to persuade him to make a distinction between his political functions and the humanitarian ones that he performed in the world of the International Red Cross; in light of the Arab hostility towards the UN, simultaneously carrying out duties in the service of the UN and within the Red Cross could create confusion, and complicate the activities the ICRC conducted under the Red Cross emblem, especially the safety zones project. From Ruegger's viewpoint, it would be wise if Bernadotte marked the difference between the UN and the Red Cross by renouncing the use of the Red Cross emblem in the framework of his mission as United Nations mediator.[517] Ruegger's reasoning, however, which he shared with Bernadotte when they met in Cairo, did not convince the mediator, who reproved the ICRC for misusing the red cross itself in the Israeli–Arab conflict. The issue of using the protective sign of the red cross, on one hand, and the Red Cross emblem in its symbolic dimension, on the other, would have to be re-examined in Stockholm.[518]

The ICRC safety zones were in an especially delicate situation because during the first truce (June 11–July 8), Bernadotte, in his joint capacities as UN mediator and Red Cross official, decided to set up his offices in the King David Hotel, in the middle of

[517]ICRC, procès-verbal, Bureau meeting of May 19, 1948 (AICRC, no file number). On the reasons for Ruegger's trip to Jerusalem, see also Michael Hoffman, 'Red Cross to Press Jerusalem Efforts – Aim to Set up a Security Zone,' *New York Times* (May 21, 1948). The Swiss government commented on this dispatch as follows: 'Michael Hoffmann's dispatch to the *New York Times*, which may have been inspired by a collaborator of the ICRC, is assuredly unfortunate. It is ill-timed support, and Geneva realizes this perfectly.' De Haller, 'Commentaire sur la lettre du Ministre Bruggmann en date du 21 mai 1948,' Bern, June 4, 1948 (ADPF. 2001 [E] 5). [Translation: M.G.] See also Délégation du CICR à Stockholm, 'Séances de travail, compte rendu de la 1ère séance, mardi 22 juin 1948' (AICRC, CR 25), as well as letter from Kahany, Provisional Government of Israel, Representative to European Office of the United Nations and to the International Committee of the Red Cross, Geneva, to Shertok, Foreign Ministry, Tel Aviv, June 18, 1948 (ISA/MEA/2406.6).

[518]Délégation du CICR à Stockholm, 'Séances de travail, compte rendu de la 5ème séance, 20 juillet 1948' (AICRC, CR 25).

safety zone no. I. The King David, which flew the Red Cross flag, had been entrusted to the ICRC by the Mandatory power, to be transferred eventually to the United Nations; consequently, Bernadotte considered his residence there to be perfectly legitimate. It meant, however, that the United Nations mediator would be conducting political activities for the UN in the middle of the ICRC safety zone, and, in a way, 'under the protection' of the Red Cross emblem. After some attempt to oppose the plan, the ICRC finally gave in. On June 15, 1948, Bernadotte took up his quarters in the old hotel, which the ICRC immediately cut out of the safety zone[519] in order to avoid any confusion between the ICRC and the UN.

Why did the ICRC give in? At least two plausible hypotheses can be postulated, and they are not mutually exclusive. Ruegger may not have wanted to annoy a man whose position on the issues discussed in Stockholm might influence the Committee's future, especially since the two parties to the conflict had consented to the mediator's moving into the King David. Another possibility is that Ruegger wanted to avoid giving the impression that the ICRC sought to hinder Bernadotte's peace efforts.

The Red Cross flags on the YMCA and the UN flag on the King David waved about a hundred meters from each other as the crow flies, on a cliff in the Jewish part of Jerusalem overlooking the Old City, which was then in the hands of the Arab Legion and the forces of the Arab Higher Committee. The Israeli troops were posted on the surrounding hills, except for the hill on which the King David stood. They themselves were surrounded by the Arab armies. The ICRC expected fighting to resume at the end of the truce, and if the King David should become a target, the safety zone might be fired on. Consequently, between July 3 and 5, 1948, it asked Israel and the Arab Legion to agree to the reincorporation of the King David into the safety zone if Bernadotte left it. Abdullah Tel, the local commander of the Arab Legion, accepted; it was to his advantage strategically. Israel, however, refused, and the ICRC was not in a position to insist, especially since, in order not to presume on the outcome of the truce, the ICRC had not proposed before Bernadotte moved to

---

[519]ICRC, memorandum to civil and military authorities in Palestine, Jerusalem, June 14, 1948 (AICRC, G.59/I/G.C.).

the King David that the building should be reintegrated into safety zone no. 1 if the mediator should leave it.[520]

On July 9, when the truce ended, Bernadotte and his little group of colleagues fled the King David in disorder. The Haganah moved into the building with, according to the Israeli version – which the ICRC found difficult to believe – the approval of the mediator and the UN Truce Commission[521] The King David then became a shooting target for the Arab Legion, whose army held the Old City of Jerusalem. As a result, the adjacent ICRC safety zone, now reduced to the YMCA alone, also received shells, becoming, in the opinion of the ICRC delegates, the most dangerous place in West Jerusalem.[522] Ruegger kept trying to negotiate with Shertok for the evacuation of the King David by the Haganah, convinced that the Jews – who had supposedly agreed unconditionally to the ICRC safety zones – had acted in bad faith. Relations between Ruegger and Shertok deteriorated.

The King David remained in Israeli hands.[523] The ICRC unilaterally terminated the zone on July 22, after having evacuated the administrative personnel and the few children who were staying there. Resentfully, it put the entire responsibility for the closure of the zone on the 'Jewish authorities.' For their part, the Israeli authorities could not help but feel justified in their earlier impression that the ICRC was biased – particularly de Reynier, but also the ICRC president, whom they considered to be very 'pro-British.'[524]

For several weeks the ICRC sought to renew the impetus for establishing safety zones, this time in conformity with the draft laws that would be presented in Stockholm. It envisioned, for example, setting up one in Amman and another in Tel Aviv,

---

[520] According to telegram from Shertok, Minister of Foreign Affairs of Israel, Tel Aviv, to Ruegger, President of the ICRC, Geneva, July 14, 1948 (ISA/MEA/537.1).

[521] Ibid.

[522] Note from Raoul Pflimlin, ICRC Jerusalem, to ICRC Geneva, July 10, 1948, (AICRC, G.59/I/G.C.).

[523] Telegram from Ruegger, President of the ICRC, Geneva, to Shertok, Minister of Foreign Affairs, Israel, July 12, 1948 (ISA/MEA/537.1). Telegram from Shertok, Minister of Foreign Affairs, Israel, Tel Aviv, to Ruegger, President of the ICRC, Geneva, July 15, 1948 (ISA/MEA/537.1).

[524] According to letter from Zvi Loker, Provisional Government of Israel, Division of International Organizations, Hakirya, to Kahany, Provisional Government of Israel, Representative to the European Office of the United Nations and to the ICRC, Geneva, Jan. 31, 1949 (ISA/MEA/1987.1).

and announced this plan, although negotiations for it had not seriously begun. This tentative project was never implemented.

One month away from the Conference of Stockholm, which would open on August 20, the whole safety zone enterprise now depended solely on the maintenance and proper functioning of zone no. II, which incorporated Government House. This zone was vital for ICRC activities when the second truce began on July 17, 1948. Since June, 1948, the ICRC had been acting as a neutral intermediary between Israel and the Arab countries for the benefit of the prisoners of war on both sides.[525] Due to the new configuration of the war fronts, the Government House zone was the only point through which the ICRC could freely transfer aid supplies and mail for prisoners of war between Israel and Transjordan. For the Egyptians and the Arab League in the southeast, however, and the Israelis in the north-west, the ICRC safety zone was an obstacle that prevented them from confronting each other.

Haganah soldiers disguised as UN observers entered the zone for the first time on July 19, 1948, the day after safety zone no. I was closed down. This incident was taken all the way to the Security Council, for it constituted a violation of the second truce, negotiated this time for an indefinite period. The ICRC decided not to terminate the zone, while the Arab armies took over the Jewish School of Agriculture. De Reynier was on his way to Stockholm, and Government House had been entrusted to two ICRC delegates and a nurse, under the supervision of Lehner, the interim head of the ICRC delegation in Jerusalem.

Several diversely dramatic incidents demonstrated that Government House zone was not a safe haven for the few dozen people staying there, most of them since before the institution of the safety zone. During the fighting, many Beduin were killed there.[526] Israeli soldiers under Egyptian fire asked for refuge in the zone on the morning of August 17. The ICRC agreed, on condition that they lay down their arms. Then, after long negotiations with Arab irregulars, who were ready to massacre the Jewish soldiers, and with an officer of the regular army, the ICRC took the Israelis, with their consent, to the headquarters of the

[525]See Chapter 5, pp. 212 ff.
[526]Note from Munier, ICRC Amman, to de Reynier, ICRC Delegation, Stockholm, Aug. 17, 1948 (AICRC, G.59/I/G.C.).

Arab Legion in the Old City of Jerusalem. The next day the ICRC, represented by Pflimlin (who continued to exercise his functions), noted that these prisoners had been maltreated.[527] The Israelis had also taken prisoners, whom they were holding in the Arab college in the middle of the zone. These prisoners were put at the ICRC's disposal, except for the men of fighting age.[528] Finally, the ICRC delegates discovered, the day after a battle, the unmutilated bodies of two Jewish soldiers,[529] which they were not immediately able to bury. When they returned, two days later, to take the bodies away, they saw that in the meantime the corpses had been decapitated.[530] The Government House zone did not offer the slightest guarantee of safety, to say the least – yet, for some reason, the ICRC kept it operating.

The answer must be sought in Stockholm. Israel indignantly reported the incidents mentioned above to Bernadotte and Ruegger during the Conference of Stockholm.[531] For the moment the ICRC's interests accorded with those of Bernadotte. The ICRC did not want its last remaining safety zone to fail, not did it want to withdraw hastily, as it had from the other two zones, for fear that the Israeli forces would immediately occupy the premises. By the same token, Bernadotte would gain nothing if the ICRC's safety zone were to degenerate into a battlefield, since that would detract from his credibility in respect to the success of the truce, and could lead to the resumption of hostilities.

Bernadotte, Ruegger, and de Reynier, who was also in Stockholm, thus found common ground. The ICRC undertook to keep the safety zone functioning long enough for the UN observers in Jerusalem to negotiate with the forces involved for the estab-

[527]Note from Pflimlin, ICRC Jerusalem, to ICRC Geneva, Sept. 4, 1948 (AICRC, G.59/I/G.C.).
[528]Letter from Bernard Joseph, Military Governor, Jerusalem, to Lehner, ICRC Jerusalem, Aug. 19, 1948 (ISA/MEA/2406.2).
[529]Letter from Lehner, ICRC Jerusalem, to Jewish Authorities, care of Bernard Joseph, Military Governor, Jerusalem, Aug. 18, 1948 (ISA/MEA/2406.2).
[530]Letter from Lehner, ICRC Jerusalem, to Bernard Joseph, Military Governor, Jerusalem, Aug. 21, 1948 (ISA/MEA/2406.2).
[531]Telegram from Shertok, Minister of Foreign Affairs, Tel Aviv, to Bernadotte, International Red Cross Conference, Stockholm, Aug. 22, 1948 (ISA/MEA/537.1). Letter from Katznelson, Delegation of the Provisional Government of the State of Israel to the International Conference of Stockholm, to the ICRC Delegation to the International Red Cross Conference of Stockholm, Aug. 23, 1948 (ISA/MEA/537.1).

lishment of a demilitarized belt around the Government House zone. This was conducive to Bernadotte's plan for a progressive demilitarization of Jerusalem,[532] which city, according to another plan that he had on the drawing board, he intended to hand over to King Abdullah.

From Stockholm, on August 25, 1948, de Reynier ordered his delegates in Jerusalem not to close the zone. He gave them no explanation for this decision, and informed them that for tactical reasons he would postpone the protests[533] that were in order regarding the Arabs' mutilation of the corpses of Jewish soldiers. A few UN observers were living in the safety zone, under the Red Cross flag, which irritated and worried the delegates; for the ICRC's mission was becoming increasingly confused with that of the UN, in particular because Bernadotte had not hesitated, on many occasions, to wear the uniform of the Swedish Red Cross and to use an airplane displaying a red cross in the course of his political mission for the UN.

On September 17, 1948, Bernadotte went to Government House to meet with the UN observers, and when he left the safety zone he was assassinated on the orders of the Stern group, together with the French Colonel André Sérot. The crime was committed before the eyes of an appalled ICRC delegate, Pierre Fasel.[534] ICRC delegates transported the two bodies to the Lydda airport.

Due to the possible confusion between the ICRC and the UN owing to Bernadotte's use of the Red Cross emblem and his stay in the ICRC safety zones, de Reynier considered that the threat to his delegates' safety was too great to keep the zone open after this tragedy. However, at the request of the United Nations, which wanted to take possession of the premises, he temporized for another three weeks. Finally, on October 8, 1948, the ICRC

---

[532]Amitzur Ilan, *Bernadotte in Palestine, 1948 – A Study in Contemporary Humanitarian Knight-Errantry* (Oxford, London: MacMillan, in association with St. Antony's College, 1989), p. 162.

[533]Note from de Reynier, ICRC Geneva, Stockholm, to Gaillard, ICRC Tel Aviv, Aug. 25, 1948 (AICRC, G.3/82). See also telegram from Ruegger and de Reynier, Geneva, to Gaillard, ICRC Government House, Sept. 2, 1948 (AICRC, G.59/I/G.C.).

[534]On the circumstances of this assassination, see, for example, Amitzur Ilan, *op. cit.*, pp. 193–222.

handed the former residence of the high commissioner in Palestine over to Ralph Bunche, Bernadotte's successor. The ICRC flag was taken down and replaced with that of the United Nations.[535]

---

[535]De Reynier, Central ICRC Delegation, Beirut, 'Rapport sur la deuxième inspection des délégations de Palestine du 7 au 18 octobre 1948,' Beirut, Oct. 20, 1948 (AICRC, G.59/I/G.C.).

Chapter Five

FROM HEROISM TO TRADITIONAL ACTIVITIES: THE EVOLUTION FROM IDEALS TO STRATEGY

From ideals to strategy

The big projects that de Reynier began to implement from March, 1948, on, namely the ICRC's activities on behalf of the wounded, the sick, and civilian populations, were significant to the ICRC in several ways, in the context of the accusations aimed at it at the beginning of the Cold War. By linking its actions to the Geneva Convention, the ICRC was bearing witness; it was implicitly pointing out that it was the source of the Red Cross ideal, that it was the guardian of Red Cross principles. Both locally and within the International Red Cross, the ICRC sought to present itself as a moral authority, an authority symbolized by its emblem.

Historically, however, what was the basis for the moral authority on which the ICRC prided itself? True, the organization had given rise to both the International Red Cross and the Geneva Convention. But the ICRC was not the direct heir of the act that had provided the model for the International Red Cross, Henry Dunant's philanthropic gesture at Solferino. It was a neutral intermediary more than anything else, not a good Samaritan tending to the wounded and sick in the aftermath of battle. Yet the connection with Henry Dunant was the only possible basis for the moral authority the ICRC sought to wield. And it could not claim Dunant's ideal as its inspiration unless it had delegates who actually perpetuated Dunant's gesture at Solferino, who came directly to the assistance of the suffering victims of war.

This raises the question, of course, as to whether de Reynier's subordinates were acting in that spirit, and whether they considered the value of their actions as part of the model operation in war-torn Palestine that the ICRC was so anxious to carry out before the Stockholm Conference. Were they able to reconcile the practice of direct assistance to the victims of battle with the ICRC's role as neutral intermediary?

This chapter will examine the ICRC delegates' actions and the significance they may have had for that organization in terms of its more general concerns. In the process, I will show how the ICRC delegates moved progressively from the implementation of their ideal to the implementation of the organization's strategy vis-à-vis the Stockholm Conference.

The reports from the ICRC delegates active during first the Palestine 'civil war' and then the Israeli-Arab conflict indicate that these men were not directly concerned by de Reynier's big plans; only occasionally did they take a hand in them. They were above all field workers. Instructed to maintain the best possible relations with the local authorities in the regions where they had set up their quarters, they reacted on a day-to-day basis to the tribulations of the war victims, and described them in their reports. From April to June, 1948, they dealt mostly with combatants, with ambushed civilians, with wounded and dead. Only rarely were there any prisoners – an unfamiliar situation for the ICRC envoys, since up until then their primary task had always been carrying out the ICRC's role as a neutral intermediary on behalf of prisoners of war. Until June, 1948, the delegates' reports brimmed with innumerable accounts of isolated humanitarian acts.

Two days with an ICRC delegate in Galilee

To discover the link between the mass of anecdotes recounted in the delegates' reports – if there was one – I examined a report that Jean Courvoisier, the delegate based in Nablus, wrote concerning his activities during May 9 and 10, 1948. I chose this report both for its spontaneity and because it was the least fragmented report I could find written by a rank-and-file delegate in the period preceding the Stockholm Conference.

On May 9, Courvoisier, together with the Arab driver who also served as his interpreter, went to see el-Kaukji, the head of

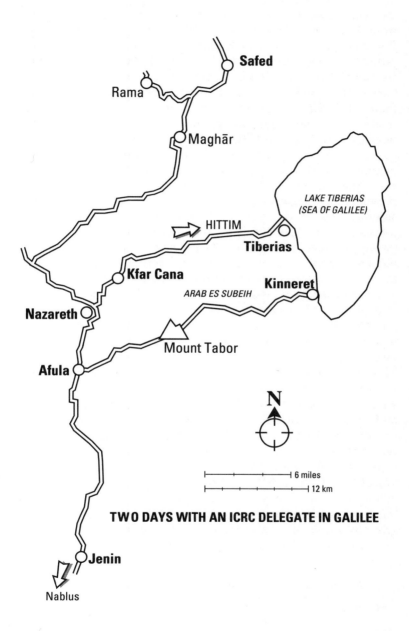

the Arab Liberation Army which had begun entering Palestine from Syria and Transjordan in January, 1948. It was the ICRC's first contact with this war leader. After accomplishing the purpose of his visit, which was to explain the ICRC's plan to 'neutralize' Jerusalem, Courvoisier talked to el-Kaukji about the 1929 Conventions and asked him to direct his armed forces to apply them. El-Kaukji promised to instruct his troops to accord humane treatment to the wounded, prisoners, and civilians – namely women, children, and the elderly. Courvoisier created the impression that the civilian population was protected by the conventions, which was inaccurate; but the fact that he did so indicates that he knew the ICRC wished to emphasize civilian populations. Regarding this category of victims, el-Kaukji asserted that he did not normally detain foreign women, but released them whenever possible, except for spies, who were promptly taken before a military court. Courvoisier made no response to this information, not considering female spies to be an issue related to the conventions of their principles.

Courvoisier then insisted on the ICRC's desire to be notified of captures and given lists of prisoners, a necessary condition if the ICRC was to be able to perform its traditional function as a neutral intermediary. El-Kaukji answered that he would have his own troops do this, but stressed that he could not speak for the Mufti's irregulars. Courvoisier commented on this to Geneva, with a reference to World War II: 'We are seeing a repetition of what happened in 1944 in France: on one side the regular troops and on the other the FFI.'[536] In making this comparison, Courvoisier was not thinking of the historical parallel, but rather of the different categories of victims defined by international humanitarian law and the ICRC's ability to act in their favor. During World War II, the ICRC had been able to justify in law its intervention on behalf of prisoners of war from the regular armies, but for captured partisans, such as FFI members, the legal grounds for intervention were much weaker, and the ICRC's representations went unheeded.[537]

---

[536]'Forces françaises de l'intérieur' (an organization of French resistance fighters). Report by Jean Courvoisier, ICRC Nablus, to ICRC Geneva, May 14, 1948 (AICRC, G.59/I/G.C.).

[537]Courvoisier confirmed this interpretation in an interview with the author on March 19, 1993.

Before taking leave of el-Kaukji, Courvoisier also asked him if he would be interested in the establishment of a safety zone in the north of Palestine. The offer was theoretical, probably dictated by de Reynier; no specific plan, based on an evaluation of local needs, had as yet been devised. El-Kaukji turned it down.

Courvoisier left the commander of the Arab Liberation Army and, in a white car bearing the ICRC emblem, drove towards Nazareth. Coming to Afula, a small Jewish town where Haganah forces were stationed, he asked the Jewish soldiers for authorization to pass through the town with his Arab driver. Obtaining it, he requested an escort to Nazareth, for despite the emblem on his car, he feared for his own safety and that of his companion. He did not seem particularly anxious to promote the red cross as such.

In Nazareth, he introduced himself to the local authorities. The representative of the Arab National Committee of Nazareth, Ibrahim Effendi Fahum, gave him a 'list of dead and mutilated who allegedly were savagely attacked by the Jews on the date of May 6, 1948.'[538] Another dignitary asked him to verify the facts, comparing them to the atrocities committed at Deir Yassin. 'Since it was a matter of certifying facts,' Courvoisier commented in his report to Geneva, 'I was cautious and circumspect.'[539] The only indication that allowed him to diagnose a confrontation between the Jewish forces and Arab civilians was the hospitalization of many Arab children in the Scottish mission in Nazareth. The ICRC delegate's caution in the face of the possibility that he might have to denounce a violation of international law and thereby risk placing the ICRC in the position of judge or arbiter reflected his 'Red Cross professionalism,' which implied the ability to control his reactions when an appeal was made to his emotions.

When he visited the Edinburgh mission hospital, Courvoisier learned that another establishment of the Scottish mission, located in Tiberias, had had to be evacuated when the Haganah took over the city. The local administrator of the Scottish mission in Nazareth wished to turn the Tiberias building over to the Magen David Adom through the intermediary of the ICRC, believing this to be the best means of safeguarding it. She joined

---

[538]Report from Jean Courvoisier, ICRC Nablus, to ICRC Geneva, May 14, 1948 (AICRC, G.59/I/G.C.). [Translation: M.G.]
[539]Ibid.

Courvoisier and his driver, and all three set off for Tiberias. They were not able to reach it, however, as the road north, through Kfar Cana and Hittim, had been mined. Accordingly, they turned towards Maghār, the center of military operations for the Arab Liberation Army. There they were received by a local military leader, who advised them to take the Jewish road through Afula and Mount Tabor, as they would run fewer risks. But it was late. Courvoisier and his two companions decided to spend the night in Rama, among the anxious Arab refugees; not far away, the battle for the control of Safed threatened them. Courvoisier, in his report to Geneva, mentioned the existence of the 'refugees,' but offered no suggestions concerning them. This silence suggests that Courvoisier did not consider the 'refugees' as 'civilian populations victimized by war,' such as the ICRC wanted to protect in the safety zones.

And so the day of May 9 came to an end. It had been full and exhausting, and had given the delegate feelings of disorientation which, according to his report, had made it interesting.

On May 10, Courvoisier and his companions left Rama, taking a woman and five small children to 'a safe place.'[540] Who and where, the report does not say; it was a case which, apparently, he would not follow up. He went back to Maghār, where he watched, impressed, the levy of thousands of combatants who were getting ready to fight in Safed. The local officer presented Courvoisier to the troops. Then the ICRC delegate returned to Nazareth.

As soon as he arrived, the mayor asked him to escort a group of wounded Arabs, hospitalized in the Scottish mission, from Nazareth to Nablus. Courvoisier led the convoy. They had to pass through Afula again, but at the entrance to the town, a Haganah officer refused to let the wounded through, arguing that Jews killed in the region of Arab es Subeih had not yet been buried by the Arab troops. Courvoisier explained to the officer that the passage of the wounded through Afula could not be made conditional on reciprocity; that would be contrary to the spirit of the Geneva Convention, the principles of which were absolute. These humanitarian operations had to be treated individually, on a unilateral basis. He asked, therefore, that the convoy be allowed to pass. The mentality of the Haganah officers

[540]Ibid.

being what it was, however, he ended up making the necessary concession: In exchange for free passage of the convoy, he promised to ask the Arab authorities to inter the dead Jews, or even to return them to the Jewish authorities. The Jewish officers accepted this proposal, and offered to release three Arab prisoners if their request was granted. In the meantime, the convoy of wounded could pass through Afula. Thus, in this instance, the presence of the ICRC delegate in that little corner of Palestine had made it possible to 'humanize the war' for a moment, and to a limited degree, by triggering a humanitarian transaction between Jews and Arabs.

Courvoisier escorted the wounded Arabs through Afula, but afterwards allowed the convoy to go on without him, towards the Arab lines. He himself set off again for Nazareth, to settle the issue of collecting the Jewish remains at Arab es Subeih. It was decided that on May 11, 1948, the local police would hand the bodies over to the Jews in exchange for three Arab prisoners. Courvoisier gave no details on the method of the operation, but the ICRC delegate had acted as a neutral intermediary between Jews and Arabs, transmitting mutual proposals and helping to organize their implementation. In a setting with which he was unfamiliar, abandoned solely to his own initiative, with the international conventions as his mental context, and the doctrine deriving from the ICRC's role of neutral intermediary as his only guide, the ICRC delegate drove back and forth through fragmented Palestine in his white car with the red crosses. At each encounter with soldiers, he tried to explain the ICRC's terms of reference: its role of neutral intermediary, the 1929 Conventions and their general spirit. Mentally, his priorities – whether reflected in speech or in action – were the civilian populations, prisoners, the wounded, and the dead, in accordance with the Committee's objectives in Palestine and the categories of existing or future law. For Courvoisier, what linked all the anecdotes and all the little gestures together was the 'Red Cross code,' or the implementation of the rules of conduct linked to the ICRC's function as a neutral intermediary and to its mandate to act in the letter and spirit of the Geneva Conventions. It was this, too, that apparently served as an ideal – in that context – for Courvoisier.

We cannot systematically examine here, on the basis of the

reports in the ICRC archives, the way that each individual ICRC delegate in the Palestine-EY conflict lived his mission. Each man integrated the ICRC rules to a different degree. For some they became second nature; other delegates had a little more trouble with them.

In general, however, the ICRC delegates who did the everyday work were strongly imbued with a sense of doctrine and law, and acted accordingly. It was their way of living the ideals of the ICRC. Their reports never refer to Henry Dunant, the source and the ideal of the Red Cross, but all the delegates were well acquainted with the Geneva Convention, which translated Dunant's ideal and to some extent organized its implementation. For these delegates, acting in the spirit of the Geneva Convention meant identifying with the ideal of the Red Cross.

Since all the tasks laid down by the Geneva Convention were within the purview of the army medical services aided by the relief societies, however, what did the convention leave for ICRC delegates to do? De Reynier recalls in this respect that when he arrived in Palestine, neither the Jews nor the Arabs had army medical services in the European sense. The ICRC delegates were therefore obliged to educate the belligerents, by setting an example and emulating Henry Dunant. According to de Reynier, this was the intent behind the delegates' individual initiatives on the battlefield, the site of all the suffering but, nevertheless, a place where they should never have been in the first place, under a strict interpretation of the Geneva Convention. He had reportedly had to make similar sacrifices himself.

We will examine the situations and incidents that de Reynier had in mind, and the way the delegates perceived and experienced them. Another interesting question is whether there was any evidence of this intention to educate the belligerents that de Reynier describes.

Promoting the ICRC in Nebi Daniel

The first incident occurred at the end of March, 1948, near Solomon's Pools and not far from Gush[541] Etzion, a bloc of four Jewish colonies located close to the road linking Hebron and Bethlehem. Gush Etzion had already been attacked several times

---

[541]The Hebrew *'gush'* means 'bloc.'

since the beginning of 1948, but had stood fast; it was a Jewish policy never to abandon settlements, owing to their importance in the eventual demarcation of borders. It was very difficult to reach the area from West Jerusalem, but from time to time an armed convoy would attempt to get through with food and other supplies – even arms, although at the time the Jews had few.

The ICRC had already launched its appeal of March 12, 1948, to obtain the belligerent parties' agreement to act according to the basic principles of the 1929 Conventions, but the Jewish Agency and the Arab Higher Committee had not yet given their written consent. De Reynier was alone in Jerusalem, and he knew that the ICRC official operation, beginning with the protection of the hospitals and the establishment of safety zones, could not begin until the Jews and Arabs in Palestine had formally agreed to respect the principles of the conventions. Such an agreement implied, in particular, that their armies would have to organize themselves so that they could collect the wounded and dead.

On March 27, not far from Solomon's Pools between Jerusalem and Hebron, the irregular forces of the Arab Higher Committee blocked a Jewish military convoy from Gush Etzion. The Jewish combatants abandoned their vehicles and took up a defensive position in a little stone house. That same evening, de Reynier received a telephone call from a Jewish Agency worker, who asked him to intervene on the battlefield. Reportedly some 25 men had been seriously wounded.[542] Conditioned by the philosophy of the conventions, de Reynier retained only one fact from this appeal: There were *wounded*. He consequently decided to go to Gush Etzion, to make sure the wounded were properly collected and cared for. He obtained the assistance of a doctor and an ambulance from the Arab Medical Association, since the Arab forces occupied the battlefield.

Before he could set out, de Reynier had to await British authorization, which was long in coming; the British army tried to dissuade him, telling him that the adventure was too dangerous, and explaining that army sappers would first have to clear the mines in the road. But it finally gave its permission, in the afternoon of March 28. De Reynier prepared to leave, but now it was the Arab Higher Committee's turn to try to discourage him; de

---

[542]Note from de Reynier, ICRC mission to Palestine, to ICRC Geneva, March 31, 1948 (AICRC, G.59/I/G.C.).

Reynier would be risking his life, the ambulance of the Red Crescent Association should go alone. The Arab doctor, whose name de Reynier could not remember, left on his own. De Reynier thought the matter over. If he stayed behind, he risked letting a member of the Red Crescent Arab Medical Association get in ahead of him. Overcoming his fear, he decided to rejoin the Arab ambulance, and explained his reasoning after the fact (though in the present tense) in his report to Geneva: 'The ICRC's work as a neutral intermediary must become known'; it must not be said that the ICRC delegates 'were afraid to go save defenseless, wounded men.' De Reynier added that he had taken responsibility for the Arab ambulance and doctor: 'If the Jews attack,' he concluded, 'I must at least share their fate' so that if the operation to evacuate the wounded failed, 'no one could accuse the ICRC of avoiding its responsibilities.'[543] Of course, in the case of Jewish aggression (very improbable under the circumstances, in any case), how could de Reynier's presence have helped to insure the safety of the Arab medical team? Perhaps he thought the emblem would have a deterrent effect.

It is interesting to note that de Reynier was apparently ready to die with the Arab medical team in order to protect the ICRC's reputation – instead of doing his utmost to stay alive in order to emulate Henry Dunant, whose objective he claimed as his own, and which should have been his only objective: to try to help the war-wounded. It was not Henry Dunant's example that inspired de Reynier's act of courage, at least not directly, but rather his own attachment to the ICRC, the institution he served and to which he attributed an intrinsic value. He raised the ICRC as a kind of screen between the Red Cross ideal, inspired by Henry Dunant's model, and its purpose in this particular context: aiding the wounded fighters in Gush Etzion.

To return to the chain of events, as far as it can be reconstructed (mainly from the ICRC archives), de Reynier himself drove his car with the red crosses, brandishing the ICRC flag through the half-open window, and rejoined the ambulance marked with the red crescent. He then took the lead, and together the two medical vehicles drove to the battlefield.

De Reynier was horrified at the sight that met his eyes. Overturned trucks burned with mutilated corpses inside them. From

[543]Ibid.

FROM HEROISM TO TRADITIONAL ACTIVITIES

a distance of 300 meters, thousands of recumbent Arabs shot at the little house where the Jews were entrenched. The latter returned fire, aiming well, but with little chance of coming out alive. Watching this unequal combat and waiting for the ICRC delegate, the British army stood by,[544] obeying the commands of neutrality. During the period of its withdrawal, the Mandatory power wanted to avoid any military engagement that might lead it to fight the Arabs and favor the Jews.[545] As soon as the ICRC delegate arrived, however, the situation changed; an officer of the British army negotiated a cease-fire to permit the besieged Jews to surrender.[546] He may have considered that the mere presence of the ICRC offered him the means of giving his act a humanitarian significance, which he could always justify if necessary. De Reynier's report says nothing of this, but it seems a plausible hypothesis.

The Jews emerged exhausted from the house, the able ones carrying the wounded, and laid down their arms (which the British left lying there). The British army put both the wounded and the unhurt Jews in its military vehicles, and asked de Reynier to lead the convoy – which would place this repatriation under the ICRC's responsibility.

De Reynier was uncomfortable. The situation was deviating from the model of the Geneva Convention, which basically provided that only vehicles used to transport war wounded could be designated with the red cross. Under the circumstances, de Reynier did not want to use the sign to protect able-bodied soldiers who could be sent back into combat. He therefore tried to offer the ICRC's services only for the evacuation of the wounded, leaving the British army the responsibility for restoring the unhurt combatants to their own territory.[547]

Clearly, the distinction that de Reynier wanted to make would put the British army in an uncomfortable position: It would have to shoulder the responsibility for saving and repatriating able-bodied Jews, men likely to fight again – an act it would not be able to justify in the face of Arab demands. The British refused

[544]Ibid.
[545]Telegram from High Commissioner for Palestine, Jerusalem, to Secretary of State, Colonial Office, London, Feb. 14, 1948 (Cunningham Private Papers, III/1/94, St. Antony's College. Middle East Library, Oxford).
[546]Note from de Reynier, ICRC mission in Palestine, to ICRC Geneva, March 31, 1948 (AICRC, G.59/I/G.C.).
[547]Ibid.

de Reynier's proposal, and the ICRC representative consequently had to resign himself to leading the convoy. The line of vehicles set off in the direction of Bethlehem under a hail of bullets, which wounded a few more men.[548] The doctor from the Arab Medical Association, for his part, acted in perfect accord with the Geneva Convention and the medical code of ethics. Attached to the Arab forces occupying the battlefield, he provided care to the wounded Jews who reached his ambulance.[549] Meanwhile, de Reynier made a final inspection of the area, as dictated by the ICRC's basic vocation: 'I wanted to see the last man taken away, to see that no wounded were left behind.'[550]

By some of the ICRC's criteria, the conduct of the operation had not been completely satisfactory; there had been too great a gap between the conventional model, in which a distinction was made between wounded and able-bodied fighters, and reality, which obliged delegates to save lives without making this distinction. Moreover, the ICRC had laid itself open to Arab hostility by repatriating uninjured Jews, just at a time when de Reynier was trying to make the Arab authorities understand that the ICRC delegates could be neither Jewish nor pro-Jews. De Reynier blamed the Jewish authorities, who had spoken only of wounded men. He felt he had been tricked.[551] In absolute terms, however, the balance was positive. By its 'mere presence,'[552] as de Reynier pointed out, the ICRC had saved human lives. The Israelis, who would remember the incident, translated this historical episode from their war of independence into the symbolism of Daniel's prophesies, naming the place where the fighters had been saved 'Nebi Daniel.'

De Reynier – if what he reported after the fact is completely reliable – did intend to educate the parties to the conflict, by trying to give them a real-life demonstration of the role of neutral intermediary that the ICRC wanted to play in the Palestine conflict. Was the same true for his colleagues?

---

[548]Ibid.
[549]Ibid.
[550]Ibid. As yet no one has studied ICRC operations in the Palestine-EY conflict from the perspective of this institution's humanitarian vocation and its delegates' desire to implement it as such.
[551]Ibid.
[552]De Reynier, report no. 3, April 1948, Jerusalem, May 1, 1948 (AICRC, G.59/I/G.C.).

Educating the belligerents in Katamon

The 1929 Geneva Convention stipulated that 'after each engagement the occupant of the field of battle shall take measures to search for the wounded and dead and to protect them against pillage and maltreatment.'[553] This duty, like the others, was to be performed by the personnel of the army medical services or of the aid societies, but not by ICRC delegates. The Geneva Convention also provided that 'whenever circumstances permit, a local armistice or a suspension of fire shall be arranged to permit the removal of the wounded remaining between the lines.'[554] The wounded could be removed thus, but not the dead. The removal of the wounded was also the task of the army medical services or the aid societies.

Nonetheless, ICRC delegates quite often went to the battlefield to remove wounded or dead combatants. They did so, for example, following the Jewish offensive against the Arab neighborhood of Katamon in West Jerusalem, which was the Jewish side of the city. The Haganah wanted to create a continuous chain of Jewish neighborhoods in West Jerusalem. On May 2, 1948, Katamon, defended by irregulars and Arab Liberation Army soldiers who were stationed there, fell into the hands of the Haganah. The British asked for a cease-fire. On May 3, 1948, Courvoisier left his base in Nablus and went through Damascus Gate, which gave access to the large Arab quarter of the Old City of Jerusalem, where he sought out his contact for the Arab Higher Committee, Musa Husseini. According to Courvoisier's report, the Arab Higher Committee wanted the dead Arabs from Katamon to be buried in an Arab cemetery, and assured the ICRC delegate that the Arabs would respect the cease-fire.

On May 4, 1948, Courvoisier received the Jewish Agency's authorization to enter the area in order to arrange for the removal of those killed in battle – a task that, according to the Geneva Convention, was incumbent on the occupant of the battlefield. In this case, that meant the Haganah. The Arab Higher Committee put trucks at Courvoisier's disposal, but Jews were to drive them: Elimelech Zelnicher, appointed by the Jewish Agency, and

---

[553]'Geneva Convention of July 27, 1929, for the Amelioration of the Condition of the Wounded and Sick in Armed Forces in the Field,' Chapter I, 'Wounded and Sick,' Art. 3, in ICRC/LRCS, *Handbook of the International Red Cross*, p. 59.
[554]Ibid.

Eliahu Mizrahi, a driver who worked for the ICRC delegation in Jerusalem. They were to serve as the medical service personnel. Courvoisier used his own car, painted white and marked with red crosses encircled by the inscription 'International Committee, Geneva,' and with the Red Cross flag flying from its front antenna, like the other ICRC vehicles in Mandatory Palestine. Three journalists followed in another car.

When they arrived in Katamon, the Jewish drivers began to carry Arab corpses out of the buildings, and Courvoisier helped them. About 300 meters from the St. Simeon Monastery, they discovered about a dozen bodies piled in a sort of cave that had been hastily covered up with branches and a sheep carcass. Courvoisier had the commanding officer called, and asked him to assign a few men to help him pick up the bodies,[555] as the Geneva Convention prescribed. Courvoisier referred to the convention, but in an impulsive, emotional outburst: 'If your people kill, you should also know that you have to remove the dead,'[556] he reportedly exclaimed, under the strain of the trying circumstances.

Courvoisier left the scene and, in a Jewish hospital, obtained the assistance of Oriental Jewish gravediggers who thought they were being asked to bury Jews according to the rites of their religion. When they saw that the bodies were Arabs, they abandoned the operation.[557] The journalists and Courvoisier continued the work on their own, but could not finish it on the same day. The ICRC delegate returned the next day, accompanied this time by Dr. Werth of the medical services of the Jewish Agency in Jerusalem and 15 Jewish sanitary workers who were prepared for the situation. This arrangement complied perfectly with the Geneva Convention which Courvoisier had resolved to promote.

Courvoisier had secured a promise from both the Arabs and the Jews to observe the local cease-fire, but suddenly the ICRC delegate and the Jewish health-care workers were caught in a volley of infantry fire coming from the Arab front lines near Bethlehem. It was a debacle. Courvoisier and his companions, caught on open ground, sought refuge behind trees or in shell-craters. After two hours, on the advice of a Haganah officer

---

[555]Note from Courvoisier, ICRC Nablus, to ICRC Geneva, May 22, 1948 (AICRC, G.59/I/G.C.).
[556]Report by Elimelech Zelnicher, Jerusalem, May 5, 1948 (CZA.S.25.8943).
[557]Ibid.

who informed him that the Arabs were attacking the position, Courvoisier decided to evacuate the premises with the Jewish workers, 'not being able to take the risk they would run of being captured by the Arabs.'[558] The two Jewish drivers each drove one of the mortuary trucks, which carried only some of the Arab remains. Courvoisier and Werth, in the ICRC car with the Red Cross emblem, led the convoy to the Arab lines. There the Jewish drivers were replaced by Arab ones, who drove the bodies into their sector.

Courvoisier then went to the headquarters of the Arab Higher Committee and strongly protested the violation of the cease-fire, which had nearly cost him his life. Now fearing for his safety, he refused to return to Katamon, but instead asked the Jewish Agency to make its own arrangements for the burial of the remaining bodies.[559]

The ICRC delegate had risked his life to demonstrate theoretical criteria on the battlefield; acting in the spirit of the Geneva Convention he knew so well, he had seized the opportunity of a local cease-fire to take Jewish sanitary workers to remove the dead from the territory controlled by the Haganah. In this respect, he had put his ideal into practice.

All the same, the operation presented a problem: Courvoisier and the Jewish workers had almost died under the 'protection' of the Red Cross emblem. If they had been killed, it would, of course, have been a human tragedy; but it would also have been extremely damaging to the emblem's credibility, leading some people, perhaps, to lose respect for it. De Reynier learned a lesson from the incident. On May 10, 1948, he announced by radio to the Jewish and Arab civil and military authorities in Palestine that the ICRC was

> a neutral intermediary aiming to obtain from the two parties respect for the organizations protected by the Red Cross emblems and the application of the Conventions to the wounded and sick. Under no circumstances does its role consist in replacing or substituting for the responsible bodies ... of the two parties. In this respect, the removal and inter-

---

[558]Note from Courvoisier, ICRC Nablus, to ICRC Geneva, May 22, 1948 (AICRC, G.59/I/G.C.). [Translation: M.G.].

[559]Ibid. Also, 'Red Cross Take Out Arab Dead,' *Palestine Post* (May 6, 1948): 1.

ment of corpses are the exclusive responsibility of the military medical services of the parties involved.[560]

Consequently, the ICRC would at most be prepared, in cases of absolute necessity and in accordance with its mission of neutral intermediary, to intervene between the combatants and try to obtain from them the cease-fires necessary for the removal of the dead.[561] It is interesting to note that this communiqué was sent out at a time when de Reynier still believed that all of Jerusalem would be placed under the 'protection' of the Red Cross emblem. It was therefore understandable that he attached great importance to insuring that the Red Cross flag continued to command respect.

A model operation in Gush Etzion

Four days after this memorandum was sent out, on May 14, 1948, the ICRC received a request from the Jewish Agency. With de Reynier's consent, two ICRC delegates, Otto Lehner and Pierre Fasel, went to Gush Etzion, where three civilian settlements were being besieged by Arab irregulars. The ICRC delegates were needed to negotiate a cease-fire for the evacuation of the wounded, a task within the powers that the ICRC had declared itself prepared to assume in its public statement of May 10, 1948.

Lehner had previously been an ICRC delegate in Berlin and in the Nazi protectorate of Bohemia-Moravia. During the death march of the Orianenburg deportees to Lubeck, he had done all he could to assist the Jews, whom he had tried to provide with food. The Chief Rabbi of Prague, a survivor of that torturous trek, did not forget him, and at the end of the war invited him to his wedding. When Lehner left for Palestine, the Rabbi recommended him to the Jewish Agency.[562] Fasel was a Catholic doctor from Fribourg, Switzerland, who had arrived the previous day to begin his first mission for the ICRC.

---

[560] De Reynier, memorandum to civil and military authorities, Jerusalem, May 10, 1948 (AICRC, G.59/I/G.C.). [Translation: M.G.]

[561] Ibid. On several occasions the ICRC ordered its delegates to stop exposing themselves to danger in such situations.

[562] Katznelson, 'Tizkoret bidvar pinui nashim, yeladim, vezkenim meha'ir ha'atika' (Memo in re evacuation of women, children, and old people from the Old City), May 25, 1948 (CZA.S.25.8943).

FROM HEROISM TO TRADITIONAL ACTIVITIES

The delegates' report gives the sequence of events. With the support of Krikorian, formerly employed by the health service of the government of Palestine and now apparently attached to the embryonic Transjordanian Red Crescent society, the ICRC delegates drove to Gush Etzion accompanied by Arab doctors and health-care workers, and one Jewish doctor. The team had five ambulances displaying the red cross. When they reached the area, the delegates saw that the Jews were being sniped at by Arab irregulars and civilians posted on the hills. From the outpost of the Ein Tzurim settlement, the Jews returned fire.

According to Lehner and Fasel's joint report, Krikorian asked the ICRC delegates to advance towards the Jews in order to demand a cease-fire. But since the delegates did not want to expose themselves to Arab bullets, they went first towards the Arab lines in order to explain their intentions and to insure their immunity would be respected. At the same moment, two Jewish scouts carrying a white flag came towards the ICRC delegates and joined them by the Arab front lines. Talks began between Jews, Arabs, and ICRC delegates, but suddenly shooting burst forth from all sides. There were wounded. Lehner and Fasel jumped into a car and drove back up towards the Jewish outpost, thereby interposing themselves between the Jews and the Arabs. The shooting ceased; the delegates were unhurt, but shortly afterwards they discovered that one of the Arab doctors, who had remained with his colleagues in an ambulance about 500 meters from the front formed by the irregulars, had been seriously wounded.

In Ein Tzurim, the residents were afraid. The day before the delegates arrived, they had already concluded a cease-fire with a unit of the Arab Legion posted not far away, in order to permit both the evacuation of the women and the surrender of prisoners of war to the Legion. But this truce had not been observed; instead, there had been a massacre.[563] The inhabitants of Ein Tzurim did not want to run such a risk again, and they were sure that if certain of their number were to fall into the hands of the Arab irregulars, they would be murdered. The ICRC delegates were equally convinced of this, and whatever the outcome of the negotiations they were ready to conduct, they could not

[563]On this subject, see Netanel Lorch, *Israel's War of Independence, 1947–1949* (Hartford, Connecticut: Putnam, 1961), pp. 138–143.

offer any guarantee to the residents of Ein Tzurim that their lives would be spared. It seemed to them that the least dangerous solution was to seek out the local commander of the Arab Legion; with him they negotiated the evacuation of the Jews of Ein Tzurim, in Transjordanian army trucks. The prisoners of war, in one group, and the women, children, and wounded, in another group, took their places in the Legion's trucks.

The ICRC delegates and the Arab Legion soldiers then proceeded to the settlement of Revadim, where, menaced by thousands of fast approaching irregulars, they repeated the same procedure they had carried out at Ein Tzurim. One more settlement remained, Massuot Yitzhak, at some distance from the others. The Arab Legion discouraged the ICRC delegates from going there, since the irregulars were very close to Revadim and the Legion trucks were full. Lehner and Fasel resigned themselves to leaving the area, certain that they could do no more.[564] They retained from this operation the memory of what they had accomplished.

The delegates allowed the Arab Legion to evacuate 137 prisoners of war, 85 from Ein Tzurim and 52 from Revadim, including women and children. The prisoners were initially interned in Hebron and later transferred to the Mafraq prisoner-of-war camp in Transjordan.[565] In accordance with the Geneva Convention, the ICRC delegates, with the aid of the Arab Legion, evacuated only noncombatants and medical personnel: two wounded, 21 women, and 2 medical workers from Ein Tzurim, and 8 wounded, 23 women, and 7 medical workers from Revadim. Owing to the condition of the road, however, they could not drive them all the way to Jerusalem, so they turned them all over to the doctor in charge of the French hospital in Bethlehem – except for one Jewish doctor who, suffering a nervous breakdown, was taken to the Bethlehem mental hospital, where he joined the other Jewish patients who had remained interned there, despite the conflict, under the care of the Arab Medical Association. In order to give the evacuated Jews the greatest guarantee of safety they could, Lehner and Fasel went to the

---

[564]Lehner and Fasel, 'Mission in Kfar Etzion, Gebiet zwischen Bethlehem und Hebron,' Jerusalem, May 15, 1948 (AICRC, G.59/I/G.C.).

[565]Ibid. See also, 'Etzion Settlers Taken P.O.W.,' *Palestine Post* (May 16, 1948): 1. See also Katznelson, 'Haheskem im ha'aravim al hahzarat petzu'im, nashim veyeladim' (Agreement with the Arabs on the return of wounded, women, and children), June 8, 1948 (CZA.S.25.8943).

mayor of Bethlehem, Isa Bandak, and asked him to consider the wounded Jews as under the ICRC's responsibility.[566]

The delegates' action in Gush Etzion would be inscribed in the annals of the ICRC as a model operation. Because it was carried out on the battlefield, as close to the victims of war as possible, and because it called on the ICRC delegates' courage and sense of self-sacrifice, it followed Henry Dunant's model, while at the same time emphasizing the ICRC's role as a neutral intermediary between the belligerents.

The strengths and weaknesses of dedication

Gush Etzion was not the only occasion on which the ICRC delegates negotiated a local cease-fire; they were to do this many times over, usually – despite de Reynier's orders – in order to remove wounded and dead. Unfortunately, however, the Red Cross emblem did not inspire the desired respect on the part of the Arab irregulars. The delegates kept trying to remove the wounded and dead themselves, despite repeated orders not to do so. Such dedication cost delegate André Durand his arm. On July 17, 1948, at the very beginning of the second Arab-Israeli truce and at the request of the Arab authorities, this delegate, armed with the Red Cross flag, went between the lines to locate wounded men. In the process, he stepped on a landmine and at the same time came under fire. The source of the shots was never established, since de Reynier, not wishing to compromise the ICRC's position, wanted to avoid an inquiry.[567]

---

[566]Lehner and Fasel, 'Mission in Kfar Etzion, Gebiet zwischen Bethlehem und Hebron,' Jerusalem, May 15, 1948 (AICRC, G.59/I/G.C.). See also Lehner, 'Besuch bei den Militarischen Behoerden von Bethlehem. Betrifft: Kriegsgefangenen und Verletzte von Kfar Etzion,' Jerusalem, May 27, 1948 (CZA.S.25.8943).

[567]Letter from Zvi Loker, Ministry of Foreign Affairs, Hakirya, to Kahany, Geneva, July 28, 1948 (ISA/MEA/1987.1). Also letter from André Durand, Geneva, to author, March 8, 1993. The ICRC did never succeed in getting body-removal operations carried out in the way it wished. The Arabs nearly always fired on the Red Cross emblem. The Jews continued to request the presence of ICRC delegates, who went to the battlefield reluctantly. Finally, on Sept. 10, 1948, the liaison officer, Steinberg, laid the situation before the ICRC officials in Geneva, Gallopin and Wolf. Steinberg proposed a direct, formal agreement with the Arabs, but the ICRC would not consider it. He then asked that the ICRC delegates participate in the removal of the wounded. Gallopin replied that local truces were intended only for the removal of the dead, not the wounded. Steinberg pointed out that from a distance it was hard to tell the difference. According to in-house note from de Bondeli, Sept. 10, 1948 (AICRC, G.59/I/G.C.).

Durand's accident was not the first. On May 17, 1948, Gaillard was returning from Jericho, where, in a car displaying the ICRC emblem, he had been escorting two representatives of the UN Truce Commission, Azcarate and the consul-general of Belgium, to a meeting with King Abdullah. In order to return to the ICRC delegation headquarters at the YMCA hostel from the Old City, Gaillard obtained a pass from the Arab Legion. When he came to the Jewish lines, a Haganah soldier stopped him and proposed to escort him to the YMCA. Gaillard opened the door of his car and immediately the window was shattered by Arab fire. Wounded, Gaillard was taken to the Jewish hospital of Sha'are Tzedek ('gates of charity').[568]

Another incident occurred on May 22, 1948. Courvoisier and his colleague Gouy from Tel Aviv had decided to try to exchange two Arabs held by the Haganah for three Jewish teenagers (a fourth had died) who had been taken hostage by Hassan Salameh's men on the Petah Tikva road. Negotiations were conducted on both sides of the lines, by Gouy and Courvoisier respectively. According to Israeli sources, the young Jews had been entrusted to an Arab woman in a house belonging to the brother of the mayor of Lydda.[569] The Jews were to be handed over to the ICRC delegate on Saturday morning, May 22, between 11:00 and 12:00, on a road between Kfar Yehuda and Ramle.

Gouy was at the rendezvous at the appointed time with an ICRC nurse named Florence Cousin, but their Arab contact did not come. Tired of waiting, Gouy and Cousin left the place. The Arabs fired on them, wounding Cousin in the head. Gouy took her behind the Jewish lines, where she had to be trephined in Beilinson Hospital. Courvoisier and Gouy nevertheless did not abandon the planned humanitarian operation. The exchange of hostages took place the following day, at a point between Kfar Saba and Kalkilya, where Courvoisier came forth from the Arab lines with the

---

[568]Note from Gaillard, ICRC Jerusalem, to ICRC Geneva, May 22, 1948 (AICRC, G.59/I/G.C.).

[569]'Doch al peulot hatzlav ha'adom mi 15 mai al 31 mai' (Report on Red Cross actions from May 15 to May 31), (ISA/MEA/1987.1). In this document the name 'Lod' is used instead of 'Lydda.'

FROM HEROISM TO TRADITIONAL ACTIVITIES

Jewish teenagers and Gouy from the Jewish lines with the Arab prisoners.[570]

These emissaries of the ICRC were dedicated and courageous, but undeniably reckless, and their trust that the belligerents would respect the Red Cross flag was very unrealistic, especially in the case of the Arab irregulars. Yet they persisted. De Reynier provided some indication of their state of mind in his comments, in his report to Geneva, on ICRC operations and the use of the flag in Gush Etzion, Katamon, Kfar Saba, and Jerusalem:

> Since May 14 a heroic page in ICRC history has been written, a pale imitation of the efforts of Henry Dunant, but exactly in his spirit. The veteran delegates and the novices, the boys and the nurses, all have thrown themselves boldly into the hard, bloody *mêlée* to carry the flag of the Red Cross, the only salvation for thousands of people. Every day, each man and woman has calmly risked his or her life without any other intent but to serve the flag.[571]

'To serve the flag' was the significance that the head of the ICRC in Palestine, preoccupied with thoughts of the Stockholm Conference, attributed to his subordinates' sacrifices. De Reynier seemed, however, to have established an emotional, even mystical relationship with the Red Cross emblem, of which he confused the protective function and the symbolic significance. For de Reynier, concerned as he was with the prestige of the institution to which he devoted himself, bearing the flag high was an end in itself, encompassing all his other motivations. This will be confirmed much later in his final mission report where he states in the Preamble: 'The three crosses of the National Exhibition of 1939 [the Christian Cross, the Swiss Cross, and the Red Cross] have constantly presided over our destinies.'

De Reynier's subordinates, however, made no explicit references to the flag. They apparently worked without thinking about it, trying, out of humanitarian motives and a sense of

---

[570]Report from Gouy, ICRC Tel Aviv (posted in London on July 3, 1948) to ICRC Geneva, June 2, 1948 (AICRC, G.3/82). Note from Courvoisier, ICRC Nablus, to ICRC Jerusalem, June 7, 1948 (AICRC, G.59/I/G.C.). See also CICR, 'Le Comité international de la Croix-Rouge en Palestine,' *RICR* (June 1948): 398.

[571]De Reynier, ICRC Jerusalem, monthly report no. 3, May 1948, to ICRC Geneva, June 3, 1948 (AICRC, G.59/I/G.C.). [Translation: M.G.]

sacrifice, to perform acts of charity here and there, the conventions in hand and the ICRC's role of neutral intermediary on their minds – a role which they did indeed, as de Reynier said, intend to promote by example. For them, the humanitarian action itself, conducted according to ICRC procedures and principles, took precedence over the institution and its flag. In general, they did the opposite to de Reynier: They did not serve the ICRC, but rather used the ICRC, the Geneva Convention, and the Red Cross emblem as means for aiding the victims of war.

Heroism or not, the delegates' reckless disregard for their own safety was not appreciated by the belligerents, who saw it as unrealistic and unorganized. In this respect, the delegates' accidents tended to damage the ICRC's credibility in the Arab-Israeli conflict.

Putting an end to heroism

On May 25, after Florence Cousin's accident, de Reynier warned Geneva that 'the heroic individual work must stop and give way to organized, methodical teamwork. . . .' If it did not, he wrote to Geneva, 'the ICRC in Palestine will collapse.' At the time, he was preoccupied with the establishment of the safety zones in Jerusalem, the success of which depended primarily on the belligerents' disposition to respect the Red Cross emblem. His communications to Geneva reflected a need to justify the commands to exercise caution that he gave his subordinates. He emphasized the delegates' courage, their selflessness, and commented: 'We do not have the right to get them killed for nothing, and that is where we are rapidly heading. Miracles do not last forever.'[572]

The accidents described above – except for Durand's – occurred during the days preceding Bernadotte's appointment as United Nations mediator. Ruegger's reaction was to go to Palestine, for the reasons described in the previous chapter.[573] As mentioned, one of the ICRC president's aims was to dissuade Bernadotte from using the Red Cross emblem for his UN mission; any confusion between the UN and the ICRC, between a political mission and a humanitarian mission, would be damaging to the International Red Cross. All the ICRC operations conducted

[572]Note from de Reynier, ICRC Jerusalem, to ICRC Geneva, May 25, 1948 (AICRC, G.59/I/G.C.). [Translation: M.G.]
[573]See Chapter 4, p. 180.

under the Red Cross symbol were liable to suffer: the protection of hospitals, the safety zones, the negotiation of local cease-fires.

Since the real reasons that led the president of the ICRC to rush to Jerusalem could not be revealed to the public during the conflict, the various accidents suffered by ICRC delegates provided justification for the presidential mission. Officially, Ruegger was going to Jerusalem to provide moral support to the ICRC delegation in response to the 'alarming news' of delegates' accidents that had been appearing in the press.[574] The ICRC delegates' heroism on the battlefield gained even greater notoriety as a result. Ruegger may also have been thinking about how the news would appear to the USSR; since 1946, the Committee had hoped that by showing greater interest in actions that used the red cross and upheld the Geneva Convention and Henry Dunant's ideal it would win greater understanding from the Soviet signatories of that convention than by emphasizing its own role as neutral intermediary on behalf of prisoners of war.

Once in Jerusalem, Paul Ruegger endorsed Jacques de Reynier's decision to stop the acts of heroism. By now the public was widely informed about the ICRC's activities in the Arab-Israeli conflict, the Red Cross flag flew over the hospitals and the safety zones, and it was familiar everywhere as the emblem of the ICRC. It was important not to detract from the respect it had won, but rather to make it the symbol of the ICRC's moral authority and actions as a neutral intermediary on behalf of prisoners, the wounded, and noncombatant civilian populations.

From the heroic period to traditional activities

Liberation of civilians from the Jewish Quarter of the Old City of Jerusalem

The plight of the Jewish Quarter of the Old City, surrounded as it was by Arab forces under the authority of the Transjordanian Arab Legion, gave Ruegger the opportunity to highlight the ICRC's role and emblem with a designedly imposing gesture: On 29 May, a day after the Jewish Quarter had surrendered and

---

[574]ICRC, procès-verbal, Bureau meeting of May 24, 1948 (AICRC, no file number). ICRC, press release no. 364b, 'The President of the International Committee of the Red Cross Leaves for the Near East,' Geneva, May 25, 1948 (Press Release Collection, ICRC Library).

following a request for a cease-fire by the ICRC delegation, the ICRC president walked to the firing line with the flag in his hand. There, he was present at the evacuation of the 2,000 or so inhabitants, which had been negotiated by the ICRC delegates. De Reynier's report of this operation[575] gives the impression of a miraculous event:

> The fall of the Jewish Quarter in the Old City, taken by the Arabs, ought to have ended in a general massacre. The President's presence and his advice allowed the delegation to obtain an absolutely incredible chivalrous gesture from the Arabs, namely the handing over to the ICRC of all the women and all the children, the elderly and the wounded, to be conducted to the Jewish quarter of the New City. More than 2,000 people were saved in this way, thanks exclusively to the presence of President Ruegger. . . .[576]

In reality, the evacuation of civilians from the Jewish Quarter of the Old City, requested by Katznelson, the health minister of the Israeli provisional government, was the outcome of negotiations begun with the Arab Legion ten days previously, through the intermediary of the ICRC delegates de Reynier and Lehner. These negotiations had given rise on May 25, 1948, to an oral agreement of principle between the parties concerned, covering various exchanges of prisoners and wounded, combatants and hostages, from both camps. The liberation of civilians from the Jewish Quarter of the Old City was one of the operations stipulated, but up until May 28, the date the Jewish Quarter surrendered, Abdullah Tel, the Arab Legion commander for the Jerusalem area, hesitated to implement it, for strategic reasons[577]: The presence of the civilian population made defending the quar-

---

[575]De Reynier, ICRC Jerusalem, monthly report no. 3, May 1948, Jerusalem, June 3, 1948 (AICRC, G.59/I/G.C.). [Translation: M.G.]
[576]Ibid.
[577]According to author's telephone interview with Netanel Lorch, Jerusalem, May 3, 1993. Kohn, 'Tohen pgisha im anashim hatzlav ha'adom veasoar ha'adom shenitkaima beimka beyom gimmel' (Substance of meeting with people from the Red Cross and the Red Crescent that took place at the YMCA on Tuesday), May 18, 1948, de Reynier, Basel, Krikorian, Katznelson, and Gaulan (CZA.S.25.8943). Letter from Kohn, JA Jerusalem, to de Reynier, ICRC Jerusalem, May 19, 1948 (CZA.S.25.8943). 'Negotiations under Way for Exchange of War Prisoners,' *Palestine Post* (May 21, 1948): 3. Katznelson, 'Tizkoret bidvar pinui nashim yeladim ve zkenim meha'ir ha'atika' (Memo regarding evacuation of women, children, and elderly from the Old City), May 25, 1948 (CZA.S.25.8943).

ter more difficult for the Haganah.[578] Once the Legion had conquered the area, however, it no longer had anything to gain by retaining the Jewish civilians, and could therefore afford to let Ruegger liberate them.

It seems significant, too, that on his way to Jerusalem the ICRC president stopped in Cairo and then in Amman; in the Transjordanian capital, he met with King Abdullah, and following that meeting, the ICRC asked the international community for medicines for Jerusalem.[579] When the Jewish Quarter of the Old City surrendered, the Hashemite sovereign was in Jerusalem with his troops. With the Legion in a position of strength, the circumstances could not have been more favorable for the ICRC to obtain from it the liberation of the inhabitants of the Jewish Quarter. It seems possible that Ruegger promised the Transjordanian king to provide increased material aid to the Arab Palestinians and asked for a favor in return – in this case, the liberation of the Jewish civilians of the Old City. If so, the ICRC had managed to link the two branches of its activities, assistance and protection, as it had intended to do in February, 1948, when it devised its plan of action for Mandatory Palestine.[580] This, however, is only a guess, since no minutes from the meeting between Ruegger and King Abdullah have been found.

Once the operation had been carried out, Ruegger could be satisfied, but he was a little angry with the Jews; the cease-fire necessary for the evacuation of the Old City had been more difficult to negotiate with the Jews than with the Arabs. Israeli military commanders had hesitated to sign the agreement immediately, on the grounds that the Sabbath, during which Jewish religious law forbids writing, had already begun. The ICRC president's resentment was reinforced by another annoying experience: He had been manhandled by a Haganah soldier armed with a machine-gun – though defended by another. Despite his displeasure, Ruegger refrained from publicizing the incident.[581] As will be seen, he considered the liberation of

---

[578]According to author's telephone interview with Netanel Lorch, Jerusalem, May 3, 1993.

[579]ICRC, press release no. 365b, 'The President of the International Committee of the Red Cross in the Near East – Medical Supplies for Jerusalem,' Geneva, May 28, 1948 (Press Release Collection, ICRC Library).

[580]See Chapter 3, p. 113.

[581]Paul Ruegger, 'Instructions à M. Wolf, Conseiller du CICR, pour sa mission spéciale à Tel Aviv,' Geneva, Oct. 31, 1948 (AICRC, G.59/I/G.C.).

the Jewish civilians of the Old City of Jerusalem to be merely the beginning of a larger operation, for which he wished to keep all his options open. Indeed, Ruegger would take advantage of this first success to inaugurate the ICRC's traditional activities as a neutral intermediary in the Arab-Israeli conflict, first of all, and its material relief operation as well.

Inauguration of the ICRC's activities as neutral intermediary

The ICRC began by acting as a neutral intermediary in exchanges of wounded prisoners. There were, of course, wounded among the inhabitants of the Jewish Quarter, many of them survivors of the Arab Legion's bombing raids on the Misgav Ladach Hospital. The hospital had been destroyed despite the red cross it displayed, and the survivors evacuated to a house nearby. These wounded had been held provisionally by the Arab Legion, and on May 29, 1948, the day after the civilian inhabitants of the Jewish Quarter were evacuated, the president of the ICRC issued, from Jerusalem, a press release announcing that these wounded could be 'returned unconditionally to the Jewish forces.'[582] The Prisoners of War Convention of 1929 in fact obliged the belligerents to repatriate seriously ill or wounded prisoners as soon as possible, regardless of their rank or number.[583] The prisoners eligible for repatriation were to be chosen by mixed medical commissions comprising a doctor appointed by the detaining power and two neutral doctors, according to the criteria and procedure set forth in a model draft agreement annexed to the Prisoners of War Convention.[584] Since that agreement did not give the ICRC a role to play, the Committee had included a provision in the draft conventions to be presented in Stockholm stipulating that the ICRC, together with the protecting power and at the request of the detaining power, would designate the

---

[582]ICRC, press release no. 366b, 'Jerusalem, May 29, 1948,' Geneva, June 1, 1948 (Press Release Collection, ICRC Library).

[583]'Geneva Convention of July 27, 1929, Relative to the Treatment of Prisoners of War,' Part IV: 'End of Captivity,' Section I, 'Direct Repatriation and Accommodation in a Neutral Country,' Art. 58, par. 1, in *Handbook*, p. 88.

[584]Ibid., Art. 69, in ICRC/LRCS, *Handbook*, p. 88, and 'Accord-type concernant le repatriement direct et l'hopitalisation en pays neutre des prisonniers de guerre pour raison de santé,' in CICR/LSCR, *Manuel*, pp. 146–153.

neutral members of the mixed medical commissions.[585] There was nothing to exclude an ICRC doctor from being a neutral member.[586]

In the Old City, according to the local press, an Arab doctor and an ICRC doctor (Lehner, as it happened)[587] formed a sort of mixed medical commission that identified the wounded Jews who could be repatriated to the Jewish side of the front. On May 29, 1948, the ICRC publicly announced the evacuation of these wounded in terms meant to be instructive and which put great emphasis on the Arab Legion's conduct. The ICRC was presented as a moral authority and a neutral intermediary, the active partners in humanizing the war being the belligerents themselves:

> The Arab Command, wishing to give proof to the International Committee of their desire to observe Red Cross and Red Crescent principles, have agreed to hand over 140 Jewish wounded to the Jewish authorities, with the Committee's co-operation. To that effect, the parties have promised the delegation to cease fire locally for this operation, at which M. Ruegger will be present. It is presumed that the Jewish authorities will make a similar offer, in particular to hand over to the Arab Legion the wounded in the French Hospital and some captured Arab women.[588]

By the word 'similar,' the ICRC wanted to convey the message that the wounded and, by extension, civilians had to be liberated without compensation, as was consistent with the spirit of the Geneva Convention. In reality, however, the ICRC was merely repeating and presenting in its own way – which was intended to be didactic – certain terms of the major transaction agreed upon between the Jewish Agency and the Arab Legion through the intermediary of de Reynier and Lehner. Under that agreement, Israel essentially undertook to release 40 Arab women detained by Israel at Neve She'an and about 20 other Arab civilians. The Arab Legion, for its part, promised to release the

---

[585] 'Draft Regulations Relative to Mixed Medical Commissions,' Art. 2, in XVIIth International Conference of the Red Cross, Stockholm, 1948, *Draft Revised or New Conventions for the Protection of War Victims*, Annex II, pp. 142–144, p. 142.
[586] Ibid.
[587] Drs. Canaan and Laufer, according to 'Last Out of the Old City,' *Palestine Post* (May 31, 1948): 1.
[588] ICRC, press release no. 367b, Geneva, June 2, 1948 (Press Release Collection, ICRC Library).

women captured in Gush Etzion, who were being held in Bethlehem.[589]

Transmitted by radio in English, Hebrew, and Arabic to all of former Mandatory Palestine, the ICRC press release was also sent to the press in Geneva[590] and Lake Success,[591] New York, where the UN debates on the war between Israel and its Arab neighbors were taking place.

The Israeli health service handed over 60 wounded Arabs at the French Hospital, selected by a mixed medical commission including Lehner and Fasel, and a group of about 20 Arab civilians – women, elderly, and children – to representatives of the Arab Medical Association. The transfer took place in Suleiman Street, at the guardpost between the French Hospital and the New Gate, in the presence of Musa Husseini and Katznelson. Katznelson, incidentally, seized the opportunity to propose other dealings to Musa Husseini.[592] De Reynier had negotiated a local cease-fire, as was customary for all such prisoner releases.[593]

Before moving on to new, concrete proposals, the Israelis wanted the Arabs to carry out what they had already promised to do in the negotiations mentioned above.[594] On June 1, 1948, for

---

[589]Katznelson, 'Haheskem im ha'aravim al hahzarat petzuim, nashim veyeladim' (Agreement with the Arabs on the return of wounded, women, and children), June 8, 1948 (CZA.S.25.8943).

[590]ICRC, press release no. 366b, Geneva, June 1, 1948 (Press Release Collection, ICRC Library).

[591]Urgent message from the President of the ICRC to the ICRC delegation at Lake Success, May 31, 1948, through the intermediary of the US Consul (AICRC, G.59/I/G.C.). 'Evacuation offered by Arab Command at our request of 2,000 women, children, ill people surrendered Jewish area old city and their handing over to Jewish authorities carried through last night. Have expressed appreciation of humanitarian measures taken carried out with greatest discipline by Arab Legion. De Reynier was incessingly (sic) negociating and Lehner present in Arab area. Desirous offering to intercross proof of Red Cross Crescent spirit Arab command offered further hand over Jewish authorities under ICRC control of 140 wounded Jews. De Reynier arranged cease fire for this evening. I intend to be present with Wolf and him at return Jewish wounded I hope now similar gesture from Jewish side following our now repeated request regarding handing back to Arab Legion wounded Arab from French hospital and captured women. You may inform press. Ruegger.'

[592]'POW Exchange in Jerusalem,' *Palestine Post* (June 2, 1948): 1.

[593]Katznelson, 'Haheskem im ha'aravim al hahzarat petzuim, nashim veyeladim' (Agreement with the Arabs on the return of wounded, women, and children), June 8, 1948 (CZA.S.25.8943). 'POW Exchange in Jerusalem,' *Palestine Post* (June 2, 1948): 1.

[594]See above, p. 210.

FROM HEROISM TO TRADITIONAL ACTIVITIES

example, the Israelis were expecting wounded prisoners from Gush Etzion whom the Arab Legion had agreed to release, but many other issues remained in abeyance, and Israel was dissatisfied. Exasperated by the way the ICRC was singing the Legion's praises, and not seeing the positive aspects of this encouragement of the Arab armies to good behavior, Nahum Gaulan, the Israeli Defense Force's liaison officer with the ICRC in Jerusalem, protested to Katznelson. Why was the ICRC giving the Transjordanian army so much publicity? The ICRC, which had been the intermediary in the negotiations, should be firmly reminded of the Arab Legion's promise to furnish the Israelis without delay, through the ICRC, with a list of the Jewish wounded, women, and other prisoners captured by Transjordan, particularly in the Gush Etzion battles. It should also be reminded that the Jewish women of Etzion were still imprisoned in Bethlehem, despite the Arab Legion's undertaking to release them as soon as possible. Finally, shouldn't a protest be registered with the ICRC concerning the fact that the Jews killed at Etzion had still not received a religious burial?[595]

Katznelson followed this up, and on June 5, responding to the Israeli complaint, Lehner began to act as an ICRC neutral intermediary for the wounded and prisoners of Gush Etzion. Accompanied by three members of the Arab Medical Association, he went to Bethlehem, where he went to visit the wounded Jews whom, on his return from Gush Etzion, he had entrusted to the French Hospital. He discovered that the Arab Legion had transferred those considered by the local doctor to be only lightly wounded to the Mafraq prisoner-of-war camp in Transjordan, together with the women. He was also assured by a Legion officer that the Jews killed at Gush Etzion had been buried, although without religious rites and without any record being made of their names and places of burial.[596]

At the same time, Courvoisier was visiting the Israeli prisoners in the Mafraq camp. On June 7, he brought back the 83 women

---

[595]To A. Katznelson, from Gaulan, Jerusalem, May 30, 1948 (CZA.S.25.8943).
[596]Lehner, 'Besuch bei den Militarischen Behoerden von Bethlehem. Betrifft: Kriegsgefangenen und Verletzte von Kfar Etzion,' Jerusalem, May 27, 1948 (CZA.S.25.8943). See also Katznelson, 'Haheskem im ha'aravim al hahzarat petzuim, nashim veyeladim' (Agreement with the Arabs on the return of wounded, women, and children), June 8, 1948 (CZA.S.25.8943).

from Gush Etzion, along with other women captured in the Jisr Mejama electricity plant on the Jordan River, for a total of 89 people.[597] This repatriation was carried out under peculiar conditions. The women were taken, with their eyes blindfolded, to the Nablus Triangle, escorted by Arab Legion and Iraqi soldiers. In 'Arab Palestine,' to use the ICRC delegates' expression, they were handed over to Courvoisier, who took them through Tulkarem up to the Jewish position at Kfar Yona. All the way the local population shouted abuse at them and tried to lynch them, but once they had gotten through, the formerly hostile Arab crowd broke into enthusiastic applause. French journalists, including one from the *Figaro*, filmed the operation.[598] On the same day, the Arab Legion returned the family of A.M. Weingarten, the head of the Jewish community of the Old City of Jerusalem, and two Jewish children who had been among the prisoners. Lehner collected them at the New Gate and took them, under the protection of the Red Cross flag, to West Jerusalem, passing through Damascus Gate.[599]

Similarly, on June 10, at the request of the Nablus authorities, the Israelis handed 30 Arab children over to Courvoisier, who restored them to their homes.[600] On June 18, in response to another request by the same authorities, Gouy and Courvoisier obtained permission from the Israelis to conduct to Arab lines 1,068 Arab women who had somehow been cut off in Israel, near Netanya. They gained the Arab side through the lines at Kfar Yona. Although the Arab Palestinians were in favor of the operation, King Abdullah's opposition apparently had to be overcome before the transfer could proceed – much to Courvoisier's displeasure; he was personally concerned for the sovereignty of the Palestinian Arabs, with whose cause he identified.[601]

These operations were the first in a long series of exchanges

---

[597]Katznelson, ibid. See also 'Jewish Captives Cross the Lines, Etzion Girls Returned,' *Palestine Post* (June 8, 1948): 1.

[598]Note from Courvoisier, ICRC Ramallah, to ICRC Geneva, July 6, 1948 (AICRC, G.59/I/G.C.).

[599]Katznelson, 'Haheskem im ha'aravim al hahzarat petzuim, nashim veyeladim' (Agreement with the Arabs on the return of wounded, women, and children), June 8, 1948 (CZA.S.25.8943). See also 'Jewish Captives Cross the Lines, Family of Five and Two Babies,' *Palestine Post* (June 8, 1948): 1.

[600]Note from Courvoisier, ICRC Ramallah, to ICRC Geneva, June 26, 1948 (AICRC, G.59/I/G.C.).

[601]Note from Courvoisier, ICRC Ramallah, to ICRC Geneva, July 5, 1948 (AICRC, G.59/I/G.C.).

and repatriations that were to be one of the main manifestations of the ICRC's role of neutral intermediary in the Arab-Israeli war, up to the armistice agreements. They included both individual repatriations and collective repatriations of sick or handicapped people – such as that of the Jewish mental patients from the hospital in Bethlehem, which took place only after many negotiations concerning payment for their upkeep by Israel. Israel was slow to pay its bills to the Arab Medical Association, since it was itself saddled with the responsibility for Arab mental patients interned in Acre.[602]

These repatriations can be interpreted as reflecting the ICRC's eagerness to confirm its tradition in this field and to highlight its statutory role as neutral intermediary on behalf of the sick and wounded (and, by extension, noncombatant civilians) – the category of victims with which the whole idea of the Red Cross began. The ICRC had carried out this type of operation in World War I and during the Spanish Civil War. If such repatriations were taken out of its hands, it would be considerably affected. This is evident from the delegate Munier's reaction when he arrived too late to organize the return to Israel of 76 disabled prisoners from the Mafraq camp; Moshe Dayan, for the Israel Defense Force, and Abdullah Tel, for the Arab Legion, had already arranged the matter through direct talks. Munier, worried about the ICRC's future as a neutral intermediary, considered this type of direct negotiation an alarm signal which should spur the ICRC on in its efforts.[603]

Perhaps as the sequel to Katznelson's informal interview with Musa Husseini on June 1 at the New Gate, on the occasion of the handing over of wounded Arabs, on June 17, 1948, Israel issued a proposal for a general exchange of the wounded of both camps,[604] following it up on June 20 with an offer for a global

---

[602]See on this subject 'Mission Courvoisier en Palestine' (AICRC, G.3/82 and CZA.S.25.8943).

[603]Munier, monthly report no. 9, February, 1949, Amman, to ICRC Geneva, March 1, 1949 (AICRC, G.59/I/G.C.). Munier, 'Rapport du rapatriement de 76 Juifs malades et blessés du camp d'Um el Djemal le 3 février 1949, Amman,' to ICRC Geneva, Feb. 7, 1949 (AICRC, G.59/I/G.C.). On the Israeli side, these direct negotiations were encouraged by the fact that the ICRC, for reasons that will be explained later, had left Jerusalem to establish a central delegation in Beirut. *Cf.* note from Zvi Loker, Hakirya, to Kahany, Geneva, Feb. 9, 1949 (ISA/MEA/1987.21).

[604]De Reynier, ICRC Jerusalem, monthly report no. 4, month of June, 1948, Jerusalem, July 20, 1948 (AICRC, G.59/I/G.C.).

exchange of able-bodied prisoners of war.[605] Asked to act as neutral intermediaries, the ICRC delegates began to make arrangements,[606] but were forced to back out. They had received doctrinal instructions from Geneva that all such exchanges were to be forbidden. The Prisoners of War Convention provided that wounded and sick prisoners were to be repatriated unconditionally, once they had been selected by the mixed medical commissions.[607] As for able-bodied prisoners repatriated on the basis of reciprocity, they could be sent back into battle; the ICRC delegates were therefore ordered not to act on the Israeli proposal.[608] Israel turned instead to Bernadotte, and the ICRC ceased to take part in negotiations for prisoner exchanges – except for one, which I will describe later, involving a group of Jews imprisoned by the Egyptians in the Abassieh camp.[609]

At the end of the war, the ICRC delegates attended the meetings of the mixed commissions on the armistices between Israel and the Arab countries; these commissions would take into account the mixed medical commissions' conclusions in selecting the wounded and ill prisoners of war who were to be repatriated first.[610] The armistice accords assigned the task of monitoring the repatriation of able-bodied prisoners to the United Nations, but the ICRC delegates took de facto responsibility for part of the monitoring and for the practical execution of these operations,

---

[605]Munier, ICRC Amman, report no. 1, month of June, 1948, Amman, July 2, 1948 (AICRC, G.59/I/G.C.).

[606]Personal note from Munier, ICRC Amman, to Voegeli, ICRC Geneva, June 30, 1948 (AICRC, G.59/I/G.C.).

[607]Note from de Bondeli, ICRC Geneva, to Gouy, ICRC Tel Aviv, July 5, 1948 (AICRC, G.59/I/G.C.). See also reference given by ICRC: 'Geneva Convention of July 27, 1929, Relative to the Treatment of Prisoners of War,' Part IV: 'End of Captivity,' Section I: 'Direct Repatriation and Accommodation in a Neutral Country,' Art. 68, par. 1, in ICRC/LRCS, *Handbook*, p. 88.

[608]Note from de Bondeli, ibid.

[609]Note from de Reynier, ICRC Central Delegation for Palestine in Beirut, Beirut, to ICRC Geneva, Dec. 2, 1948 (AICRC, G.59/I/G.C.). Note from de Reynier, ICRC Central Delegation for Palestine in Beirut. Tel Aviv, to ICRC Geneva, Dec. 4, 1948 (AICRC, G.59/I/G.C.). See also pp. 193, 194.

[610]See texts of armistice agreements: 'General Armistice Agreement between Israel and Egypt, February 24, 1949' (p. 380); 'General Armistice Agreement between Israel and Lebanon, March 23, 1949' (p. 390); 'General Armistice Agreement between Israel and Jordan, April 3, 1949' (p. 397); and 'General Armistice Agreement between Israel and Syria, July 20, 1949' (p. 407) in John Norton Moore, ed., *The Arab-Israeli Conflict, Vol III: Documents*, sponsored by the American Society of International Law (Princeton, N.J.: Princeton University Press, 1974).

since their participation no longer had the implication of sending men to the front.

They also were occasionally led to take part in negotiations to persuade Arab countries to take in Palestinian Arab prisoners of combat age. According to the ICRC archives, some of these Arabs had been picked up in localities occupied, taken, or destroyed by Israel, and had been interned in camps and treated as prisoners of war without actually ever having belonged to a regular army force or to an organized armed corps.[611] These men were sometimes returned to their place of origin and sometimes merely taken behind Arab lines. The latter case obviously led to political and ethical complications, but the ICRC in Geneva did not dwell on them, being obsessed with its objective of acting as a neutral intermediary and emptying the camps of the last prisoners, wherever they might have come from.

The Arab countries, except for Transjordan, were not eager to accept, along with their own repatriated soldiers, contingents of Arab Palestinians. The case of 408 Palestinians from Gaza is illustrative of the difficulties the ICRC confronted in trying to resolve their fate. Egypt, which controlled Gaza, refused to allow their repatriation until, on July 18 and 19, 1949, the ICRC finally obtained permission through the local authorities for them to return home. The last repatriations were the final manifestation of the ICRC's work as a neutral intermediary, which it had been performing since the evacuation of the Jewish civilians from the Old City in Jerusalem.

Before the armistices and the repatriation of all the prisoners, the ICRC had followed the dictates of both the Prisoners of War Convention and its own tradition to perform a number of tasks on behalf of the prisoners of war: It had demanded notification of captures from the parties to the conflict; it had made regular visits to prisoners' camps, where it had tried to meet, unsupervised, with a prisoners' representative chosen by the detainees themselves; it had negotiated for improved treatment with the detaining powers; it had conveyed news between the prisoners and their families; and it had searched for missing persons.

---

[611]Wolf, report from Tel Aviv mission, Geneva, Nov. 18, 1948 (AICRC, G.59/I/G.C.).

In the case of Arab prisoners held by the Israelis, the ICRC intervened on the basis of observations by its representatives in Tel Aviv. Its delegates regularly inspected the camps of Jalil, Atlit, Sarafand, Tel Litvinsky, and Um el-Khaled. As the winter of 1948–1949 approached, it asked for more meat, warm clothes, and additional blankets for the prisoners.[612] It made sure that the latter were not being forced to do work of an unhealthy nature or for military ends. It also called for the election by the detainees themselves of prisoners' representatives, a practice which was not immediately instituted in Israel. Despite minor failings, relatively rare, noted by the delegates, such as delays in transmitting lists of Egyptian prisoners of war, and occasional cases of serious violations, such as the whipping of two Arab prisoners of war at the Sarafand camp on November 3, 1948,[613] the ICRC delegates remarked that the Israelis often applied the Prisoners of War Convention with a will.[614] The Israelis had expressed the hope that the Arabs would do the same,[615] but this hope was disappointed. On August 2, 1948, Israel notified its accession to the 1929 Conventions to the authorized depository, the Swiss government.[616] This official act by Israel provoked, as in the previous May,[617] a general outcry from the Arab states. The Arab newspapers increased their anti-Zionist propaganda, supporting it with accounts of multiple Zionist violations of the humanitarian conventions and incessantly evoking Deir Yassin.

The ICRC delegates were in an uncomfortable position. Usually they were not able to confirm these violations for the Arab authorities, and were sometimes even obliged to refute them; for the sake of their consciences they did so, although confidentially – in order to protect their own credi-

[612]Report from Moeri, ICRC Tel Aviv, 'mois d'octobre 1948,' Tel Aviv, Oct. 31, 1948 (AICRC, G.59/I/G.C.).
[613]Note from Lehner, ICRC Tel Aviv, to Ben-Gurion, Prime Minister and Minister of Defense of the State of Israel, Nov. 4, 1948 (AICRC, G.59/I/G.C.).
[614]Report from Moeri, ICRC Tel Aviv, 'mois de novembre 1948,' Tel Aviv, Nov. 30, 1948 (AICRC, G.59/I/G.C.).
[615]See, for example, telegram from Gouy, intercroixrouge Tel Aviv to intercroixrouge Cairo, Aug. 24, 1948 (AICRC, G.59/I/G.C.).
[616]Letter from Kahany, Geneva, to Carvhalo, Chargé d'Affaires of Uruguay, Bern, Aug. 2, 1948, for transmission to the Swiss government (ISA/MEA/1987.1).
[617]See Chapter 3, pp. 126–7.

FROM HEROISM TO TRADITIONAL ACTIVITIES

bility with the Arabs and, accordingly, the ICRC's role of neutral intermediary.[618]

The way the Arabs treated their Jewish prisoners was a function of their refusal to recognize Israel's legitimacy and of the anti-Zionist hatred that accompanied that refusal. The Israeli prisoners in Arab hands (except in Transjordan, as long as the ICRC's contacts there were British officers[619]) were often submitted to difficult ordeals. In Egypt, the most serious incidents occurred in the Abassieh camp, where 108 prisoners – including 7 women – were horribly tortured. The ICRC delegate in Cairo, de Cocatrix, who visited them together with Lehner on June 17 and by himself on August 14 and September 30, 1948, noticed nothing unusual. He was not able to talk alone with the prisoners' representative. However, one Abassieh detainee, William Shelley, escaped from the camp and told the Israeli authorities about the atrocities he and his comrades had undergone. De Reynier visited the camp on November 30, 1948[620] and the inmates corroborated Shelley's account, adding that the torture had ceased since September. In a report to Geneva, de Reynier compared the agony inflicted on these detainees to that undergone by the Jews in the concentration camps in Germany. In a written report to the ICRC, he described his own reaction, saying that he had reproached the prisoners' representative in the camp for his 'cowardice,' which, according to him, had prolonged the suffering of his comrades: 'One of them could really have informed the ICRC delegate and even accepted the worst retaliation to save his comrades,' he wrote. In de Reynier's eyes, 'these stories ... are disturbing first of all for the prisoners of war, then for the honor of the ICRC, and last because of the measures of reprisal that they could provoke on the part of the Jews.'[621] The Committee

---

[618]Dossier of the ICRC delegation in Egypt, 1948–1949 (AICRC, G.6/43). During 1949, after the Diplomatic Conference, the ICRC delegates discovered the existence of undeclared transit camps in Israel, at Gedera (Quatra in Arabic), Nahahal, and Jerusalem (Schneller), which they were not permitted to visit. Their Israeli contact, Officer Steinberg, asserted that the detainees there were deserters. This aroused the ICRC's suspicions, as it did not see why deserters should have to be deprived of its delegates' visits.

[619]Dossier 'Mission Munier à Amman' (AICRC, G.3/82).

[620]According to private letter from Loker, Tel Aviv, to Wolf, Geneva, Dec. 8, 1948, with Shelley report attached (ISA/MEA/1987.20).

[621]Report from de Reynier, Central ICRC Delegation for Palestine, Beirut, Dec. 2, 1948 (AICRC, G.59/I/G.C.). [Translation: M.G.]

did not react to the content of his report, which was shocking, to say the least. Yet given the numerous hostile remarks about Jews that punctuated de Reynier's reports, Ruegger, who had taken the ICRC's activities in the 1948 conflict under his own direct supervision, might well have wondered to what extent the acts of the head of the ICRC delegation might be influenced by anti-Jewish prejudices. As noted earlier, however, the Committee did not ask itself questions of this nature.[622]

To return to the Abassieh affair, contrary to what de Reynier had anticipated, the Israelis decided not to take revenge on the Arab prisoners in their hands. Instead, they did their utmost to achieve the quickest possible release of the detainees, the seven women among whom had been subjected to degrading treatment at the hands of their guards.[623] The prisoners of Abassieh were repatriated in March, 1948, through the mediation of the ICRC.

In Syria, the Jewish prisoners – men, women, children, and elderly – whose number varied between 48 and 43, were held in the Mazzé Prison in Damascus, and, contrary to the provisions of the Prisoners of War Convention, were treated like criminal offenders. Their conditions of detention were cruel: cold, dark, dirt, torture, deprivation of news. De Reynier and especially the delegate Munier, who was based in Amman and was responsible for visiting them, had already demonstrated great motivation as, spurred by the constant pressure of the Israelis, they tried to obtain for the Mazzé detainees treatment consistent with the Prisoners of War Convention and repatriation for the disabled prisoners. But the Israeli reaction to the Abassieh affair gave them an additional push, leading Munier, six days after de Reynier's visit to Abassieh, to send the Syrians an unusually solemn memorandum. After recapitulating the steps he had already taken, he complained of 'the seriousness of the methods employed' by Syria 'to hinder the ICRC delegates systematically

---

[622] See Chapter 1, p. 48.
[623] S. Rosenne, 'Short record of conversation between Shabtai Rosenne, accompanied by Dr. M. Kahany, with Monsieur de Traz, Deputy Executive Director, assisted by M. de Bondeli, Chief of the PW's Division of the International Red Cross at the Headquarters of the International Red Cross, Geneva, on Monday, 13th December, 1948, at 1700 hours' (ISA/MEA/1987.20).

FROM HEROISM TO TRADITIONAL ACTIVITIES

in the accomplishment of their traditional humanitarian mission.'[624]

Munier's memorandum antagonized the Syrian authorities, and they told de Reynier so. The latter was unmoved; he considered Munier's memo solely from the perspective of his relations with the Israelis, and he believed that this document would allow the ICRC, if necessary, 'to prove that the ICRC delegation made all possible efforts to accomplish its mission.'[625] These efforts did succeed in some measure, permitting individual exchanges.[626] On February 3, 1949, the Syrians agreed to the examination of the prisoners by a mixed medical commission. In March, 1949, following Syria's defeat in the Palestine war, the commander of the Syrian army, Husni el-Zaim, overthrew the government and established a strong regime. This simplified the relations between the ICRC and the Syrians, which took a turn for the better. The prisoners whom the mixed medical commission considered eligible for repatriation were returned to Israel on April 4, 1949. The suffering of the 39 prisoners remaining in Mazzé was ended only by their own repatriation, shortly afterwards.

In Transjordan, the prisoners in the Um el-Djemal and Mafraq camps received relatively adequate treatment as long as the Arab Legion had British officers in its ranks. But in the summer of 1948 the British were replaced by Transjordanians, and a new minister of defense was appointed who knew nothing of the humanitarian conventions or the ICRC. Consequently, these political changes held up the ICRC's negotiations, particularly those aimed at the repatriation of disabled prisoners and medical personnel.[627]

Although completed after the armistice accords, the ICRC's traditional interventions as a neutral intermediary on behalf of prisoners of war had actually begun before the Stockholm

[624]Memorandum from Munier, ICRC Amman, Damascus, to Kallas, General Chief-of-Staff of the Syrian Army, Dec. 6, 1948. Copies sent to the President of the Syrian Republic, the Prime Minister of Syria, the Chief of the 2nd Bureau of the Syrian Army, the President of the Syrian Red Crescent, and the President of the ICRC (AICRC, G.59/I/G.C.). [Translation: M.G.]

[625]Report from de Reynier, Central ICRC Delegation for Palestine, 'mois de decembre 1948,' Beirut, Jan. 28, 1948 (AICRC, G.59/I/G.C.). [Translation: M.G.]

[626]Note from de Reynier, Central ICRC Delegation for Palestine, Beirut, to Munier and Lehner, ICRC Amman, Jan. 27, 1949 (AICRC, G.59/I/G.C.). Report from Munier, ICRC Amman, 'mois de janvier 1949' (AICRC, G.59/I/G.C.).

[627]Dossier 'Mission Munier à Amman' (AICRC, G.3/82).

Conference. The timing was important to the ICRC, since for the second quarter of 1948, shortly before the Conference, it could point to the accomplishment of 53 visits to prisoner-of-war camps: twenty-two visits to 5 different camps for Arab prisoners in Palestine and 31 visits to Israeli prisoners held by Arabs – 15 in Transjordan, 9 in Syria, and 7 in Egypt.[628]

Linking relief actions to the role of neutral intermediary

The ICRC had decided not to begin its operations to provide material assistance until it had obtained the belligerents' agreement to conform to the 1929 Conventions, which it would require in order to exercise its role of neutral intermediary. In its view, relief activities were essentially linked to its traditional activities in aid of prisoners of war: Its task, as dictated by both the Prisoners of War Convention and its own tradition, was to transmit material aid to the prisoners on both sides of the front. The ICRC's work as a neutral intermediary on behalf of prisoners did not really begin until after the evacuation of the Jewish inhabitants of the Jerusalem Old City on May 28, 1948; consequently, relief operations could not begin until later.

Yet in the meantime the ICRC had not been completely idle in the business of providing material relief in Mandatory Palestine. In April 1948,[629] considering that material aid was its best ticket for winning over the Arabs, the ICRC provided medicines and supplies to the hospitals and sent in nurses to replace the British 'sisters' of former days. On May 12[630] and June 3,

---

[628]ICRC, *Report on General Activities (July 1, 1947–December 31, 1948)* (Geneva: ICRC, 1949), p. 110. From June 1948, the reports from the ICRC delegates were no longer anecdotal, but were organized systematically in terms of the principal fields of the ICRC's activity: action in favor of hospitals, action on behalf of prisoners of war and civilian internees, action for material relief.

[629]Note from Dunand, ICRC Geneva, to Marti, care of ICRC Cairo, April 8, 1948 (AICRC, G.59/I/G.C.).

[630]ICRC, Circular letter from Ruegger, May 12, 1948 (CP 314). To National Red Cross Societies of Australia, Belgium, Canada, France, Great Britain, Ireland, New Zealand, South Africa, Sweden, Switzerland, and the USA, as well as the following charitable associations: Auxilium Catholicum Internationale, Caritas, Catholica Internationalis, International Union for Child Welfare, Quakers, UNICEF, WHO, World Council of Churches, and the YMCA.

1948[631] the ICRC called on National Red Cross and Red Crescent Societies, and private charitable organizations, to solicit donations of goods and money for the hospital patients and for the as-yet hypothetical refugees of the safety zones, reserving the right to allocate these shipments in other ways depending on the way the conflict developed. These communiqués would be followed by new appeals for solidarity from the Red Cross Societies and other organizations on June 24[632] and July 14, 1948, still for the same beneficiaries.[633]

In the first appeal, on May 12, 1948, the ICRC specified the basis for its activity in Palestine – Article VII of the International Red Cross Statutes – because it did not want to appear simply as a relief agency; it wanted to bring to the fore the function of neutral intermediary that it was determined to protect from the effects of any unfortunate revision of the 1928 Statutes, or equally undesirable (in its view) amendments to those Statutes.

---

[631]ICRC, circular letter from Dunand, Geneva, June 3, 1948 (CP 335). To National Red Cross Societies of Australia, Belgium, Canada, France, Great Britain, Ireland, New Zealand, South Africa, Sweden, Switzerland, and the USA; to the Red Crescent Society of Iraq, the Red Cross of Lebanon, the Red Crescent Societies of Syria, Turkey, and Transjordan (still being organized), and the Red Lion and Sun Society of Iran, as well as the following charitable associations: Auxilium Catholicum Internationale, Caritas, Catholica Internationalis, International Union for Child Welfare, Quakers, UNICEF, WHO, World Council of Churches, and the YMCA.

[632]ICRC, circular letter, June 24, 1948 (CP 335 bis). To National Red Cross Societies of Australia, Belgium, Canada, France, Great Britain, Ireland, New Zealand, South Africa, Sweden, Switzerland, and the USA; to the Red Crescent Society of Iraq, the Red Cross of Lebanon, the Red Crescent Societies of Syria, Turkey, and Transjordan (still being organized), and the Red Lion and Sun Society of Iran, as well as the following charitable associations: Auxilium Catholicum Internationale, Caritas, Catholica Internationalis, International Union for Child Welfare, Quakers, UNICEF, WHO, World Council of Churches, and the YMCA.

[633]ICRC, circular letter, Geneva, July 14, 1948 (CP 335 ter.). To National Red Cross Societies of Australia, Belgium, Canada, France, Great Britain, Ireland, New Zealand, South Africa, Sweden, Switzerland, and the USA; to the Red Crescent Society of Iraq, the Red Cross of Lebanon, the Red Crescent Societies of Syria, Turkey, and Transjordan (still being organized), and the Red Lion and Sun Society of Iran, as well as the following charitable associations: Auxilium Catholicum Internationale, Caritas, Catholica Internationalis, International Union for Child Welfare, Quakers, UNICEF, WHO, World Council of Churches, and the YMCA.

Reaffirming Red Cross impartiality

Subsequently realizing that its material aid operation for the hospitals benefited primarily the Arabs, the ICRC judged it necessary to explain its interpretation of the principle of impartiality in allocating that aid. In its circular letter of July 14, 1948,[634] it defined its doctrine by referring the recipients of the circular to a work published by Max Huber in 1946, which the ICRC considered as 'a breviary for Stockholm'[635] This doctrinal text, written by Max Huber, specifies that impartiality does not mean quantitative equivalence, but equity, and that it does not imply simultaneousness.[636] In the matter of aid, the ICRC's motto was 'to each according to his needs.' Using this criterion, the ICRC divided and directly distributed those donations for which it had received no allocation instructions. It gave the other donations to the relief organizations of the communities concerned, leaving to them the task of distribution.[637] The most recent precedent for this modus operandi was the ICRC's practice during World War II, notably in the framework of the activities of the Joint Relief Commission of the International Red Cross.

It was not until August 16, 1948, that the ICRC's relief operation really got under way, as an offshoot of its role of neutral intermediary. The organization issued a new appeal mentioning two additional categories of beneficiaries: the prisoners of war in the Israeli and Arab camps, and the Arab Palestinian refugees[638] – a pertinent issue, since, according to de Reynier, Israeli combat

---

[634]Ibid.

[635]ICRC Delegation to the Conference of Stockholm, preparatory sessions, report of first session, Tuesday, June 22, 1948 (AICRC. CR 25).

[636]Max Huber, *Principles and Foundations of the Work of the International Committee of the Red Cross, 1939–1946* (Geneva: ICRC, 1947), p. 15.

[637]Ibid.

[638]ICRC, Circular letter, Geneva, Aug. 16, 1948 (AICRC, CP 355 [4]). To National Red Cross Societies of Australia, Belgium, Canada, Denmark, France, Great Britain, Ireland, the Netherlands, New Zealand, South Africa, Sweden, Switzerland, and the USA; to the Egyptian Red Crescent, the Iraqi Red Crescent, the Red Lion and Sun Society of Iran, the Lebanese Red Cross, and the Red Crescent Societies of Syria and Transjordan (still being organized), as well as the following charitable associations: Auxilium Catholicum Internationale, Caritas Internationalis, International Centre for Relief to Civilian Populations, International Union for Child Welfare, Quakers, UNICEF, WHO, World Council of Churches, and the YMCA. For a more complete analysis of the effect of that appeal, which also concerned Arab and Jewish Palestinian refugees, see Chapter 6, p. 259.

FROM HEROISM TO TRADITIONAL ACTIVITIES

troops were in West Jerusalem.[639] I will come back to the reasons that the ICRC began to take the Arab refugees into account only from that date on, whereas during the first months of the conflict it had not considered them as one of its traditional responsibilities.[640]

Generally speaking, the ICRC appeals were addressed to National Red Cross and Red Crescent Societies and to Christian or non-denominational charitable associations, excluding Jewish relief organizations; the ICRC undoubtedly feared that their names on appeals that were also sent to Arab charitable organizations would trigger a counter-productive reaction from the Arabs.

As regards relief actions, it should also be noted that under Article 8 of the conditions of the first truce arranged by Bernadotte, the ICRC was supposed to have assumed the responsibility for provisioning Jerusalem. But the Arab Palestinians might have interpreted such action as aid to the Jews, given the fact that the Jewish armed forces were in a strong position in Jerusalem, and the Arabs were counting on their being weakened by hunger and thirst. Courvoisier wrote that his work would probably be jeopardized in the Nablus area if the ICRC were to supply Jerusalem. On Courvoisier's advice, de Reynier preferred not to supply the whole city, and justified this refusal with an argument both theoretical and doctrinal: the ICRC could not possibly provision a city in which an armed force was stationed. He found a compromise solution, however, agreeing to furnish supplies and medicines to the city's hospitals, Jewish and Arab alike – an action which was not detrimental to the Arabs and whose neutrality could not be contested. The overall supply problem he left up to Bernadotte.[641] Despite all the organization's care, however, the rumor circulated that the ICRC had carried out this relief operation – a rumor the ICRC delegates hastened to refute in the Arab press and in radio broadcasts to the countries bordering Israel.[642]

---

[639]De Reynier, monthly report no. 4, June 1948, Jerusalem, July 2, 1948 (AICRC, G.59/I/G.C.).

[640]See Chapter 6, pp. 253 ff.

[641]Note from Courvoisier, June 14, 1948, to de Bondeli, ICRC Geneva (AICRC, G.59/I/G.C.). De Reynier, ICRC Jerusalem, monthly report no. 4, month of June, Jerusalem, July 2, 1948 (AICRC, G.59/I/G.C.).

[642]Note from Gaillard, ICRC Beirut, to ICRC Geneva, July 3, 1948 (AICRC, G.59/I/G.C.). Communiqué for the press and the radio, Amman, Beirut,

Reorganization of the plan of action

For the efficient conduct of the relief operations linked to its traditional work with prisoners of war on both sides of the front, the ICRC reorganized its delegation in June, 1948. It created an autonomous office in Tel Aviv, run by Robert Gouy – whom the Israelis, especially Arieh Steinberg (the Israeli army liaison officer for the ICRC in Tel Aviv), appreciated for his impartiality and his good humanitarian sense – and another autonomous office in Amman, directed by Munier, who had immersed himself in the local culture to the point of occasionally wearing a *keffiyeh*.[643] Munier was given the responsibility for Transjordan, Syria, and Iraq. The ICRC planned to transfer its central delegation from Jerusalem to Beirut; from there de Reynier was supposed to continue supervising the ICRC's activities 'in Palestine,' meaning on the entire territory of the former Mandatory Palestine.

After the Government House safety zone had been converted into a demilitarized zone under the control of the United Nations in October 1948, de Reynier confirmed the new organizational arrangements by announcing that he would spend, alternately, ten days in Tel Aviv and ten days in Amman. The Israelis saw this as evidence of bias. They considered that by leaving Jerusalem, the ICRC was abandoning the Jewish inhabitants of the city to their fate[644]; but even more important, the choice of Beirut as the central headquarters of the ICRC delegation 'for Palestine' shocked the Israelis, since Lebanon was at war with their country.[645]

Ramallah, and Damascus, July 2, 1948 (AICRC, G.59/I/G.C.). According to Gaillard, 'the delegation escorted two columns of trucks (one of forty trucks, the other of eight) containing stocks of medicines for the Jewish hospitals of Jerusalem.' This operation was apparently not carried out within the framework of Article 8 of the conditions of the first truce. Note from Gaillard, ICRC Beirut, to ICRC Geneva, July 3, 1948 (AICRC, G.59/I/G.C.).

[643] The *keffiyeh* is the traditional Beduin head-covering, and is formed by a square of fabric folded in a triangle and held in place by a head band. Questioned informally on several occasions by the author, Munier confirmed that his sympathies lay with the Arabs. Anxious to express himself impartially, however, he declared that he had great admiration for the Jews. He said that the *keffiyeh* that he sometimes wore had been given to him by Abdullah Tel.

[644] Note from de Reynier, ICRC Jerusalem, 'Fin de la zone de sécurité no I,' Jerusalem, to ICRC Geneva, July 18 and 19, 1948 (AICRC, G.59/I/G.C.).

[645] Letter from Eytan, Director-General, for the Minister of Foreign Affairs, Hakirya, to Paul Ruegger, President of the ICRC, Geneva, Oct. 10, 1948 (ISA/MEA/2406.6).

For a long time de Reynier's attitude had wounded the Israelis: He had tried to put all of Jerusalem under the Red Cross emblem, against the wishes of the Jewish Agency; he treated his Jewish contacts with scant consideration, if not the outright contempt he had shown Kohn over the issue of the safety zones. To these irritants were added the Abassieh affair, then in its initial stages, and the recall to Geneva of Gouy, an ICRC delegate whom the Israelis particularly esteemed.

The choice of Beirut as the headquarters of the ICRC's central delegation 'for Palestine' was an occasion for the Israelis to express their dissatisfaction with the head of the ICRC delegation and to request his recall.[646] Shertok, the Israeli minister of foreign affairs, decided to invite Wolf (Ruegger's advisor, who had married the third daughter of Warburg, the Jewish banker) to come and hear Israel's grievances. If Israel did not obtain de Reynier's recall through Wolf, it would declare the head of the ICRC delegation *persona non grata*.[647] Shertok did not want, however, to base his request on arguments that were subjective or difficult to prove, such as Israel's feeling that de Reynier was prejudiced against Jews. The Israelis therefore drew up a list of objective grounds for displeasure:

- Gouy's recall;
- the choice of Beirut as the headquarters for the ICRC central delegation 'for Palestine';
- the fact that under de Reynier's orders, the ICRC delegates did not visit the camps often enough, and obtained too few improvements;
- the fact that the ICRC's inquiries regarding missing persons were ineffective. The minister of foreign affairs and his colleagues in charge of relations with the ICRC did not understand how de Reynier could content himself with asking the opposing side what had become of a Jew who had disappeared

---

[646] According to letter from Zvi Loker, Provisional Government of the State of Israel, Division of International Organisations, Hakirya, to Kahany, Geneva, Oct. 27, 1948 (ISA/MEA/1987.1).

[647] According to letter from Zvi Loker, Ministry of Foreign Affairs, Division of International Organisations, Hakirya, to Kahany, Representative of the Provisional Government of the State of Israel to the European Office of the United Nations and to the International Committee of the Red Cross, Geneva, Nov. 1, 1948 (ISA/MEA/1987.1).

on the Arab side, and accept the answer he was given without trying to verify it.[648]

Wolf went to Tel Aviv at the beginning of November, and responded to the Israelis' grievances as Ruegger had instructed him to when he left Geneva:

- Concerning Gouy's recall, Wolf pointed out that if the Israelis valued this delegate, they should realize that he would be very useful in an Arab zone, where he could come to the assistance of Jewish victims;
- Concerning the central delegation in Beirut, Wolf reaffirmed the Committee's choice, citing logistical reasons: It would be easier to deploy a relief operation from Beirut than from Cyprus or Rhodes. However, Wolf assured them that the Beirut delegation would not be 'central' from Geneva's point of view, but simply an aid center and a place for storing archives. The ICRC delegates in Tel Aviv and Amman would enjoy considerable freedom of initiative and authority.[649]
- Concerning the ICRC's method for providing protection and assistance to prisoners of war and for seeking missing persons, it reflected the way the organization perceived the exercise of its role as a neutral intermediary.

Shertok did not manage to get de Reynier recalled; Ruegger instructed Wolf to tell him that the ICRC was an independent organization that could not be pressured over the choice of its delegates, and to insist on de Reynier's complete impartiality.[650]

As for the ICRC's operational methods, Kahany, in Geneva, had already presented the problem to the minister of foreign affairs some time previously:

there is a [sic] little chance for us to reform the ICRC and to make their services more effective than they really are. Either we need the Red Cross with all the deficiencies inherent to

[648]Letter from Zvi Loker, Ministry of Foreign Affairs, Division of International Organisations, Hakirya, Israel, to J. Brunschwig, office of Jean Brunschwig and Marius Lachat, Sept. 27, 1948, with memorandum attached for transmission to Professor Carry (ISA/MEA/2406.6).

[649]Paul Ruegger, 'Instructions à M. Wolf, Conseiller du CICR, pour sa mission spéciale à Tel Aviv,' Geneva, Oct. 31, 1948 (AICRC, G.59/I/G.C.).

[650]Ibid. See also Wolf, report of mission to Tel Aviv, Geneva, Nov. 18, 1948 (AICRC, G.3/83).

it, then we have to see how to compromise with all the principles and neutral manners, or we are of the opinion that we can well manage our interests without their help, then we better tell them this straight away.[651]

Israel opted for compromise, but kept a very close eye on the ICRC delegates' activities on behalf of prisoners – perhaps all the more so because just after Wolf's visit the disgraceful affair at the Abassieh camp came to light. For the Israelis, few in number, every Jew able to fight was precious. Traditionally, moreover, the Jewish people had always considered aid to prisoners and the ransom of captives as a primordial duty. The ICRC delegates were perturbed by this attitude; they had the impression that to the Israelis a Jew counted for more than an Arab. They did not understand the Israeli feeling about Jewish prisoners, nor did they try to comprehend the military or cultural reasons for it.

The operation in Palestine: an asset in Stockholm

At the end of June, 1948, the ICRC had begun – though no more than that – all the activities it planned to conduct in the Palestine conflict before the Stockholm Conference. A pamphlet that it published in July 1948 to distribute to the conference participants neatly summed up the steps taken by the organization. The ICRC began by underlining the danger the Palestine conflict represented in the international arena,[652] then pointed out that in April, 1948, the Jewish Agency and the Arab Higher Committee had undertaken to respect the essential principles of the Geneva Conventions.[653] It stressed that these principles had been accepted at a time when the events taking place in Palestine did not constitute an armed conflict between states,[654] or, in other words, when the conflict was still in the nature of a civil war. Next, it emphasized its own efforts to establish safety zones,

---

[651]Letter from Kahany, Provisional Government of the State of Israel, Representative to the European Office of the United Nations and to the International Committee of the Red Cross, Geneva, to Loker, Division of International Organisations, Ministry of Foreign Affairs, Tel Aviv, Oct. 25, 1948 (ISA/MEA/1986.8).

[652]ICRC, The International Committee of the Red Cross in Palestine (Geneva, July 1948), p. 1.

[653]Ibid.

[654]Ibid., pp. 5–7.

asserting that it had received the belligerents' consent to this on May 9 and 17, 1948. It declared that since two of those zones had been closed, it hoped to create others, one in Amman and one in Tel Aviv[655] – this, in my view, indicates the importance it attributed to keeping the Stockholm Conference participants' attention on the safety zones. It then mentioned the appeal of May 12, 1948, with which it launched its medical relief action.[656] Broaching the subject of the hospitals, 'protected by the flag of the Committee,'[657] it stressed the priority given the Arabs, who were less well equipped – according to the ICRC – than the Jews.[658] Next, the organization rendered homage to its delegates' heroic dedication, pointing out the individual character of their initiatives,[659] probably in order to dissociate itself from the resulting picture of disorganization. Finally, it asserted that it had managed to persuade the Arab states and the Arab League to respect the red star of David, even though this emblem had no official legal status.[660]

This last claim is astonishing, and merits some comment. Since the ICRC's policy was to avoid, if possible, the addition of the red star of David to future conventions, it was not in its interest to stress something that could be considered as a precedent. Why, then, did it volunteer this information? One possible reason comes to mind. In July, Katznelson asked an emissary from the League of Red Cross Societies, sent to Israel by Bernadotte, to go to Cairo and ask the Egyptians to respect the red star of David.[661] Now this proceeding, in the middle of a war, should have been the task of the ICRC. De Reynier responded by going to Cairo immediately himself to conduct the negotiations that Israel had requested – a request all the more urgent from its point of view, since the Egyptians were bombing buildings that

[655] Ibid., p. 6.
[656] Ibid., p. 7.
[657] Ibid., p. 8.
[658] Ibid.
[659] Ibid.
[660] Ibid.
[661] According to telegram from Gouy, ICRC Tel Aviv, to ICRC Geneva, June 31, 1948 (AICRC, G.59/I/G.C.). See also telegram from de Reynier, ICRC Cairo, to ICRC Geneva, July 2, 1948 (AICRC, G.59/I/G.C.); note from de Reynier, ICRC Cairo, July 14, 1948 (AICRC, G.59/I/G.C.); and confidential letter from Henry W. Dunning, Secretary-General, LRCS Geneva, to Jacques Chenevière, ICRC Geneva, July 26, 1948 (AICRC. CR 195).

FROM HEROISM TO TRADITIONAL ACTIVITIES

displayed the red star of David.[662] Perhaps by underlining the fact that it had obtained respect for the red star of David, the ICRC wanted to show that the issue of the protective emblem was its own domain rather than that of the League of Red Cross Societies, since the situation was 'wartime' and not 'peacetime.' Whatever the case, the ICRC had not abandoned its intention of opposing any increase in the number of protective signs sanctioned in the future revised Geneva Convention. In this respect, it was not taking any risks by saying that its delegate had persuaded the Arab armies to respect the red star of David, for it knew the chances were slim that the Arab states would accept the addition of the Israeli emblem to the revised or new conventions – especially since the leaders of the League of Red Cross Societies shared its view.

To return to the pamphlet put out by the ICRC, although it avoided any discussion of the transition to an international war and the measures the organization had taken at the end of May, 1948, to insure that the states at war, including Israel, respected the conventions, the ICRC did describe at length the appeal it had sent out to the belligerent armies on May 21 asking them to spare the safety zones.[663] It then mentioned President Ruegger's mission to Jerusalem and the evacuation of the civilian population of the Jewish Quarter of the Old City.

Next, it listed different categories. The first, entitled *Wounded, Sick and Prisoners*, briefly described the delegates' intervention in Deir Yassin, Solomon's Pools (Nebi Daniel), and Gush Etzion.[664] The second, *Camp Visits*, focused on the traditional work the ICRC had begun in this sphere, and highlighted the exchanges of 'civilian internees'[665] – the ICRC was apparently referring to the exchange of Jewish teenagers for Arab prisoners not far from Kalkilya, and other individual exchanges.

---

[662] According to note from de Bondeli, ICRC Geneva, citing a passage from a report by the ICRC delegation in Cairo, to Gouy, ICRC Tel Aviv, July 21, 1948 (AICRC, G.59/I/G.C.). See also 'List of Egyptians [sic] violations to honour the Magen David Emblem with effect from 13th July, 1948' (ISA/MEA/537.1). See also letter from Pflimlin, ICRC Jerusalem, to Gaulan, 'Jewish Agency, Jerusalem,' July 11, 1948, and letter from Pflimlin, ICRC Jerusalem, 'Aux hautes autorités juives, Agence juive, Jérusalem' (ISA/MEA/537.1).
[663] ICRC, *The ICRC in Palestine*, pp. 9–10.
[664] Ibid., pp. 11–12.
[665] Ibid., p. 12.

THE IMPERILED RED CROSS

Finally, it is noteworthy that the ICRC included a category entitled *Refugees*. Not long before, like the rest of the international community, it had realized the burgeoning political importance of the Arab Palestinian refugee problem.[666] In the context of its aid to the refugees of Palestine, the ICRC took credit for the fact that the day after the Jaffa attack, its delegate had intervened on behalf of 'more than 30,000 people [who] were able to cross the Jewish lines over a space of about six miles. . . .'[667] Under the *Refugees* heading, the ICRC also included the evacuation of 170 Egyptians from Jerusalem to the Egyptian border, the embarkation at Jaffa of some 3,000 Egyptians, and the evacuation to Tulkarem of about 1,100 Arab women, children, and old people. In order to balance the Arabs and the Jews, the ICRC felt it necessary to refer again, in the *Refugees* section, to the evacuation of able-bodied settlers from Gush Etzion and to that of the civilians from the Jewish Quarter in the Old City.[668] The way the ICRC wrote about refugee operations at the end of June and beginning of July, 1948, indicates that the Committee in Geneva had not yet realized the full significance of the Palestinian refugee issue. The ICRC finished its summary with an initial assessment of its relief action to date: On June 21, one of its delegates was able to escort 50 trucks filled with food and medicines to the Jerusalem hospitals.[669]

This little report on the ICRC's activities in Palestine was the only printed document concerning an operation in progress that the ICRC presented to the participants of the Stockholm Conference. The ICRC's operations in other parts of the world were not mentioned except in a few mimeographed pages stapled together. The pamphlet on Palestine, then, joined the ICRC's major reports – a three-volume report comprising more than 2,000 pages on its activities during the Second World War[670] and a White Paper of some 200 pages on the ICRC's efforts to aid the victims of the German concentration camps, which it was issuing for the third time.[671]

[666]See Chapter 6, pp. 221 *ff*.
[667]ICRC, *The ICRC in Palestine*, p. 12.
[668]Ibid.
[669]Ibid., p. 13.
[670]ICRC, XVIIth International Red Cross Conference, Stockholm, 1948, *Report of the ICRC on Its Activities during the Second World War (September 1, 1939–June 30, 1947,* 3 volumes (Geneva, May 1948).
[671]ICRC, *The Work of the ICRC for Civilian Detainees in German Concentration Camps from 1939 to 1945.*

FROM HEROISM TO TRADITIONAL ACTIVITIES

As far as documentation was concerned, the ICRC was all ready. Now all that was needed was the tactical preparation for that conference at which the future of the ICRC and of the entire International Red Cross would probably be at stake.

Chapter Six

FROM STOCKHOLM TO TORONTO: THE RED CROSS RECOVERS ITS BALANCE

The ICRC on the eve of the Stockholm Conference

From mid-June to August 20, 1948, the ICRC in Geneva tried to anticipate the debates that might arise at the Stockholm Conference and prepare for them. Would the USSR attend? Bernadotte, as chairman of the Standing Commission of the Conference, had the honor of sending out the invitations. The ICRC, as guardian of the Red Cross principles – including that of the organization's universality – made a final attempt to open up a dialogue with the USSR. On March 31, 1948, at the instigation of O'Connor, the American chairman of a fragile League of Red Cross Societies, it sent a telegram to Stalin to propose that he meet the ICRC president in Moscow.[672] The reply came from a minor Soviet diplomat, who simply told ICRC officials, in person, that it was still too early. This was not an absolute refusal.[673] The Swiss government, which had tried to sound out the Soviets' intentions through other channels, let the ICRC understand that the USSR might come.[674]

The ICRC therefore entertained some hope, but it was still worried; if the Soviets came to the conference, the diplomatic contest for its own future and that of the International Red Cross would be very close. The debate over the composition of the

[672]Telegram from Gloor and Bodmer, ICRC Vice-Presidents, Geneva, to Stalin, March 31, 1948 (IZG, Zurich, 28.3.1. Fonds Ruegger).

[673]'Bref exposé sur les relations générales du CICR avec les autorités de l'Union des Républiques Socialistes Soviétiques et avec l'Alliance des Sociétés de la Croix-Rouge et du Croissant-Rouge de l'URSS depuis 1939,' Geneva, Nov. 27, 1953, unsigned (AICRC, D. 318).

[674]Letter from de Haller, Federal Council's Delegate for Mutual International Aid, Bern, to Ruegger, Minister of Switzerland to London, March 10, 1948 (IZG, Zurich, Fonds Ruegger).

ICRC had not been buried, even if the Red Cross could now count on a few states, including Britain, that believed the ICRC should be kept independent and neutral, and to that end should continue to recruit its membership by co-optation among Swiss citizens. The USSR and its satellites had not yet said their last word. As for Bernadotte, he continued to support the idea that the ICRC and the League should be placed under the authority of an international body, which could be constituted from the Standing Commission of the IRC, of which he was the chairman. Naturally, under the current circumstances, the ICRC wanted the Red Cross world to be in harmony; but it feared that such unity would be realized at its own expense, at the price of its internationalization or of its subordination to an international body.

Humanitarian conventions to unite a divided world

In the ICRC's view, the most important documents of the conference were the 'Draft Revised or New Conventions for the Protection of War Victims, Established by the International Committee of the Red Cross with the Assistance of Government Experts, National Red Cross Societies and Other Humanitarian Associations.'[675] The ICRC was the main author of the drafts, but at every stage of their elaboration, it had scrupulously consulted the most representative range of experts possible, and had for the most part heeded their advice. In any case, the ICRC drafts, which were designed to be presented at Stockholm and to become Geneva Conventions at the next diplomatic conference – scheduled for the spring of 1949 – could not be universally binding unless the USSR and its allies ratified them and then acceded to them, together with the Western countries.

The USSR had been invited to each meeting of experts, and to increase the chances that it would attend, the ICRC had not invited jurists from the countries defeated in World War II. Instead, it discreetly asked them to send in their comments in writing, a procedure that many of them accepted. The USSR did not respond to the ICRC's invitations, however. The ICRC sent

---

[675]XVIIth International Conference of the Red Cross, Stockholm, August 1948, *Draft Revised or New Conventions for the Protection of War Victims, established by the International Committee of the Red Cross with the assistance of government experts, national Red Cross societies and other humanitarian associations* (Geneva: ICRC, May 1948), 245 pp.

it the drafts formulated by the experts for its perusal, but the USSR did not react.

The documents that were to constitute the 1949 Geneva Conventions had been thought up and drafted to satisfy both the Western camp and the Soviet camp. The ICRC drafts drew on the organization's experiences during World War II and its perception of them. Their main legal focus was the protection of civilian individuals and populations, partisans and members of resistance groups – categories of victims of particular concern to the countries of the Communist East.

Thus, the 'Draft Revised or New Conventions' provided for the protection of civilian wounded and sick; the revised version of the 1929 Prisoners of War Convention took into account, in addition to the soldiers of regular armies, various other categories of combatants, including the members of organized militias – which was a way of extending the convention's protection to partisans and resistance fighters.[676]

Finally, a new convention, protecting civilians in wartime,[677] imposed humane treatment of civilians who were not nationals of the power in whose hands they found themselves, meaning aliens and stateless people.[678] This draft convention also recognized the immunity of civilian populations, and contained provisions intended to protect them against the consequences of warfare – for example, the possibility that signatory states could reach an agreement regarding the establishment of safety zones and localities which would be respected by combatants just as hospitals were.

This provision was an indirect (and very weak) – way of condemning weapons of mass destruction, since it was based on the distinction between combatants and noncombatants which is fundamental to the philosophy of the Geneva Convention – a

---

[676] In designating the beneficiaries of the revised convention, the ICRC drafters eliminated all reference to The Hague law. The new convention for the relief of prisoners of war could therefore be correctly termed a 'Geneva Convention,' whereas the old one had been a 'convention concluded at Geneva.'

[677] 'Convention for the Protection of Civilian Persons in Wartime,' Part I: 'General Provisions,' Art. 3, in XVIIth International Conference of the Red Cross, Stockholm, August 1948, *Draft Revised or New Conventions for the Protection of War Victims*, p. 154.

[678] The ICRC did not succeed in extending the protection of the conventions to nationals under the power of their own state; these civilians remained under the exclusive jurisdiction of the latter.

distinction that such weapons do not make.[679] In this respect, the ICRC was responding to the wishes of the USSR, which, through its Alliance of Red Cross and Red Crescent Societies and the relief societies of the countries of the East, had conveyed its opinion that the International Red Cross should condemn the use of atomic weapons.[680] This had put the ICRC in an awkward position, since it was anxious not to provoke the US. Under these circumstances, the possibility of establishing safety zones for the protection of civilian populations seemed to be an acceptable compromise.

As for the application of the future Geneva Conventions, the ICRC had learned a lesson from World War II; it proposed that the conventions be applicable in occupied territories. Moreover, in the expectation of generalized hostilities in future, which seemed to be heralded by certain burgeoning civil wars, a provision was included which prescribed the integral application of the conventions to all non-international armed conflicts.[681] Thus, the ICRC had taken the liberty of going beyond the draft article endorsed by the Conference of Government Experts in 1947, which had provided merely that in cases of civil war the essential principles of the 1929 Conventions were to be respected – the same article that had inspired the Committee to issue its appeal of March 12, 1948, urging the parties to the Palestine conflict to respect the principles of the conventions.[682] It should be noted that this article's definition of an armed conflict – of the civil-war type – did not include the case of unilateral aggressive action by an armed power against an unarmed population. An example was the incident known as *Kristallnacht*, the night in November, 1938, when the Nazis in Germany wreaked systematic havoc on Jewish businesses and burned the synagogues.[683]

---

[679]For the ICRC's official position on weapons of mass destruction, see CICR, 'La fin des hostilités et les tâches futures de la Croix-Rouge,' Sept. 5, 1945, *RICR* 321 (Sept. 1945): 657–662.

[680]Croix-Rouge yougoslave, Conférence régionale des Croix-Rouges européennes, Belgrade, 24 septembre-1er octobre 1947, *Compte rendu*, 'Résolution no 9,' pp. 116–117.

[681]XVIIth International Conference of the Red Cross, Stockholm, August 1948, *Draft Revised or New Conventions*, Art. 2/2/2/2, pp. 5, 34–35, 52, 153–154.

[682]See Chapter 3, pp. 117 ff.

[683]Gerhardt Riegner, the representative of the World Jewish Congress who was invited to the conference in an advisory capacity, proposed an amendment to extend the applicability of the conventions in cases of 'internal conflicts in a country where one of the parties is not able to resist.' The proposal was defeated

Wanting to return to the use of a single emblem, the ICRC had thought of doing away with the red crescent and the red lion and sun; but given the international context and the necessity of rallying the states from all points of the globe to the conventions, it decided not to take the risk. It retained the crescent, the sign used by most of the Arab states and those Soviet republics with a Moslem majority. It did suggest, however, eliminating the red lion and sun in the revised Geneva Convention, since this symbol was used by only one country, Iran; and it invited the conference participants to show their 'constant determination not to furnish an argument for the use of other exceptional emblems.'[684] By implication, it was asking the states to block the Israeli request to include the red star of David in future conventions.

The revised and new draft conventions were coordinated so that they could be totally or partially merged.[685] The revised conventions and the new one were also linked together by common articles. The future Geneva Conventions thus formed a whole, making it difficult for a state to sign one and not the others, as the USSR had done in World War II – it had been a party to the Geneva Convention for the protection of sick and wounded soldiers, but not to the Prisoners of War Convention.

The future Geneva Conventions: protection for the ICRC

The ICRC's drafts, which made good use of the organization's past experiences while trying to anticipate wars to come, constituted a major advance for international humanitarian law, notably because they extended the protection of the conventions to civilian victims of war. They were equally important for the ICRC itself, for they incorporated a major reinforcement of its

---

by ten votes against and three abstentions. Invited to give his opinion, the ICRC jurist, Claude Pilloud, responded, 'by wanting to be too precise, one always weakens the provisions. That is our general tendency, but we have not had enough time to consider this delicate question.' XVIIème Conférence internationale de la Croix-Rouge, Stockholm, 1948, Commission juridique, stenographic record, meeting of Aug. 24, 1948, pp. 37 and 41 (ICRC Library). [Translation: M.G.]

[684]'Revision of the Geneva Convention of July 27, 1929, for the Relief of the Wounded and Sick in Armies in the Field,' in XVIIth International Conference of the Red Cross, Stockholm, August 1948, Chapter VII: 'The Distinctive Emblem,' Art. 31, Remarks by the ICRC, in *Draft Revised or New Conventions*, p. 23.

[685]XVIIth International Conference of the Red Cross, Stockholm, August 1948, *Draft Revised or New Conventions*, p. 221.

legal grounds for intervention. In fact, in them the ICRC had explicitly stipulated the tasks it wanted to be given.

First of all, it would be able to assume the role of the protecting powers in humanitarian matters, a role it had already exercised during World War II and its aftermath when it tried to help prisoners of war who had no one to speak on their behalf. Since protecting powers assumed responsibility not only for prisoners, but also for the wounded and sick, civilians, and civilian populations, the ICRC would extend the scope of its own activities to these same categories of victims.[686] The ICRC was not in a position to present itself as the only body able to substitute for the protecting powers; during the Conference of Government Experts in April, 1947, the participants, remembering the debate concerning the ICRC's inadequacies during World War II, had noted that should Switzerland be occupied, the ICRC would no longer be able to operate.[687] The French expert Georges Cahen-Salvador then proposed that the convention allow for the possibility of creating a competent international body able to take the ICRC's place if the ICRC should become either incapable of acting or unsuited to meeting the needs of the victims. An international body of this kind, benefiting from the support of the states, would be in a better position than the ICRC to fight against war crimes or large-scale massacres, according to Cahen-Salvador.

The ICRC opposed this proposal.[688] Indeed, precisely because such a body would be international in composition, its operations could easily fall prey to political motives and bias. Yet impartiality was a fundamental principle of the Geneva Convention, and the most important of the Red Cross principles of which the ICRC was the guardian. Instead of openly opposing any mention of a competent international body in the revised or new conven-

[686]XVIIth International Conference of the Red Cross, Stockholm, August 1948, *Draft Revised or New Conventions*, Art. 8/9/9/9, pp. 809, 36–37, 57, 157.

[687]J.N.B. Crawford (Lt. Col.), National Defence, W.B. Amstrong (Capt.), National Defence, K.J. Burbridge, External Affairs, Ottawa, 'Report of the Sub-Committee of the Interdepartmental Committee of Ottawa on the Revision of the 1929 Convention for the Amelioration of the Condition of the Wounded and Sick in Armies in the Field.' Confidential, Ottawa, May 28, 1948. Annex to letter from Commonwealth Relations Office (signature illegible), London, to Under-Secretary of State, Foreign Office, London, July 6, 1948 (FO 369/3969.K.7957). See also ICRC, procès-verbal, Commission juridique, Jan. 16, 1948 (AICRC CR 211).

[688]See in particular ICRC, procès-verbal, Commission juridique, meeting of Jan. 16, 1948. (AICRC, CR 211).

tions, the ICRC came up with the idea of a 'lightning rod' article,[689] that would prevent humanitarian actions carried out in accordance with these conventions from becoming politicized or biased; the tasks allotted to the protecting powers or the ICRC could also be entrusted to 'an impartial body such as the International Committee of the Red Cross.'[690] If this formula – which avoided the qualifier 'international' – were accepted, the ICRC would be recognized in international law as impartial by nature in the format it held at the moment the draft conventions were presented in Stockholm – that is, with its uninational, Swiss composition; and any other body eligible to replace it would have to offer the same guarantees of impartiality. Up until then, impartiality had been a principle to be observed in the course of a humanitarian action. Now, however, given the threats to the ICRC's future, the competition the organization faced, and its desire to avoid the risk of humanitarian actions becoming politicized, the authors of the convention presented impartiality as a constitutive quality of the ICRC.

The ICRC, recognized as the model for impartial organizations, was to be granted, besides the role of substitute for the protecting powers, a right of initiative in respect not only of prisoners of war – which it already had under the Prisoners of War Convention – but of all the persons protected by the new or revised conventions to come.[691]

If these draft conventions were accepted at Stockholm – and subsequently, in Geneva – they would serve, for the components of the International Red Cross, as a kind of cement around the organization's common values and around the ICRC itself. They would also anchor in international law the recognition of specific services that the ICRC believed it would be able to render by virtue of its Swiss, uninational character. In this way, they would be a rampart against the internationalization of the Committee,

---

[689]Ibid.

[690]XVIIth International Conference of the Red Cross, Stockholm, August 1948, *Draft Revised or New Conventions*, Art. 8/9/9/9, pp. 8–9, 36–37, 57, 157.

[691]Ibid., Art. 7/8/8/8, pp. 8, 36, 56, 156–157. Besides permitting the ICRC to offer its services as a substitute for the protecting power and confirming and extending its right of humanitarian initiative, the 'Draft Revised or New Conventions' submitted to the Stockholm Conference included many provisions intended to give the ICRC specific tasks and attributes. See in particular Art. 13, 18, and 36 of the revised version of the 1929 Geneva Convention and Art. 59, 61, 62, 64, 65, 99, 113, 115, and 116 of the revised Prisoners of War Convention.

A breach in the rampart

while sanctioning the name 'International Committee of the Red Cross.'

There was, however, a breach in this rampart. In order to maximize the draft conventions' chances of winning the approval of the Stockholm Conference, the ICRC had decided not to introduce a provision stipulating its own funding by the signatory states. Some states might have hesitated to ratify such a provision.[692] This meant that the proposal to universalize the financing of the ICRC would have to be examined when and if the 1928 Statutes of the International Red Cross were revised. The risk was that the states of Eastern Europe – followed, perhaps, by others – would make their undertaking to contribute to the regular upkeep of the ICRC conditional on the internationalization of its membership.[693]

The ICRC had no procedural means of parrying such a risk. The only solution was to rally a maximum of votes before the conference, by convincing the states of its usefulness as a neutral, independent intermediary, and by showing the powers to which it was already useful that they would be wise, in both the short and long run, to maintain the ICRC in its Swiss format and continue to allow it to recruit its members by co-optation. The only activity it could point to for this purpose was the one it had undertaken in the former Mandatory Palestine. In other places – Greece, Indochina – it had not been authorized by governments considered legitimate by the community of states to act on both sides of the battle lines and, consequently, to present itself as a neutral, independent intermediary. Moreover, its financial situation was so precarious that in order to continue its activities in Palestine and elsewhere, it was obliged to rely on the fund that the Swiss federal government had agreed

---

[692] ICRC Delegation to the Conference of Stockholm, work sessions, report on 7th meeting, Tuesday, Aug. 3, 1948. Present: Gloor, Odier, van Berchem, Carry, Chenevière, Cramer, Pictet, Dunand, Siordet, Mlle Jung, Marti, Kuhne, Borsinger, Perret, Schoenholzer, Wilhem, Horneffer, Robert-Tissot. Absent: Ruegger, Bodmer, Boissier, Chapuisat, Gallopin, Duchosal, Wolf, von der Mühll (AICRC CR 25).

[693] Memorandum from D.L.O. Davidson, to Secretary of State, Foreign Office, Aug. 9, 1948 (FO 369/3969.K.2000).

to put at its disposal in 1946 in case a new world war broke out.[694] Urgently seeking sources of funding other than Switzerland, the ICRC turned first to the United States, where Ruegger spent the days from June 17 to 30, 1948, accompanied by Wolf, who was well-known in financial circles, and by Jean Pictet, the ICRC's primary specialist on the International Red Cross Statutes and the humanitarian conventions.

The ICRC's action in Palestine: arguments for the defense

Ruegger met with President Truman on June 30, and, during his stay, with various officials of the State Department and the American Red Cross. Ruegger and his colleagues gave each one two memoranda,[695] designed to be sent to Britain as well, which revealed the tenor of their concerns and advocated solutions: essentially, in the short term, the rapid release of the frozen Japanese funds, which would save the United States and Britain from burdening their own budgets; and active support by the American and British governments and their National Societies for the preservation of the ICRC's Swiss composition.

In its memorandum on the structure of the International Red Cross, the ICRC stressed the operation it was conducting in 'Palestine,'[696] implicitly highlighting – through the facts it chose to stress – its acceptance by both the Arabs and the Jews: The ICRC had persuaded both sides to apply the humanitarian conventions; it had established two large safety zones and planned to create two more, one in Amman and one in Tel Aviv; it had evacuated civilians, notably the inhabitants of the Jewish Quarter of the Old City; it had protected and aided prisoners and wounded from both camps; and it had supplied material relief to both sides.[697]

The ICRC did not send a similar mission to Britain. Bevin being already well-informed, Ruegger settled for sending him a long

---

[694]According to letter from Ruegger, President of the ICRC, Geneva, to Petitpierre, head of the Federal Political Department, Bern, March 30, 1949 (AICRC CR 59).

[695]According to letter from Ruegger, President of the ICRC, Geneva, to George Marshall, US Secretary of State, and annexes A and B, July 13, 1948 (IZG, Zurich, Fonds Ruegger).

[696]Ibid., Annex A.

[697]Ibid.

letter enclosed with the same two memos he had given his American hosts. Ruegger made no allusion to the political implications – advantageous for the British, given their favorable orientation towards the Arabs – of its aid to the Mandatory power's hospitals and of the establishment of safety zones around the English administrative buildings in Jerusalem. In my view, the ICRC's impartiality obliged it to keep silent about the political aspects. It simply stressed the importance of finding a solution to the Committee's financial difficulties so that it could continue its actions in Palestine – in other words, unfreezing the Japanese funds, a move that would be less of a burden for Britain than granting a direct credit.[698]

Max Huber, the former ICRC president, was again at the forefront of the struggle for the ICRC. In July, 1948, the review *Foreign Affairs* published an article he had written which gave a theoretical demonstration of the utility of an independent, neutral ICRC in the role of the guardian of Red Cross principles, principles which the article promoted.[699] Ruegger mentioned the article to the American and British officials.[700]

Before the conference, the ICRC had highlighted its action 'in Palestine' to persuade the United States, the United Kingdom, and perhaps the Commonwealth countries as well to finance it and to take a stand favoring the status quo regarding any structural modification of the International Red Cross. During the conference, however, it preferred not to discuss the subject of Palestine, fearing that the issue of the safety zones might be too closely examined. Its fear was motivated by at least two factors.

First of all, the safety zone affair was liable to give rise to an ill-timed debate on the use of the red cross emblem. The ICRC was proposing to include in the revised Geneva Convention authorization for itself – and the other bodies of the International

[698]Letter from Ruegger, President of the ICRC, Geneva, to Bevin, Principal Secretary of State for Foreign Affairs, Foreign Office, London, July 24, 1948, with Annexes A and B (FO 369/3969.K.9000).

[699]Max Huber, 'The Principles of the Red Cross,' *Foreign Affairs. An American Quarterly Review* 26, no. 4 (July 1948): 723–727.

[700]Letter from Ruegger, President of the ICRC, Geneva, to Bevin, Principal Secretary of State for Foreign Affairs, Foreign Office, London, July 24, 1948, with Annexes A and B (FO 369/3969.K.9000).

Red Cross – to use the red cross to designate both itself and whatever activities it might decide to conduct on behalf of the military and civilian sick and wounded war victims.[701] At the same time, however, the ICRC staunchly maintained that the use of the distinctive sign should be reserved solely for the protection of the war wounded and sick, both military personnel and civilians; this simple message was intended to prevent the red cross from becoming commonplace and to encourage the belligerents to show greater respect for the persons, supplies, and buildings displaying the symbol. Extending its use to multiple categories of victims would mean exposing medical personnel, buildings, and vehicles marked with the protective sign to an increased risk of violations. The only chance of eventually returning to the exclusive use of the red cross lay not only in preventing an increase in the number of protective symbols, but also in insuring that the red cross and the emblems considered as its equivalents under the Geneva Convention conveyed a simple message to combatants: to spare the wounded and sick in wartime and, by the same token, the personnel and supplies that aided them.[702]

Contrary to this principle, however, de Reynier had used the Red Cross emblem for the safety zones in Jerusalem, arbitrarily assigning it – without any juridical basis – the protective function of the red cross that was normally reserved for the sick and wounded. He used it to indicate activities benefiting civilian populations, and the Committee had not dissuaded him from doing so. The ICRC, not having abided by the rules it had promoted, was not in a position to defend them. If the issue of the safety zones should come up, it might lead to a discussion of the use of the emblem. Bernadotte would be in a strong position to defend his own view that working for peace was not incompatible with the performance of his official duties within the International Red Cross, a view shared by the Alliance of Red Cross and Red Crescent Societies of the USSR and by the

[701] XVIIth International Conference of the Red Cross, Stockholm, August 1948, *Draft Revised or New Conventions*, Art. 36/-/-/-, p. 26.

[702] For a contemporary synthesis of the ICRC's position on the question of the emblem, see ICRC, *Revised and New Draft Conventions for the Protection of War Victims. Remarks and Proposals Submitted by the International Committee of the Red Cross, Document for the Consideration of Governments Invited by the Swiss Federal Council to Attend the Diplomatic Conference at Geneva (April 21, 1949)* (Geneva: ICRC, Feb. 1949), pp. 15–17.

other relief societies of the Communist countries of Eastern Europe. The ensuing discussions might be complex, and could delay the Stockholm Conference's adoption of the revised and new draft conventions. The ICRC, of course, wanted the drafts approved quickly, so that the diplomatic conference in Geneva where they would be definitively adopted could be convened as soon as possible.[703]

The other, less important, reason that the ICRC hoped the safety zones would not be discussed was that on the whole the experiment attempted in Jerusalem, as seen earlier,[704] had not conformed to the provisions for such situations set forth in the drafts that were to be presented in Stockholm. The ICRC therefore hastily put together a document to be held in reserve in case the subject of the safety zones should come up, in connection with the use of the emblem. This document was entitled 'Rules Relative to Neutralized Zones in Combat Zones,' and was based on de Reynier's experience in Jerusalem. In this document, the ICRC suggested that in emergency situations it should be authorized to establish safety zones unilaterally, and to place them under the sign of the red cross.[705] This provision could be added to the revised or new draft conventions after they were approved at Stockholm, so that it could be introduced at the Geneva Diplomatic Conference.

The safety zone enterprise in Jerusalem had been conceived partly because Switzerland wanted something with which to counter Anderegg's proposal,[706] and it was intended to be used as a showpiece at the Stockholm Conference; yet now, on the eve of the conference, it had become, paradoxically, a subject best avoided, since it might spark difficult and interminable debates.

Meanwhile, Anderegg continued to agitate in favor of turning Switzerland into a country of refuge. On August 13, 1948, Ruegger wrote him a quick message, thanking him for his interest in

[703]ICRC Delegation to the Conference of Stockholm, work sessions, report on 7th meeting, Tuesday, Aug. 3, 1948. Present: Gloor, Odier, van Berchem, Carry, Chenevière, Cramer, Pictet, Dunand, Siordet, Mlle Jung, Marti, Kuhne, Borsinger, Perret, Schoenholzer, Wilhem, Horneffer, Robert-Tissot. Absent: Ruegger, Bodmer, Boissier, Chapuisat, Gallopin, Duchosal, Wolf, von der Mühll (AICRC. CR 25).
[704]See Chapter 4, pp. 159 ff.
[705]'Réglement relatif aux zones neutralisées en zone de combat,' annexed to Hans Popper, note to the Legal Division, Geneva, July 19, 1948 (AICRC CR 201).
[706]See Chapter 4, p. 157.

the promotion of safety zones and hoping that the Stockholm Conference would 'be able to prepare, in a decisive manner, the codification desired in this matter.' He underlined the fact that the ICRC had 'succeeded in putting to the test, in Jerusalem, the system of safety zones under the ICRC flag.'[707]

The conference of Stockholm

Five days before the conference opened, on August 15, 1948, the Alliance of Red Cross and Red Crescent Societies of the USSR informed Count Bernadotte that it was not coming to Stockholm. The reasons cited were confused and reflected Soviet ignorance of the Red Cross world and the humanitarian conventions. During World War II, the 'Red Cross Conventions' had not been respected by the Fascist governments, namely Germany, Japan, and Italy. The Soviets believed that the ICRC's duty, as specified in the International Red Cross Statutes, was to supervise the strict application of the conventions, and that the organization had therefore failed in its task; according to the Alliance, it had known about the atrocities committed by the Fascists but had not made the slightest attempt to prevent or warn against these criminal violations of the conventions. And it had done nothing for their victims after the war, either; it did not protest the plight of the displaced persons who were still being held against their will, in the former Fascist camps. Since the end of the war, the Alliance added, the ICRC had not raised its voice against the 'banditry of the Fascist Greek monarchy', nor against the bloodbaths in Indonesia and Vietnam. According to the Soviet thesis, however, the ICRC was not the only guilty party. The Standing Commission of the International Conference of the Red Cross was at fault as well, since it had made the mistake of inviting to the conference associations like the Automobile Club, the Scouts Organization, the Order of Malta, and the Pax Romana, which had nothing to do with the ideas and fundamentals of the Red Cross; it had also invited Franco's Spain, a regime which had been censured by the United Nations on December 12, 1946. On the basis of this collection of accusations, the Alliance

---

[707]Personal letter from Ruegger, Geneva, to Anderegg, National Councilor, Aug. 13, 1948 (AICRC, CR 201). [Translation: M.G.]

announced it would not come to the XVIIth International Conference of the Red Cross in Stockholm.[708]

The Soviet government also declined to attend, voicing only two complaints: that one of the conference's organizers was the ICRC, which had not protested against Fascist crimes; and that Spain was to participate.[709] Following the Soviet example, the Eastern European Communist bloc boycotted the proceedings as well.[710]

Ruegger refuted all the accusations in a restrained speech during the first session of the conference.[711] He asserted that the ICRC was not hostile to the Soviets, as evidenced by the Committee's efforts since 1946 to establish a dialogue with the Alliance of Red Cross and Red Crescent Societies of the USSR. As to the reproaches regarding the ICRC's silence in the face of Fascist crimes during the war, Ruegger simply referred the critics to the relevant pages of the ICRC report on its activities during World War II, which in particular explained, with examples, the organization's doctrine on protest and cases where conventions were violated.[712] He did not allude to the presence of the Spaniards, since that was the responsibility of

[708]Letter from Dr. Chodlokoff, Chairman of the Working Committee of the Soviet Union Red Cross and Red Crescent, Moscow, to Count Folke Bernadotte, Chairman of the Standing Committee of the International Red Cross Conference, Aug. 15, 1948 (FO 369/3969. K.9831).

[709]Letter from S. Basarov, Acting Chargé d'Affaires of USSR in Sweden, to Count Folke Bernadotte, Chairman of the Central Committee of the Swedish Red Cross, Aug. 17, 1948 (FO 369/3969.K.9831).

[710]Hungary and Czechoslovakia, which had already communicated the names of their participants, withdrew without explanation. See letter from Chancery, British Embassy, Stockholm, to Northern Department, Foreign Office, London, Aug. 26, 1948 (FO 369/3969. K.9831). However, in public statements made in Prague, Dr. Pavliç of the Czech Red Cross wondered what the ICRC had done to help the victims of the concentration camps, and where its sympathies lay in Greece, Malaysia, Spain, and Palestine. According to letter from Anthony Rumbold, British Embassy, Prague, to Bevin, Aug. 25, 1948 (FO 369/3969. K.9878). Romania and Poland did not respond to the invitation. Bulgaria sent its excuses; it lacked foreign currency. Yugoslavia contested the Standing Committee's right to invite it. Albania refused without explanation. See letter from Chancery, British Embassy, Stockholm, to Northern Department, Foreign Office, London, Aug. 26, 1948 (FO 369/3969. K.9821).

[711]Speech by Ruegger, first plenary meeting, Aug. 20, 1948, in Seventeenth International Red Cross Conference, Stockholm, August 1948, *Report*, Stockholm, 1948, p. 31.

[712]ICRC, XVIIth International Conference of the Red Cross, Stockholm, 1948, *Report of the International Committee of the Red Cross on Its Activities during the Second World War (September 1, 1939–June 30, 1947)*, Vol. I, *General Activities*, pp. 18, 173, 427, and 608.

the Standing Commission. Ruegger's sober response was disseminated through the press.[713]

The Australian and Indian delegates proposed to put a motion of support for the ICRC to the vote, but the United States and Sweden skillfully dissuaded them.[714] They doubtless felt it best not to make too much of the matter, in order not to discourage the USSR from coming to the Diplomatic Conference of Geneva – especially since the Swiss government, which had approached the Soviets itself, believed it detected in them a disposition to attend.[715] Another auspicious sign was that two representatives of the Alliance of Red Cross and Red Crescent Societies of the USSR were in Stockholm during the conference to participate in a meeting of the Board of Governors of the League of Red Cross Societies, which was being held at the same time in the Swedish capital. To everyone's surprise, these representatives discreetly attended the debates from the second session on, in the observers' gallery.[716]

In the absence of the USSR and the Communist countries of Eastern Europe, the great issues that had preoccupied the ICRC during the period leading up to the Stockholm Conference did not give rise to the debates the ICRC had feared. The main points of the conference may be summed up as follows:

– The conference adopted the *Draft Revised* or *New Conventions for the Protection of War Victims, Established by the International Committee of the Red Cross with the Assistance of Government Experts, National Red Cross Societies and Other Humanitarian Associations*, with a few amendments, and recommended that

---

[713]'Reply of the International Committee of the Red Cross to the Chargé of the Soviet Government,' Geneva, Aug. 25, 1948, communiqué no. 374 b. (FO 369/3969. K.9784).

[714]First plenary meeting, Aug. 20, 1948, in Seventeenth International Red Cross Conference, *Report*, p. 34.

[715]Letter from de Haller, Federal Councilor for Mutual International Aid at the Federal Political Department, Bern, to C. Rezzonico, Councillor of the Legation of Switzerland, Paris, March 10, 1948, annexed to letter from Haller, Bern, to Ruegger, Minister of Switzerland in Great Britain, March 10, 1948 (IZG, Zurich, Fonds Ruegger).

[716]Report to the Federal Council by the Swiss governmental delegation to the XVIIth International Conference of the Red Cross in Stockholm, Aug. 20–30, 1948, confidential, Sept. 17, 1948 (ADPF 2800.1967/59.-28/4).

a diplomatic conference be held as soon as possible,[717] to which it clearly hoped the major absentees would come.[718]

- Examination of the safety zone issue could not be avoided; there were Shertok's protests concerning the disgraceful incidents in the Government House zone, and the agreements concluded in Stockholm between Bernadotte, in his capacity as UN mediator, and the ICRC in order to establish around that zone a demilitarized belt under the control of the United Nations.[719] The ICRC turned the situation to its advantage, however – at its instigation, the Legal Commission of the Stockholm Conference approved an article[720] that would 'establish, in the regions where fighting is taking place, neutralized zones intended to shelter from the effects of war'[721] the wounded, the sick, and the persons 'taking no active part in the fighting, as, for example, the personnel responsible for the administration, supervision and food-supply of the said zones.'[722] But it would be up to the parties to the conflict to propose the establishment of such zones, through the intermediary of a neutral state or a humanitarian body, which could be the ICRC, but did not have to be. Neither Switzerland nor

---

[717]'Resolution XIX, Draft International Conventions,' in ICRC, Seventeenth International Red Cross Conference, Stockholm, August 1948, *Report*, pp. 92–93.

[718]'Resolution XVI, Appeal to Governments and National Societies Which Did Not Attend the Conference,' in ICRC, Seventeenth International Red Cross Conference, Stockholm, August 1948, *Report*, p. 91.

[719]See Chapter 4, pp. 184–5.

[720]Addenda to the *Draft Revised or New Conventions for the Protection of War Victims:* 'In view of practical experience gained in Spain, China and quite recently in Palestine, where neutral zones were set up in the immediate neighbourhood of fighting areas, the ICRC has thought it proper to introduce here a new Article, providing for the possibility of constituting such zones in similar conditions.' This Article 12A, added to the draft of the Convention for the Protection of Civilian Persons in Time of War, provided for the establishment of neutralized zones in combat regions to shelter without distinction the wounded and sick, whether combatants or noncombatants, and any other person not participating in the fighting. XVIIth International Conference of the Red Cross, Stockholm, 20–30 August 1948, *Draft Revised or New Conventions for the Protection of War Victims, Addenda and Amendments, Report of the International Committee of the Red Cross (Under Item III of the Agenda of the Legal Commission)* (Geneva: August, 1948), pp. 13–14.

[721]'Convention Relative to the Protection of Civilian Persons in Time of War,' Part II: 'Protection of Populations against Certain Consequences of War, Art. 12A, in ICRC, *Revised and New Draft Conventions for the Protection of War Victims. Texts Approved and Amended by the XVIIth International Red Cross Conference* [Revised Translation] (Geneva: ICRC, 1948), p. 118.

[722]Ibid.

the ICRC was mentioned in the article, in accordance with the low profile that Max Petitpierre had advised in response to Anderegg's proposal.[723] It was a tactical success for the ICRC.
- As for the provision extending the application of the conventions to non-international conflicts such as civil wars,[724] the ICRC succeeded in carrying the principle of the integral application of these conventions by the parties to the conflict.
- In the absence of the Soviets, the 1928 Statutes of the International Red Cross were not revised. The Americans and the British, following the anxious measures taken by Ruegger and Pictet, paid homage to the usefulness of a neutral, independent ICRC. The Stockholm conference did recommend that the Standing Commission be given a stronger role in coordinating league activities with those of the ICRC, but it added the cautious rider that the components of the movement were not to lose their autonomy as a result. It suggested that the cooperation between the two bodies could be exercised by means of regular meetings between the chairman of the League, the president of the ICRC, and the chairman of the Standing Commission.[725]
- The question of the regular funding of the Committee ran into difficulties. For one, many National Societies refused to commit themselves, since their own budgets were already strained. Moreover, some governments were given pause by the ICRC's attitude: To preserve its independence and prevent the donors from exerting any influence over its actions, the organization had declared itself the sole arbiter as to the assignment of the funds it was allocated.[726] The conference settled for turning the matter over to a commission of experts.[727] The issue thus remained unresolved, posing the risk

[723]See Chapter 4, pp. 157 ff.
[724]ICRC, *Revised and New Draft Conventions for the Protection of War Victims. Texts Approved and Amended*, common article 2/2/2/2, last paragraph, pp. 10, 32, 51–52, 114.
[725]'Resolution XIII, Strengthening of the Constitutive Bodies of the International Red Cross,' in Seventeenth International Red Cross Conference, Stockholm, August 1948, *Report*, p. 90.
[726]Report to the Federal Council by the Swiss governmental delegation to the XVII International Conference of the Red Cross in Stockholm, August 20–30, 1948, confidential, Sept. 17, 1948 (ADPF 2800.1967.59.-28/4).
[727]The experts were to be members of the National Societies of Belgium, Canada, France, Norway, and the United States. 'Resolution VIII, 'Regular Financing of the International Committee of the Red Cross,' in ICRC, Seventeenth International Red Cross Conference, Stockholm, *Report*, p. 88.

of a future revision of the International Red Cross Statutes, which could take place in 1952, during the next international conference of the Red Cross.

As Max Petitpierre correctly pointed out to Carl Burckhardt in a personal letter written in October, 1948, 'The ICRC's success in Stockholm is indisputable, but illusory in part, in the sense that the difficulties the ICRC was facing have not been either resolved or overcome, but merely avoided.' It was to be feared that 'the States of the East [might] decline the invitation made them to participate in the diplomatic Conference.'[728] On a separate sheet of paper, in a pessimistic, telegraphic style, Petitpierre had jotted down what he was really thinking: 'Anxiety, Red Cross perhaps condemned. . . .'[729]

For the ICRC, the moment had never been more critical, nor the future more uncertain. The organization had no more conventions to draft or substantial revisions to make. The diplomatic conference was now the exclusive business of the Swiss government, at least officially. The Statutes of the International Red Cross could not be revised until the XVIIIth International Conference of the Red Cross in 1952, at the earliest. The ICRC absolutely had to hold on somehow until then, and what ensured its survival was either work aimed at developing humanitarian law, or operations in the field. In ex-Mandatory Palestine, however, the site of the ICRC's only important operation at the time, the second truce, then in effect, seemed likely to lead to the termination of hostilities between the Arabs and the Israelis – bringing an end as well to the ICRC's activities as a neutral intermediary on behalf of the prisoners of war there, which had only just begun.

The refugees of Palestine and the Red Cross's quest for balance

Keeping active

The ICRC had to continue its activities in the former Mandatory Palestine; as justification, it could point to Article VII of the ICRC

---

[728]Personal, confidential letter from Petitpierre, head of Federal Political Department, Bern, to C.J. Burckhardt, Minister of Switzerland in France (ADPF.E 2800 1967/61/100). [Translation: M.G.]

[729]Manuscript by Pertitpierre, head of Federal Political Department, Oct. 15, 1948 (ADPF.E 2800 1967/61/100).

Statutes, which stipulated that in peacetime the ICRC 'shall work for the relief of distress considered to be a result of war.'[730] The victims of the aftermath of the Arab-Israeli war were likely to be the Arab refugees, in whom the ICRC had begun to take an interest in July, 1948. To understand the circumstances of this new focus, we must go back to the middle of June, 1948. At that time, the ICRC sent a delegate who had specialized in relief work, Pierre Calpini, to Palestine to evaluate, at the donors' request, the exact needs of the hospitals and dispensaries there. During his mission, which lasted from mid-June to mid-July, 1948, Calpini studied the possibility of setting up a system to take delivery, store, and transport relief supplies from Beirut. For Israel, such supplies could be sent via Haifa, while for Arab Palestine (the Nablus Triangle, the Hebron region) they would pass through Amman.

In July, 1948, the Arab League countries began to draw international attention to the plight of the Arab Palestinians who had found refuge either in what used to be Mandatory Palestine itself or in other Arab countries. During the same period, Calpini told the ICRC that the Arab authorities were showing interest in the Palestinian refugees. Calpini suggested to the ICRC that it put part of the large donations received for the hospitals at the disposal of these refugees, and pointed out that this gesture would be appreciated for its true value when the time came; to the Arab states, the ICRC would appear as the only organization to have undertaken such a move spontaneously.[731] Calpini admitted that an ICRC action on behalf of the Arab refugees of Palestine did not fall into the traditional purview of that organization – namely, the activities of a neutral intermediary – but he thought the Committee should assist the refugees all the same, because of the positive impression it would make on the Arab states 'from the humanitarian as well as the political point of view. . . .'[732] At about the same time, ICRC nurses, motivated by compassion, drew the Committee's attention to the general destitution of these refugees, for whom they themselves, here and

---

[730]'Statutes of the International Red Cross,' Article VII, in ICRC/LSCR, *Handbook*, p. 307.

[731]Note from Calpini, ICRC Delegation in Syria and Lebanon, 'Rapport sur l'activité dans le domaine des secours du 15 juin au 15 juillet 1948,' Beirut, to ICRC Geneva, July 24, 1948 (AICRC, G.59/I/G.C.).

[732]Note from Calpini, ICRC Beirut, to Dunand, ICRC Geneva, July 16, 1948 (AICRC, G.59/I/G.C.). [Translation: M.G.]

there, had undertaken little initiatives based on scanty means and the strength of their devotion.[733]

Politically, the issue began to loom large from the beginning of August, 1948. On August 2, Alexander Cadogan of the United Kingdom delegation to Lake Success took the problem of the Palestinian refugees to the Security Council.[734] He suggested that 'the Security Council might ask the International Red Cross to send' a study mission to Palestine with instructions to make recommendations, and stated that if, 'as is almost certain to be the case,' it was 'found that extra funds [would] be required by the International Red Cross,' his government, 'for its part, [would] be willing to provide its due share, on the assumption that other countries also made appropriate contributions.'[735]

Rivalry with Bernadotte

The ICRC was ready to go ahead, but so was Bernadotte. In July, 1948, he sent an emissary of the American Red Cross, Wilfred de St. Aubin, to Palestine to make a preliminary study of the refugee problem. In response to Cadogan's proposal, he dispatched a second specialist, Sir Raphael Cilento, to the Near East, this time for the United Nations.[736]

After having instructed de Reynier to make inquiries about the mediator's initiatives,[737] the ICRC decided not to let Bernadotte steal a march on it, but to maintain its own advantage with respect to Arab refugees; it, after all, had been the first to under-

---

[733]See, for example, note from Madeleine Weber, ICRC nurse, Gaza, to Lehner, ICRC Gaza, July 3, 1948, on the poverty of some 50,000 utterly destitute refugees who had arrived by sea from the Jaffa area. Sent on to the ICRC enclosed with a note from de Cocatrix, ICRC Cairo, to ICRC Geneva, July 12, 1948 (AICRC, G.59/I/G.C.). Note from Juliane Beauverd, ICRC Ramallah, to Odier, ICRC Geneva, Aug. 3, 1948, proposing that some tents left at the YMCA by the departing British could be used to set up a little refugee camp, an initiative which could be expanded (AICRC, G.59/I/G.C.).

[734]For the ICRC's perception of his speech, see note from Straehler, ICRC Delegation to the United Nations, Lake Success, to ICRC Geneva, Aug. 3, 1948, and enclosure: United Kingdom Delegation to the United Nations, 'Advance text of statement to be delivered by Sir Alexander Cadogan in Security Council on the question of refugees and the Palestine problem' (AICRC, G.59/I/G.C.).

[735]Remarks by Alexander Cadogan, United Nations, Security Council, *Official Record*, Third Year. 343rd meeting, 2 August 1948, no. 10, Lake Success, New York, pp. 6–7.

[736]Intercroixrouge telegram from Dunand, ICRC Geneva, to de Reynier, c/o ICRC Amman, Aug. 9, 1948 (AICRC, G.59/I/G.C.).

[737]Ibid.

take charitable activities on their behalf, providing material aid to the hospitals, dispatching nurses, and instituting measures to prevent disease. On August 16, 1948, it sent out an appeal to international charities on behalf of the victims of the conflict in Palestine. After congratulating itself on the achievement of a truce and the hope of a peaceful solution, and having explained that its 'essential task ... [was] to help prisoners of war and to ensure the supply service, protection and proper working of the hospitals,'[738] it announced the intention of extending its relief operations to benefit the Arab and Jewish refugees.[739]

Two days later, on August 18, 1948, at a meeting of the League Board of Governors held in Stockholm just before the conference, Bernadotte expressed his own intention of taking the refugee problem in hand, in his several capacities as president of the Swedish Red Cross, chairman of the Standing Commission of the International Conference of the Red Cross, and United Nations mediator for Palestine. Mentioning his obligation as mediator to monitor the well-being of all the inhabitants of Palestine, he announced that he would propose to the United Nations a large-scale operation on behalf of the refugees, Arabs and Jews. As usual, he fostered confusion between the UN and the International Red Cross, by appealing to the National Red Cross and Red Crescent Societies, as well as the ICRC, for help with his project.[740]

Bernadotte's decision posed a danger for the ICRC in terms of the future revision of the International Red Cross Statutes. In the framework of his project, the pyramidal structure that Depage had envisioned for the International Red Cross and which Bernadotte supported in principle might be put into practice on the concrete level. An operation by the ICRC and the League of Red Cross Societies, all their goals merged, on behalf of the refugees could come under the authority of the Standing Commission of the International Conference of the Red Cross, of which Bernadotte was the chairman. Such an operation might also be super-

---

[738]ICRC, Circular letter, Geneva, Aug. 16, 1948 (AICRC, CP 335 [4]).
[739]Cilento reported 7,000 Jewish refugees.
[740]'Count Bernadotte Appeal for Assistance to the Palestine Refugees, Board of Governors, Stockholm, August 18, 1948, in LRCS, *Report of the Relief Operation in behalf of the Palestine Refugees Conducted by the Middle East Commission of the League of the Red Cross Societies in conjunction with the United Nations Relief for Palestine Refugees. 1949–1950* (Geneva: LRCS, 1951), Appendix 1, p. 110.

vised by the UN, since Bernadotte exercised concurrent functions in the International Red Cross and the United Nations.

The ICRC could not allow itself to be carried towards a precedent so risky for its own future independence and its ability to act impartially, as well as for the future of the International Red Cross as a whole. In particular, it had to try to maintain one of the elements responsible for the International Red Cross's structural balance and harmony – namely, the agreement distributing powers between itself and the League of Red Cross Societies. It should be recalled that this agreement rested on the distinction between wartime and peacetime, the ICRC being the body empowered to deal with the problems of war and its immediate aftermath, while the League's mandate operated in peacetime. The ICRC, while preparing for the Stockholm Conference, had clearly set out to preserve, in any revised version of the Red Cross Statutes, this essential difference, which was stipulated by Article IX of the 1928 Statutes and was consecrated notably when the International Red Cross Joint Relief Commission was set up in 1941.[741]

Humanitarian understanding on a delicate subject

In the corridors of the Stockholm Conference, fierce negotiations began among the three executive officers: Ruegger, the president of the ICRC; O'Connor, the American chairman of the League; and Bernadotte, the chairman of the Standing Commission of the International Conference of the Red Cross. The problem was to define key words: What did 'peacetime' and 'wartime' mean, in ex-Mandatory Palestine? Was the truce to be considered a state of peace during which the League would be the body competent to act? For obvious reasons, it was in Bernadotte's interest to lean towards this interpretation.[742] Divisions and

[741] ICRC Delegation to the Stockholm Conference, working sessions, report of 4th session, Tuesday, July 13, 1948. Present: Ruegger, Gloor, Bodmer, Odier, Carry, Chenevière, Chapuisat, Siordet, Wolf, Marti, Mlle Yung, von der Mühll, Borsinger, Perret, Schoenholzer, Wilhem, Horneffer, Robert-Tissot. Absent: Boissier, van Berchem, Cramer, Dunand, Gallopin, Pictet, Duchosal, Pilloud, Kuhne (AICRC. CR 25).

[742] AICRC, 'Memorandum covering the meeting of Count Bernadotte, Mr. Ruegger and Mr. O'Connor on Sunday, 22nd August 1948.' Attached to note from Dunand, ICRC Delegation to Stockholm, 'Palestine, secours matériels notamment aux personnes déplacés,' to Chenevière, ICRC Geneva, Aug. 29, 1948 (AICRC, G.59/I/G.C.).

power struggles were evident, but it was imperative to find a harmonious solution, for on August 25, at the second plenary session, Ahmed Kadry, under-secretary of state in the Syrian health ministry and president of the Syrian Red Crescent, placed the issue of the Palestinian refugees before the conference, even though it had not been on the day's agenda. He was followed by the Egyptian plenipotentiary minister Hussein Rady Bey, extraordinary envoy from Egypt to the conference, who underlined the interest in these refugees that Bernadotte had already shown at the meeting of the Board of Governors in Stockholm.[743]

The debate threatened to turn stormy. Before the conference opened, the parties to the Arab-Israeli conflict had submitted to the conference secretariat documents containing their respective arguments concerning the refugees. Syria, in its paper, claimed that the Arab Palestinians had been deported by force, and established a parallel with the Jewish victims of Nazi persecution. It also declared that the atrocities of Deir Yassin were worse than Hitler's crimes.[744] Israel rejected these comparisons and allegations. According to the Hebrew state, the Arab Palestinians had not been forcibly deported, but had left or fled their homes, in some cases frightened by the Arab propaganda against the 'Zionist atrocities' – even though the Israelis had tried to persuade them to stay. In Haifa, for instance, the Jewish mayor had sought to retain the Arab residents. Moreover, Israel continued, those refugees who wanted to return home had been dissuaded by the Arab Higher Committee.[745]

Bernadotte, the ICRC, and the League all had an interest in insuring that the disputes between Israel and the Arab countries did not spoil or politicize the atmosphere of the conference; it was important to show the USSR a united front, in order to encourage it to attend both the diplomatic conference[746] and,

[743] Seventeenth International Red Cross Conference, Stockholm, *Report*, p. 40.

[744] According to document by Ahmed Kadry, President of Syrian Red Cross, no. 2.1.F, Aug. 5, 1948, cited in 'Note on the Refugee Problem in Palestine submitted to the International Red Cross Conference in Stockholm by the Delegation of the Government of Israel,' Aug. 1948 (ISA/MEA/1986.8).

[745] 'Note on the Refugee Problem in Palestine submitted to the International Red Cross Conference in Stockholm by the delegation of the Government of Israel,' Aug. 1948 (ISA/MEA/1986.8).

[746] According to note from Kahany, Representative of the Provisional Government of Israel to the European Office of the United Nations and to the International Committee of the Red Cross, Geneva, to Ministry of Foreign Affairs, Dec. 22, 1948 (ISA/MEA/1987.1).

perhaps, the XVIIIth International Conference of the Red Cross in four years. Whether speaking to the USSR or to the Arab states, Bernadotte, the ICRC, or Switzerland, depending on circumstances, all had a single, identical message to pass on: the Red Cross was neutral. Participants in the international conferences of the Red Cross attended for strictly humanitarian reasons, and the International Red Cross was not to become a forum for political debates. For the time being, the subject of the Palestinian refugees, a breeding-ground for propaganda, would have to be contained within the limits of propriety.

To that end, it was indispensable that the ICRC and the League come to an understanding based on a single concern: offering together a worthy humanitarian response to the problem confronting them. Together they would have to render aid to hundreds of thousands of Arab Palestinian refugees, and to thousands of Jewish refugees.[747]

The ICRC and international aid to the Palestinian refugees

The ICRC and the League finally came up with a written agreement which had the advantage of presenting that united front, on one hand, and, on the other, of not lending itself to the logic of a pyramidal structure for the International Red Cross – the ICRC had seen to that. The ICRC and the League recognized in each other distinct, independent powers. Until a peace treaty was signed and ratified between the Arab countries and Israel, 'Palestine' would be defined, for purposes of humanitarian action, as a single territory comprising Israel within its de facto borders and the regions of the former Mandatory Palestine under Arab control. Within this territory, the ICRC would be empowered to act as long as a peace treaty had not yet been signed. It would serve as an intermediary between the donors and the beneficiaries of the aid.

The League, in accepting this arrangement, had not renounced

[747] 7,000 Jewish refugees, according to Cilento; some 40,000 according to Israel. As for the Arab Palestinians: 550,000 according to Syria, 300,000 according to Israel, 330,000 according to Cilento. The differences apparently were not polemical but rather derived from calculations based on non-uniform criteria. Dossier 'Mission Calpini au Proche Orient' (AICRC, G.3/82). See also letter from Kahany, Representative of the Provisional Government of Israel to the European Office of the United Nations and to the International Committee of the Red Cross, to Dunand, ICRC Geneva, Dec. 6, 1948 (ISA/MEA/537.1).

the resolution it had taken in 1946 in Oxford, which stipulated that aid was to pass directly from one Red Cross society to another.[748] It had simply noted that in this 'humanitarian Palestine' there was no recognized National Society – neither the Magen David Adom nor the Palestinian Arab Medical Association. For that reason, it had accepted the idea that the ICRC could, in this case, act as a substitute 'national Red Cross' for the purpose of receiving and distributing aid. In the Arab countries surrounding the former Mandatory Palestine, however, the League would be the sole competent body, responsible for the coordination and distribution of aid by the National Societies. The Transjordanian Red Crescent was still in the process of being organized, for Transjordan had not as yet acceded to the 1929 Conventions; but this would not take long,[749] and it was no obstacle to the agreement between the ICRC and the League. The two bodies agreed that if strife broke out again in Palestine, the ICRC would be primarily concerned, while the League would render support if needed. If peace were established between Israel and the Arab countries, the ICRC would give way to the League. In the meantime, the ICRC and the League would offer the UN mediator their support and synchronize their activities with his.[750]

Under this agreement, Bernadotte, chairman of the Standing Commission of the Red Cross and United Nations mediator, would not lead an action 'of the International Red Cross' for the victims of the Arab-Israeli conflict. The ICRC and the League would carry out the operation in complete independence and a spirit of cooperation and mutual esteem, respecting their different roles.[751]

The 1948 accord between the League and the ICRC to aid victims of the Palestinian conflict was very important in terms of the revision of the Statutes of the International Red Cross.

---

[748]See Chapter 1, p. 22.
[749]Dossier 'Mission Munier à Amman' (AICRC, G.3/82).
[750]'Red Cross Relief in the Near East,' memorandum, Aug. 31, 1948, in LRCS, *Report of the Relief Operation in behalf of the Palestine Refugees Conducted by the Middle East Commission of the League of the Red Cross Societies in conjunction with the United Nations Relief for Palestine Refugees. 1949–1950*, Appendix 2, p. 113. See Annex 2.
[751]Dunand, ICRC Delegation to the Stockholm Conference, aide-mémoire, 'Secours de la Croix-Rouge au Proche-Orient,' Stockholm, Aug. 27, 1948 (CRI 1). See also 'Red Cross Relief in the Near East,' memorandum, Aug. 31, 1948, ibid.

FROM STOCKHOLM TO TORONTO

The Stockholm Conference had passed a resolution giving the Standing Commission the mission of 'insuring the coordination and harmony of the efforts of the International Committee of the Red Cross and of the League of Red Cross Societies'[752] in the periods between Red Cross international conferences. The 1948 agreement between the League and the ICRC eliminated the need for any intervention by the Standing Commission in their activities, if only the two organizations adhered to it.

Though the agreement allowed the ICRC and the League to prevent the Standing Commission from helping to coordinate their activities, it was nonetheless consistent with two other resolutions passed in Stockholm. One of these considered that it was 'essential to coordinate the relief operations undertaken in the spirit of the Red Cross' and recommended 'that the two international Red Cross institutions develop their mutual exchange of information, with a view to better coordination of Red Cross relief in their respective fields of action, it being understood that the freedom of action of the national Societies shall be fully respected.'[753] The other resolution supported 'the appeal made by the United Nations Mediator for Palestine, as well as by representatives of Middle East Governments, Red Cross and Red Crescent Societies for assistance to the victims of the hostilities in the Middle East,' and urged 'all Governments, and all national Societies to do their utmost through normal governmental and Red Cross channels to alleviate the suffering of the victims of hostilities, irrespective of race, creed, or political status.'[754]

For destitute Arabs: a major enterprise

When the Stockholm Conference ended, the ICRC and the League began to implement an operation to aid the Palestinian refugees. Their collaboration was completely disrupted, but at the same time reinforced, by Bernadotte's assassination on September 17, 1948. On September 23, the ICRC and the League

---

[752]'Resolution XIII, Strengthening the Constitutive Bodies of the International Red Cross,' in Seventeenth International Red Cross Conference, Stockholm, *Report*, p. 90.

[753]'Resolution XXXVI, Coordination of the Relief Work of the International Committee of the Red Cross and the League of Red Cross Societies,' in Seventeenth International Red Cross Conference, Stockholm, *Report*, p. 96.

[754]'Resolution XLIII, Relief Work in the Middle East,' in Seventeenth International Red Cross Conference, Stockholm, *Report*, p. 98.

issued a first worldwide, joint appeal on behalf of the victims of the Palestinian conflict, in which the two organizations explained their respective spheres of competence and gave potential donors information allowing them to direct their donations to either the ICRC or the League, as they chose.[755] The joint appeals from the ICRC and the League informed the donors that their contributions would not go only to the refugees, but also to the hospitalized wounded and sick and to the prisoners of war from both camps.[756] Consequently, from September to November, 1948, the ICRC not only continued its usual activities as a neutral intermediary on behalf of the prisoners of war, it also distributed 50 tons of supplies worth approximately 1,150,000 Swiss francs.[757]

On November 19, 1948, after studying an interim report from the mediator, the UN established the United Nations Relief for Palestine Refugees (UNRPR), a body responsible for implementing the program of UN cooperation with other qualified bodies, including those of the International Red Cross, to assist Palestinian refugees.[758] Trygve Lie, the UN secretary-general, put the entire administration of the program in the hands of Stanton Griffis, former US ambassador to Beirut. At this point, the ICRC and the League parted ways, each of them concluding a separate agreement with the United Nations.[759]

To the ICRC it was essential to remain as independent and distinct as possible from the United Nations. On December 16, 1948, it established with Stanton Griffis the modalities of its participation in the UN operation. From the ICRC's perspective, the UN would act as an ordinary donor; the ICRC would transmit and distribute all aid received in complete independence, adhering to its principle of impartiality. It would carry out its activities

[755] CICR/LSCR, 'Secours de la Croix-Rouge aux victimes du conflit de Palestine,' Geneva, Sept. 23, 1948 (Collection of Appeals, ICRC Library).

[756] Ibid. See also ICRC/LSCR, appel cojoint no. 2 (CP 402), 'Palestine, secours matériels aux victimes du conflit,' Geneva, Oct. 1, 1948 (Collection of Appeals, ICRC Library).

[757] ICRC, *Report on General Activities (July 1, 1947–December 31, 1948)*, Geneva, 1949, p. 114.

[758] United Nations, General Assembly, third session, 163rd plenary meeting, Nov. 19, 1948 (Doc A/731).

[759] On League action on behalf of the Palestinian refugees in the Near East and on the mechanics of its collaboration with the UN, see LRCS, *Report of the Relief Operation in behalf of the Palestine Refugees Conducted by the Middle East Commission of the League of the Red Cross Societies in conjunction with the United Nations Relief for Palestine Refugees. 1949–1950.*

in the territories under Israeli control and in the regions of Jenin and Hebron.[760] In the Gaza Strip, then under Egyptian control, the distribution of United Nations relief would be entrusted to the American Friends Service Committee (Quakers). The League, for its part, would distribute UN relief to the refugees in Syria, Iraq, Lebanon, and Transjordan.[761]

Thus, the agreement concluded between the ICRC and the United Nations in December, 1948, preserved the principle of a separation of powers based on the distinction between 'war' and 'peace' that the League and the ICRC had established at the Conference of Stockholm. Nonetheless, the ICRC considered that its joint operation with the UNRPR to aid refugees should remain an exception, distinct from its traditional activities as a neutral intermediary.

To conduct the refugee operation successfully, the ICRC created a Commissariat of the International Committee of the Red Cross for Refugees in the Near East, and entrusted its management to a Swiss, Alfred Escher,[762] in accordance with the wishes of de Haller, who represented the Swiss Confederation in the field of international aid.[763] From that point the Commissariat developed an enormous operation, much greater than the one the ICRC would have had to deploy at the beginning of the conflict in order to run the government hospitals in Mandatory Palestine itself, as the British had wished. Marti, it will be recalled, once remarked that, even if the ICRC had wanted to administer the hospitals, it would not have found the necessary personnel.[764] At the time, the ICRC had actually wanted to act as a neutral intermediary; but now things had changed. Cost what it might, the Committee had to maintain a presence in the Near East, even if the Arab-Israeli conflict subsided.

Politically resolute, certain of receiving donations, it found the

[760]'Agreement between the Director of United Nations Relief for Palestine Refugees and the President of the International Committee of the Red Cross' (CP 441b), Dec. 16, 1948. Annexed to note from G. Milsom, Undersecretary-General of the LRCS, and J. Duchosal, Secretary-General of the ICRC, Geneva, to the Standing Commission, Dec. 18, 1948 (CR 243/Pal).
[761]ICRC, *Report on General Activities (July 1, 1947–December 31, 1948)*, p. 115.
[762]ICRC, press release no. 382b, Dec. 7, 1948 (Press Release Collection, ICRC Library).
[763]Personal letter from de Haller to Ruegger, Nov. 3, 1948 (ADPF.3 2800 1967/59. BD. 91–92).
[764]See Chapter 3, p. 101.

necessary personnel: 92 Swiss delegates, doctors and nurses, 2 Danish nurses, and 3,395 local Arab workers. The number of people assisted rose to some 500,000. The main donor was the UNRPR, but UNICEF was also a substantial contributor. This ICRC action, undertaken for motives of institutional survival, was also the most authentically humanitarian and the most visible that it had conducted for the victims of the conflict since the arrival of its first delegates in Palestine. It was impossible to do justice to an operation of such magnitude in a few lines, and the ICRC did not try, compiling instead five voluminous reports containing primarily a quantitative appraisal of the aid provided. The reports were not published.[765]

Action on behalf of non-refugees in Jerusalem

At the beginning of 1949, not long before the Diplomatic Conference of Geneva was to open, the ICRC's only large-scale operation was the one being conducted by its Commissariat to assist the refugees of the Palestine conflict – and in which it did not act as a neutral intermediary. Its activities on behalf of prisoners – which were all that allowed it to maintain a delegation in Tel Aviv and another in Amman in the unstable Near East – were coming to an end. In the absence of a peace treaty, the ICRC wanted to remain present on both sides of the front for as long as possible.

The president of the ICRC found a solution to this problem in February, 1949, while traveling through the countries of the Near East. The solution was closely related to negotiations that his assistant, Wolf, was conducting in the United States to unblock the Japanese funds: The ICRC would take charge of the indigent Arab Palestinian population of Jerusalem that had come under Transjordanian control. The UN did not actually consider these people as refugees, and no organization was taking care of them.

---

[765]CICR, *Rapport général d'activité du Commissariat pour l'aide aux réfugiés de Palestine (Période du 1er janvier au 31 mai 1949)*, mimeographed (Beirut, 1950). CICR, *Deuxième Rapport général d'activité du Commissariat pour l'aide aux réfugiés de Palestine (Période du 1er juin au 30 septembre 1949)*, mimeographed (Beirut, 1950). CICR, *Quatrième Rapport général d'activité du Commissariat pour l'aide aux réfugiés de Palestine (Période du 1er janvier au 30 avril 1950)*, mimeographed (Beirut, 1950). Commissariat of the International Committee of the Red Cross for Relief to Palestine Refugees, *General Report on the Activities of the Medical Service* (Beirut, 1950).

FROM STOCKHOLM TO TORONTO

Their resulting destitution was heartbreaking. This operation to aid the people living in the neighborhood of the holy places would not only permit the ICRC to keep a foot in Transjordan, but it would also arouse public interest and provide a new argument for the financial negotiations Wolf was conducting in the US, something he could use to persuade the authorities to unfreeze the Japanese funds.

Accordingly, the ICRC embarked on the operation, and since it did not have the necessary budget, it drew on its own meager resources and on the donations made to the Commissariat.[766] It soon informed the American officials with whom Wolf was negotiating that it would not be able to continue the operation without additional funds, and in March, 1949, it finally received the 10 million francs that the Emperor of Japan had donated to it just before Japan surrendered. It was able to pay its debt to Switzerland and set up a permanent fund of its own which would insure its survival[767] until the XVIIIth International Conference of the Red Cross in 1952.

The operation on behalf of the Jerusalem poor[768] also allowed the ICRC to re-establish itself in the International Red Cross as a distributor of aid, and to regain the position it had lost when the Joint Relief Commission of the International Red Cross was dissolved by vote of the League Board of Governors at its Oxford session in 1946. On that occasion, it will be recalled, the Board of Governors had expressed the desire that the National Societies should begin to transmit aid directly from one to another – which was a way of ousting the ICRC from operations that involved supplying material assistance to civilian populations. In the ICRC's view, the Oxford resolution posed other problems as well: Countries without National Societies might lack the necessary transmission link, and aid distribution in general was more likely to become politicized.[769]

---

[766]ICRC, XVIII International Red Cross Conference, Toronto, July-August 1952, *Summary Report on the Work of the International Committee of the Red Cross (1st July 1947–31 December 1951)* (Geneva: ICRC, 1952), p. 52.

[767]According to letter from Ruegger, President of the ICRC, Geneva, to Petitpierre, head of the Federal Political Department, Bern, March 30, 1949 (AICRC CR 59).

[768]For a description of the humanitarian acts realized by the ICRC in the course of this operation, see ICRC, *Relief Scheme for the Poor of Jerusalem* (Geneva: ICRC, 1950), 14 pages.

[769]See Chapter 1, p. 22.

In August, 1948, the Stockholm Conference had taken formal note of the intention articulated at Oxford, and referred to it[770] in passing two resolutions that reflected its spirit. One of them advocated a more active role for the National Societies in assisting war victims,[771] and the other reinforced the task of the League of Red Cross Societies, which was to do everything in its power to facilitate the aid exchanges between the said societies.[772]

Confronted with the initiatives of the League and the ICRC, respectively, in favor of the refugees of the Arab-Israeli conflict, the National Societies showed a tendency to send their donations to the League, which was in charge of the refugees living in the territory of the former Palestine Mandate. By mobilizing the goodwill of the National Societies and other organizations suited to lend a hand with the action undertaken on behalf of those the ICRC called the 'poor of Jerusalem,'[773] the Committee was, in fact, thwarting the League's attempt to exclude Red Cross actions of solidarity towards civilian war victims. In this way, the ICRC established around itself, in the Old City of Jerusalem – a highly symbolic place – a 'Red Cross spirit,' which in principle tended towards a universal solidarity in the exercise of international charity.

The ICRC Commissariat's efforts on behalf of the refugees of Palestine and the ICRC delegates' work among the Arab poor of Jerusalem began to take on considerable dimensions: The ICRC set up 36 polyclinics, 12 mobile units serving villages, and 24 fixed units in the refugee camps. It opened 14 pediatric centers, 4 childcare centers, and 10 maternity hospitals. It organized the operation of the Augusta Victoria Hospice on the Mount of Olives, where it instituted a service for tubercular patients, together with a central pharmacy and a clinical testing laboratory. It set up a clinic in Bethany, a clinic and maternity hospital in

[770]'Resolution XXXVII, Relief Actions and Appeals by National Societies,' in Seventeenth International Red Cross Conference, Stockholm, *Report*, pp. 96–97.

[771]'Resolution XXV, Extension of the Activities of the National Societies to All Victims of War,' in Seventeenth International Red Cross Conference, Stockholm, *Report*, p. 94.

[772]'Resolution XXXV, Intensification of Relief Work of National Societies and the Role of the League of Red Cross Societies in the Exchange of Relief between the Societies,' in Seventeenth International Red Cross Conference, Stockholm, *Report*, p. 96.

[773]ICRC, XVIII International Red Cross Conference, Toronto, *Summary Report on the Work of the International Committee of the Red Cross*, p. 52.

Kalkilya, and infant welfare clinics in Tulkarem and Nablus. It subsidized the operation of the Austrian Hospice and the Arab women's clinic in the Old City of Jerusalem, as well as two hospitals in Nazareth. It supervised hygiene in the camps, fought against malaria, and, finally, reopened and administered 28 schools. At the end of 1949, it also created 22 sewing workshops to provide vocational training for Arab girls. These workshops employed several hundred workers and apprentices, who made clothes for refugees. For young people, the ICRC opened fifteen training workshops with UNESCO support: seven carpentry shops, five cobbler's shops, two tinsmith's shops, and one stonemason's shop. It provided milk for babies.[774] And this is only a sample. The ICRC also operated in northern Galilee, on the basis of an agreement it had concluded at the end of March, 1949, with the health ministry of Israel.

Staying in the Near East while waiting for the USSR in Toronto

The ICRC was going to try to remain in the Near East. It could not continue the operations of its Commissariat for Palestinian refugees, which was a non-traditional activity, nor its operation to assist the destitute Arabs of Jerusalem, without at the same time taking some kind of action as a neutral intermediary, since this had to remain the motivation and justification for its presence in a country at war or undergoing the direct consequences of war. Everything depended on Israel. Without a delegation there, the ICRC had no pretext for maintaining delegations in the Arab countries around it.

Accordingly, in September, 1949, the ICRC wrote to Moshe Shertok, Israel's minister of foreign affairs (who had recently taken the name Sharett), that it would be obliged to close its delegation in Tel Aviv, together with the corresponding ones in the Middle East, now that its traditional activities in the area were drawing to an end. But it had the feeling, following conversations with Israeli officers, that the Israeli army would like to see it prolong its mission.[775] The Israeli minister of foreign affairs confirmed this; the ICRC was still useful to Israel, because its

[774]Ibid., pp. 52–54.
[775]Letter from Wolf, Advisor to the President of the International Committee, Geneva, to Moshe Sharett (Shertok), Minister of Foreign Affairs, Tel Aviv, Sept. 14, 1949 (ISA/MEA/2406.6).

delegates, having access to both sides of the front, helped resolve individual cases.[776] To the ICRC, this was admittedly a minor activity, but one which allowed it to remain in the Near East and to conduct, at the same time, its Commissariat's operation for aid to Palestine refugees.

This immense operation, however, was jeopardized in December, 1949, by the Clapp Report to the United Nations, which recommended reducing funds by one-third – cutting the rations the ICRC allocated to the refugees by one-third as well. The refugees were likely to suffer considerably, and so was the ICRC's image in the Arab countries. Ruegger went to Lake Success, accompanied by David de Traz, a Committee executive, and Alfred Escher, who directed the Commissariat's activities, and pleaded the refugees' cause before the UN General Assembly. He obtained a reprieve.[777] On April 30, 1950, however, the ICRC was obliged to end its Commissariat's activities for the refugees of Palestine, which were taken over by the United Nations Relief and Work Agency for Palestinian Refugees (UNRWAPR). On the same date – which marked the end of winter – it also terminated its operation on behalf of the 15,000 indigent residents of Jerusalem who were not registered as refugees by the United Nations. It did not abandon them, however, but obtained from the UNRWAPR an undertaking to integrate 11,000 of them into the latter's refugee program. The other 3,000 were taken in hand by the World Lutheran Organization.[778]

Epilogue

The end of the ICRC's activities in the Near East

The ICRC still did not want to leave the Near East, which was the only terrain, as it were, where it could act as a neutral

---

[776]Letter from Eytan, Director-General of Ministry of Foreign Affairs, to Wolf, Advisor to the President of the International Committee, Sept. 27, 1949 (ISA/MEA/2406.6).

[777]'A Lake Success, M. Ruegger adjure la commission politique de l'ONU de ne pas réduire l'aide aux réfugiés de Palestine,' *Tribune de Genève* (Dec. 3–4, 1949): 1.

[778]Note from Gaillard, ICRC Geneva, 'Action du Comité international de la Croix-Rouge en Palestine et au Proche-Orient (été 1948–printemps 1951),' May 4, 1951, D.148 (AICRC, G.59/I/G.C.).

intermediary. It reopened a delegation in Jordan, in Amman,[779] the existence of which was justified only by the existence of the delegation in Tel Aviv.[780] In Tel Aviv and Amman, the ICRC concentrated its efforts on activities pertaining to the Central Tracing Agency, which were typical of a neutral intermediary: family reunification, searching for missing persons, transmitting civilian messages. It also tried to look after the Arabs who entered Israel without passing through the obligatory checkposts on the armistice lines, whom the Israeli authorities termed 'infiltrators' and normally imprisoned.

On July 31, 1950, however, Israel informed the ICRC that its presence was no longer deemed useful, since, in Israel's view, the organization's activities could be taken over by the armistice commissions and the Magen David Adom relief society.[781] But also and above all, Kahany pointed out to Ruegger, Chenevière, Gallopin, de Traz, Gaillard, and Wolf – who had met to receive him and to try to convince him of the necessity of maintaining a delegation in Israel – that the Hebrew state took a dim view of the local ICRC delegation's concern for the 'infiltrators,' considering that 'the movement of Arab infiltrators towards the territory of Israel is a true threat' to its security. In this case, it deemed the activities that the ICRC delegate in Tel Aviv – none other than Munier – was conducting to assist the infiltrators were 'undesirable, for the problem there is a political-military one, not at all a humanitarian one.'[782]

Kahany maintained that most of the Arab infiltrators were 'smugglers or looters who do not hesitate to kill Jewish settlers or Arabs living in the territory of Israel.'[783] Some of them may have been refugees trying to return to their former homes, 'but

---

[779] Note from de Cocatrix, Jerusalem, to ICRC Geneva, April 13, 1950 (AICRC, G.59/I/G.C.).

[780] According to memo no. 148, 'Le budget du CICR en Israel et notre contribution au budget du CICR,' from Kahany, Geneva, to E. Gordon, Ministry of Foreign Affairs, Tel Aviv, Sept. 22, 1948 (ISA/MEA/1987.12). The ICRC also had its two permanent delegations in Cairo and Beirut, respectively, which had no task other than to wind down the activities undertaken in Egypt and Lebanon during World War II.

[781] Letter from Sharett, Minister of Foreign Affairs, Hakirya, to Ruegger, President of the ICRC, Geneva, July 31, 1950 (ISA/MEA/2406.6).

[782] Confidential memo no. 148 from Kahany, Representative of the Government of Israel to the European Office of the United Nations, Geneva, to Gordon, Ministry of Foreign Affairs, Sept. 22, 1950, copy to Sharett, New York (ISA/MEA/1986.8). [Translation: M.G.]

[783] Ibid.

it is very clear that such a movement, if it were tolerated, would soon present a genuine threat of invasion.'[784] Kahany then reminded Ruegger of 'the very rigorous measures taken by Switzerland during the war against the illegal entry of refugees into Swiss territory.'[785] He underlined the difference, however: 'while the [Jewish] refugees not admitted or turned back at the Swiss border were thereby condemned to a certain and cruel death, nothing of that sort threatens the Arab refugees in the Arab countries, under the protection of their brothers. . . .'[786]

Nonetheless, Ruegger insisted on maintaining an ICRC delegation in Tel Aviv. He dropped the subject of the infiltrators to focus instead on the ICRC's transmission of civilian messages between separated family members, its inquiries about missing civilians or soldiers, family reunification, and civilian repatriation.[787] But Ruegger's arguments were not enough. At the end of August, 1951, the ICRC had to give in to Israel; it closed its offices in Tel Aviv and, simultaneously, in Amman.

The world gathers around the Geneva Conventions of 1949

The Diplomatic Conference opened on April 21, 1949, in Geneva, presided over by Max Petitpierre. The USSR was present, together with its satellites, in the same room with Spain and the Holy See. Israel was one of the 64 sovereign states in attendance. Greece was there too, together with Albania and Bulgaria. The Arab states had also accepted the invitation. This universality was an exceptional feat, given the state of international relations then, at the beginning of the Cold War.

The Diplomatic Conference adopted four Geneva Conventions, after discussing them on the basis of the Stockholm drafts and incorporating certain amendments. The four were as follows:

---

[784]Ibid. Probably without realizing he was addressing an advocate of energetic measures to turn back Italian Jews at the Swiss border during the Mussolini era in 1938.
[785]Ibid.
[786]Ibid.
[787]Letter from Ruegger, President of the ICRC, Geneva, to Moshe Sharett, Minister of Foreign Affairs, Tel Aviv, Jan. 29, 1951, and attached memorandum (ISA/MEA/2406.6). See also the publicity the ICRC gave this activity – emphasizing that it came into the category of its traditional neutral intermediary role – in its Feb. 1 press release, 'Le CICR et le Proche Orient,' cited by Kahany, Israel's delegate to the European Office of the United Nations, Geneva, to Eliav Pinkas, Tel Aviv, Feb. 1, 1951 (ISA/MEA/1986.8).

- the Geneva Convention for the Amelioration of the Condition of the Wounded and Sick in Armed Forces in the Field (or 'first convention');
- the Geneva Convention for the Amelioration of the Condition of Wounded, Sick, and Shipwrecked Members of Armed Forces at Sea (or 'second convention');
- the Geneva Convention Relative to the Treatment of Prisoners of War (or 'third convention');
- the Geneva Convention Relative to the Protection of Civilian Persons in Time of War (or 'fourth convention').

The Diplomatic Conference of Geneva did not accept a pure and simple extension of the application of the conventions to situations of civil war or comparable conflicts. Instead, it adopted an article common to all four Geneva Conventions (Article 3) which was a sort of miniature convention in itself. According to this article, in all non-international conflicts the belligerents would apply a series of principles expressing a minimum degree of humanity via-à-vis the victims. 'An impartial humanitarian body, such as the International Committee of the Red Cross, may offer its services to the Parties...'[788] to conflicts of this nature.

The fourth convention protected civilians who were not nationals of the power in whose hands they found themselves. This convention was applicable in occupied territories, and contained provisions prohibiting the occupier from changing the status quo, from carrying out deportations, and from taking hostages. These principles, in the ICRC's view, reflected the lessons that international humanitarian law had learned from the tragedies that had affected civilians, including the Jews, during World War II – tragedies with which the ICRC believed it had been unable to contend, lacking legal bases for intervention at the time.

The adoption of the Geneva Conventions by states which were divided by the deepest antagonisms was an indisputable success, largely due to the efforts of the ICRC. The conventions reinforced

---

[788]'Text of the Geneva Conventions as Adopted by the Diplomatic Conference on August 12th, 1949, with the Names of Signatory States and Particulars of the Reservations Made,' common article 3/3/3/3. In Federal Political Department, *Final Record of the Diplomatic Conference Convened by the Swiss Federal Council for the Establishment of International Conventions for the Protection of War Victims and Held at Geneva from April 21st to August 12th, 1949* (Bern, 1950), Vol. I, pp. 205–206, 225–226, 243–244, 297–298.

its own legal grounds for intervention, as it had desired. Article 10/10/10/11, shared by all the conventions, obliged the detaining powers, in the absence of a protecting power, to choose a substitute, which was to offer 'all guarantees of impartiality.' If they could not find one, they were to turn to 'a humanitarian organization, such as the International Committee of the Red Cross,' and would be obliged to accept its offers of service.[789]

Another desirable feature from the ICRC's point of view was that the Geneva Conventions confirmed, generalized, and extended the ICRC's right of initiative, as well as that of 'any other impartial humanitarian organization,'[790] while stipulating that these provisions would not constitute any obstacle to the activities that the ICRC might undertake on behalf of the victims protected by the Geneva Convention.[791]

As a sequel to the ICRC's experience of setting up safety zones in Jerusalem, the Diplomatic Conference of Geneva introduced in the fourth convention a provision allowing any party to the conflict to propose, either directly or through the intermediary of a humanitarian body, the creation of neutralized zones intended to shelter civilian populations from the effects of the war.[792] The ICRC was not given any explicit role, and the sign of the red cross (or its equivalents) was not to be used unless the zones were hospital zones – that is, created for the purpose of sheltering the sick and wounded.[793] Finally, the 'international Red Cross organizations' would be 'permitted to make use, at all times, of the emblem of the Red Cross on a white ground.'[794]

---

[789]Ibid., common article 10/10/10/11, Vol. I, pp. 206–207, 227, 245–246, 299.

[790]Ibid. common article 9/9/9/10, Vol. I, pp. 206, 226, 245, 299.

[791]Ibid.

[792]'Geneva Convention Relative to the Protection of Civilian Persons in Time of War of August 12, 1949.' Part II, 'General Protection of Populations Against Certain Consequences of War,' Art. 15, in 'Text of the Geneva Conventions as Adopted by the Diplomatic Conference on August 12th, 1949,' in Federal Political Department, *Final Record of the Diplomatic Conference . . . Held at Geneva*, Vol. I, p. 300.

[793]'Geneva Convention Relative to the Protection of Civilian Persons in Time of War,' in 'Text of the Geneva Conventions as Adopted by the Diplomatic Conference on August 12th, 1949,' Annex I: 'Draft Agreement Relating to Hospital and Safety Zones and Localities,' Art. 6, in Federal Political Department, *Final Record of the Diplomatic Conference*, Vol. I, pp. 336–337.

[794]'Convention for the Amelioration of the Condition of the Wounded and Sick in Armies in the Field,' Chapter VII, 'The Distinctive Emblem,' Art. 44, in 'Text of the Geneva Conventions as Adopted by the Diplomatic Conference,' in Federal Political Department, *Final Record of the Diplomatic Conference*, Vol. I, p. 215.

On the issue of the plurality of emblems, the Diplomatic Conference maintained the 1929 article authorizing the use of the red crescent or the red lion and sun by the countries that were already employing them.[795] This decision was reached following an impassioned debate that arose when the Israeli representative tabled an amendment to have the red star of David accepted as an emblem equivalent to those of the cross and the crescent. The ninth plenary meeting, chaired by Max Petitpierre, had met to examine this amendment, as well as proposals by India and Burma to introduce in the Geneva Convention a red sign on a white background with no religious significance, the design of which remained to be studied.[796] This would have delayed the adoption of the conventions. To everyone's surprise, Ruegger took the floor to make an unscheduled speech. The speech was ready, in French, and was immediately followed by an oral translation in English, also prepared in advance.[797] According to Emile Najar, who was presenting the Israeli position, Ruegger made a 'pathetic appeal against accepting any new emblem' and 'positively shouted, "The Red Cross is in peril!"'[798]

This exclamation was not recorded in the proceedings of the conference, but the rest of his speech was. Ruegger pleaded against the increase of protective emblems in order to avoid the progressive weakening of the sign denoting aid to the victims of war, but he especially emphasized the symbolic value of the red cross: 'If, on account of the multiplication of symbols, the emblem of the Red Cross were to lose its universal value, the word 'Red Cross,' which is itself perhaps equally, if not more important, would lose part of its universal significance.' The president of the ICRC beseeched the conference participants to 'make a common effort to avert such a disaster.' In conclusion, he said of the Red Cross: 'A kind of mysticism has grown up around the Red Cross, and innumerable lives have been sacrificed in the service of the idea which it represents. The Red Cross is borne

---

[795]Ibid., Art. 38, Vol. I, p. 213.

[796]Federal Political Department, *Final Record of the Diplomatic Conference*, Vol. II, Section B, Ninth Meeting, Thursday, 21 July 1949, 3.30 p.m., p. 223.

[797]According to author's telephone interview with Zvi Loker, Jerusalem, May 3, 1993.

[798]According to memorandum from Emile Najar, Ambassador of Israel to France, Israel's representative to the Diplomatic Conference of 1949, Paris, to Ezechiel Gordon, Director of the Division of International Organizations, Ministry of Foreign Affairs, July 24, 1949 (ISA/MEA/1987.6). [Translation: M.G.]

by vast spiritual forces and invisible legions.'[799] Perhaps these words were inspired by the recent example of the ICRC delegates in Mandatory Palestine and by the way that de Reynier had presented their heroic efforts to him, as sacrifices performed solely to serve the flag. They were, in any case, the product of the same state of mind. It should be noted, moreover, that the fact that Ruegger, president of a Swiss private organization, should intervene in an international diplomatic conference was reason to astonish the participants, particularly the representatives of Israel, who compared the incident to a government calling for a vote of confidence in its institutions.[800]

Like Ruegger, Najar, the delegate from Israel, fostered confusion between the protective sign – the 'label' on the hospitals – and the symbol; he talked of the Jewish people's deep-rooted attachment to the 'shield of David,' as it was called in the canticle in the Book of Samuel.[801] He pointed out that since biblical times this symbol had been linked to the existence of the Jewish people, and that it was the patrimony of all humanity. He emphasized that it was 'against this emblem that Nazism rose in the name of its racial dogma. Had this assault triumphed, it would have overwhelmed not only Judaism, but Christianity too, and all those who defend the cause of the equality of man and a universal conception of humanity.' His government, he declared, could not ask the Israeli people to renounce the red star of David and replace it with one of the signs recognized by the Geneva Convention. Moreover, added the Israeli delegate, the signs of the cross, the crescent, and the star, or shield, all being imbued with a moral force anchored in reality, should coexist. Although the Israeli delegation was ready to vote in favor of considering a neutral sign, as proposed by India and Burma, it still had not abandoned the immediate challenge of obtaining the recognition of the red star of David on the same basis as the other distinctive signs. 'We are not advocating a purely nationalistic point of view; we are endeavoring to help to assemble ... those forces without

---

[799] Federal Political Department, *Final Record of the Diplomatic Conference*, Vol. II, Section B, Ninth Meeting, Thursday, 21 July 1949, 3.30 p.m., pp. 223–224.

[800] Memorandum from Emile Najar, Israel's Representative to the Diplomatic Conference of 1949, Paris, to Ezechiel Gordon, Director of the Division of International Organizations, Ministry of Foreign Affairs (ISA/MEA/1987.6).

[801] See Chapter 4, p. 146.

which a truly universal institution cannot be built up,' Najar declared.[802]

Just before this vote, during a recess, the Italian delegate confided to Najar that 'the pressure by Ruegger, the Holy See, and the Swiss government' was such that he would not be able to vote for the adoption of the red star of David.[803] The Soviet delegate, at first opposed to adopting the red star of David, withdrew his opposition, according to Israeli documents.[804] But the Red Cross had the support of the Church – served by Catholic influences in the world – Switzerland, the English-speaking countries, and the Arab countries.[805]

The Australian delegate proposed a vote by secret ballot. Fifty-four delegations present were called upon to vote. The Israeli amendment was defeated by 22 votes against 21, with 7 abstentions, making a total of only 50. One of the Israeli delegates to the conference, Zvi Loker, expressed his perplexity regarding the results of the vote; by his calculation, there had been 4 blank ballots. Max Petitpierre discouraged him from trying to unravel the mystery, and from challenging the vote. India's draft resolution was also rejected, by 16 votes against 9, with 20 abstentions.[806]

'If you had succeeded,' Ruegger declared later, according to an Israeli representative,

> we would have had a throng of requests for new insignia from countries which, now that your demand has been dismissed, will adopt the red cross. Pakistan [which had

[802]Federal Political Department, *Final Record of the Diplomatic Conference*, Vol. II, section B, Ninth Meeting, Thursday, 21 July 1949, 3.30 p.m., pp. 224–227.

[803]Memorandum from Emile Najar, Ambassador of Israel to France, Israel's Representative to the Diplomatic Conference of 1949, Paris, to Ezechiel Gordon, Director of the Department of International Organizations, Ministry of Foreign Affairs, July 24, 1949 (ISA/MEA/1987.6).

[804]Letter from E. Gordon, Director of the Division of International Organizations, Ministry of Foreign Affairs, Hakirya, to Loker, care of the Permanent Representative of Israel to the European Office of the United Nations, Geneva, July 21, 1949 (ISA/MEA/1987.7).

[805]Letter from Israel Legation, Paris, to Eytan, Director-General of the Israeli Ministry of Foreign Affairs, Tel Aviv, July 29, 1949 (ISA/MEA/537.1 and 2406.1).

[806]Federal Political Department, *Final Record of the Diplomatic Conference*, Vol. II, Section B, Ninth Meeting, Thursday, 21 July 1949, 3.30 p.m., p. 232. See also Paul de la Pradelle, *La Conférence diplomatique et les nouvelles conventions de Genève du 12 août 1949* (Paris: Editions internationales, 1951), Section III, 'Les débats de la Conférence. La revendication d'Israel,' pp. 144–146, and Section IV, 'Le signe traditionnel en péril,' pp. 146–155.

allowed its National Society to adopt the Red Cross emblem] would have withdrawn its acceptance of the Red Cross, and the Indies would have asked for Gandhi's wheel. ... Now that Pakistan has accepted the red cross, and now that it has been stipulated that only those already using an exceptional sign have the right to continue using it, the Moslem countries that gain independence, such as Cyrenaica, Libya, and the other countries of North Africa ... will have to adopt the red cross. If this happens, and with secular Turkey's assistance, we are certain that all the Moslem world will soon adopt the red cross. By defeating your request, we have saved our Institution from an extremely serious danger.[807]

The Israeli representatives were not convinced by these 'illusory' arguments.[808] Since its proposal to add the emblem of the red star of David to the Geneva Convention had been rejected, Israel planned to sign the convention only with reservations, so that it could use the red star of David in situations where the convention stipulated the use of the red cross, crescent, or lion and sun.

On the whole, the ICRC had reason to be well satisfied with the results of the Diplomatic Conference of Geneva, which it had done so much to achieve. It had managed to gather together states representing the entire world and all the great ideologies, and gain their approbation for the documents of which it was the main author and promoter.

This left the Statutes of the International Red Cross. Because of a procedural matter, the risk of revising them had to be faced: It was in the framework of such a revision that the problem of regular funding for the Committee would have to be examined, in accordance with the decisions made in Stockholm.[809] The ICRC had achieved the beginning of a solution when the Diplomatic Conference recognized it as a possible substitute for the protecting power, a role which, the ICRC pointed out, would require it to be constantly available. Consequently, 'whereas the Geneva

---

[807] Letter from Israel Legation, Paris, to Eytan, Director-General of the Israeli Ministry of Foreign Affairs, Tel Aviv, July 29, 1949 (ISA/MEA/537.1 and 2406.1). [Translation: M.G.]
[808] Ibid.
[809] See above, p. 243.

Conventions require the International Committee of the Red Cross to be ready at all times and in all circumstances to fulfil the humanitarian tasks entrusted to it by these Conventions,' the conference passed a resolution in which it recognized 'the necessity of providing regular financial support for the International Committee of the Red Cross.'[810]

From this point on, the issue of a regular source of funds for the ICRC could no longer be invoked as a pretext for the revision of the International Red Cross Statutes, which diminished the risk of such a revision. And even if the revision of the 1928 Statutes had to be undertaken all the same, it could not lead to the internationalization of the ICRC's membership. Any structural reorganization of the Red Cross would have to guarantee that the ICRC could remain impartial. This postulated the preservation of the ingredients of both independence and political neutrality.

The resolution passed by the 1949 Diplomatic Conference regarding regular financing for the ICRC did not deter the International Red Cross from again taking up the issue of revising the 1928 Statutes, at the initiative of the Standing Commission, which met in Monaco on October 19, 1950.[811] The debate on the subject would take place at the XVIIIth International Conference of the Red Cross, to be held from July 26 to August 7, 1952, in Toronto. Probably to prevent the Standing Commission from taking an overly managerial role, the League and the ICRC, in the same spirit of cooperation achieved with the division of powers agreement they had signed in August, 1948, to aid the refugees of Palestine, concluded, on December 8, 1951, a detailed general agreement 'for the purpose of specifying certain of their respective functions.'[812]

The draft revision of the International Red Cross Statutes submitted to the Conference of Toronto was the product of the combined efforts of the ICRC president – still Ruegger – and the chairman of the Board of Governors of the League of Red

---

[810]'Resolution 11,' in Federal Political Department, *Final Record of the Diplomatic Conference*, Vol. I, p. 362.

[811]ICRC, procès-verbal, plenary session of May 20, 1952. (AICRC, no file number).

[812]'Agreement between the International Committee of the Red Cross and the League of Red Cross Societies for the Purpose of Specifying Certain of Their Respective Functions' (ratified by the Board of Governors of the League on Aug. 8, 1952, and by the ICRC on Aug. 27, 1952), in ICRC/LRCS, *Handbook of the International Red Cross*, 10th edition (Geneva, 1953), Annex IX, pp. 610–615.

Cross Societies, Emile Sandström;[813] the document had been endorsed by the Standing Commission of the International Conference of the Red Cross, which was presided over by a Frenchman, André François-Poncet.[814] Under this document, each organization of the International Red Cross would be conserved in its integrity.

The ICRC abandoned, however, the term 'neutral intermediary,' which had an unfavorable image in the Communist world, and defined itself more generally as 'a neutral institution whose humanitarian work is carried out particularly in time of war, civil war, or internal strife.'[815] It remained the competent body in wartime and its immediate aftermath.[816]

The League did not allow itself to be locked into a precise role, but gave itself complete latitude as to its spheres of activity. It specified its powers only with respect to the National Societies that it federated.[817]

The 1952 draft Statutes of the International Red Cross provided that the ICRC and the League would maintain contact in order to coordinate their activities.[818] The Standing Commission, for its part, granted itself the possibility of coordinating and harmonizing the efforts of the ICRC and the League, while stating explicitly that 'the independence and initiative of the various bodies of the International Red Cross in their respective spheres shall, however, continue to be strictly safeguarded.'[819]

A new era begins for the ICRC

Since the Soviet Union had attended the 1949 Diplomatic Conference of Geneva and had signed the conventions, it was duty bound to participate in the 1952 International Conference of the Red Cross; so this time it accepted the invitation. It demanded,

---

[813]Note from Ruegger and Sandström, 'Révision des Statuts de la Croix-Rouge internationale,' Geneva, Nov. 28, 1951 (AICRC, CRI).

[814]'Statuts de la Croix-Rouge internationale et règlement de la Conférence internationale de la Croix-Rouge, projet de révision présenté par la Commission permanente de la Conférence internationale de la Croix-Rouge à la XVIIème Conférence internationale de la Croix-Rouge,' Geneva, Dec. 7, 1951 (ISA/MEA/1986.8).

[815]Ibid., Art. VII.
[816]Ibid.
[817]Ibid., Art. VIII.
[818]Ibid., Art. IX.
[819]Ibid., Art. XI.

however, through the medium of the representative of the Alliance of Red Cross and Red Crescent Societies of the USSR, that all mention of the ICRC be simply eliminated from the future Statutes of the International Red Cross. In support of this demand, it cited in particular all the old arguments presented in 1946 regarding Hitler's crimes and the ICRC; having taken the side of the Fascists, the ICRC could not be considered as an impartial or neutral body, and should not call itself international. The delegation from the USSR societies would never accept the International Red Cross Statutes as they appeared in the 1952 drafts, according to the delegate of the Alliance of USSR relief societies.[820] The representative of the Swiss government was quick to take up the cudgels in the ICRC's defense.[821] Despite the opposition of the Communist bloc, including China, the revised statutes of the International Red Cross were adopted in the proposed version by all the bodies of the International Red Cross, by 70 to 17, with no abstentions.

The ICRC again found itself the target of Communist propaganda, of course, which now extended to its problems in the Korean War; but it could respond with greater force than formerly, since the Geneva Conventions recognized its international legal personality and gave its moral authority a basis in law. The USSR acceded to the four 1949 Geneva Conventions in 1954, and the United States followed suit in 1955. With such a foundation for its future actions, the International Committee of the Red Cross was on the threshold of a new era.

---

[820]XVIIIth International Red Cross Conference, Toronto, July-August 1952, *Proceedings* (Toronto, 1952), pp. 97–98.
[821]Ibid., pp. 98–100.

CONCLUSION

The action of the International Committee of the Red Cross in the Palestine–Eretz Yisrael conflict was carried out at a time when this humanitarian organization was facing one of the most difficult challenges in its history. The ICRC, a Swiss private institution, had been criticized for its conduct during World War II, primarily for the weakness of its efforts on behalf of the victims of the Nazis. The USSR and its allies accused it of being pro-Fascist and pro-German. Other states, such as Sweden, were more restrained, maintaining that the ICRC's excessive caution with respect to the victims of Hitler's crimes could be attributed to the fact that the organization was located in Switzerland, a country surrounded by Axis countries, and to the Swiss nationality of its members.

Seeking ways to reinforce the ICRC's effectiveness in future wars, in 1946 Count Folke Bernadotte, who held a key position in the International Red Cross, proposed that the latter's composition be internationalized. This idea was supported by the Alliance of Red Cross and Red Crescent Societies of the USSR and by the relief societies of the Eastern European Communist countries – if they did not simply advocate eliminating the ICRC altogether and replacing it with the League of Red Cross Societies. Other plans involved subordinating the ICRC and the League to a higher international governing council, and merging their purposes. These plans would affect the ICRC much as the plans for its internationalization would: They would deprive it of the ability to perform the tasks that made the international community recognize it as useful, namely upholding the fundamental principles of the Red Cross, on one hand, and acting as a neutral intermediary between belligerents, on the other.

CONCLUSION

Any change in the composition of the ICRC or the structure of the International Red Cross meant revising the Statutes of the International Red Cross, by means of a Red Cross international conference. Since 1928, these Statutes had governed the structure and operation of this humanitarian association. Article VII, which defined the ICRC and the tasks allotted to it, gave the Committee a position that was crucial to the unity and permanence of the International Red Cross. Since the ICRC was a private body whose members were Swiss citizens recruited by co-optation, and which was therefore unaffected by international pressures, Article VII of the Statutes considered that the ICRC possessed all the characteristics necessary to safeguard the principles of the Red Cross. It was these principles that allowed the humanitarian movement to develop harmoniously and to remain faithful to its ideal – notably, impartial action on behalf of war victims. Article VII also confirmed the ICRC in a role that, in fact, it had already been exercising for decades: that of a neutral intermediary among belligerents for the protection of war victims, particularly prisoners.

Thus, as I showed in the first chapter of this book, any attack on the Swiss composition of the ICRC and its system of recruitment by co-optation would prevent this organization from rendering its specific services as the guardian of Red Cross principles – without which the International Red Cross would lose its unity – and as a neutral intermediary on behalf of war victims – without which Red Cross operations in wartime would inevitably be paralyzed or politicized. World War II had just proven that the multinational League of Red Cross Societies was unable to organize an action of solidarity between the National Red Cross Societies that formed its membership.

Consequently, revising the 1928 Statutes of the International Red Cross could have disastrous consequences for both the ICRC and the entire International Red Cross, all the more so since the International Red Cross had not escaped the ideological divisions that marked the start of the Cold War. In fact, depending on which camp they belonged to, the Red Cross societies had differing views on the very nature of the Red Cross ideal, the objectives they believed they could or should pursue, and the correct way to apply the principle of impartiality that was supposed to characterize the actions of all the components of the International Red Cross. If its Statutes were revised, the International Red

Cross, already showing cracks, might well break apart completely.

Although it was itself the primary target of the anticipated revision, the ICRC, conscious of its importance to the unity of the International Red Cross and to the preservation of its founding ideal, defended the endangered movement's future quietly, demonstrating a remarkable tactical sense. Without denying the need to seek ways of enhancing its effectiveness in case of future hostilities, the ICRC fought against the internationalization of its membership. It tried to persuade as many National Red Cross Societies as possible to look for a solution somewhere other than in the revision of the International Red Cross system.

From its point of view, structural reforms could only weaken it, if not annihilate it entirely, and expose the International Red Cross to the danger of schism. To abolish its attributes and functions as defined by Article VII of the IRC Statutes would not be the appropriate response to the failings for which it was reproached. If it had managed to do anything at all in World War II, maintained the ICRC defensively – speaking with a single voice – it was because it had adhered to its role as a neutral, independent intermediary, a part it could not have played if it had not been composed of Swiss citizens who were recruited autonomously, by co-optation.

In exercising its role as neutral intermediary, the ICRC had been able to rely to some extent on the belligerents' obligations towards certain categories of war victims, obligations they had undertaken when they acceded to the 1929 humanitarian conventions. The ICRC's greatest failures had been in regard to victims who were not protected by those conventions. The ICRC concluded from this experience that if its effectiveness was to be increased in future wars, the assets it already had should be preserved and improved upon. All the elements that had brought it any success had to be conserved; its Swiss membership and autonomous recruitment method had to be maintained, and the juridical foundation for its intervention needed to be consolidated, through the updating of international humanitarian law.

It was therefore desirable that the Geneva Conventions of 1949 should cover the categories of victims whom the ICRC had been most powerless to help during the war: civilians and civilian populations. These future conventions should also provide for

CONCLUSION

situations that might arise in civil or international wars to come. Last and most important, they should assign specific duties to the ICRC, compatible with its role of neutral intermediary – such as substituting for the protecting powers. They should also stipulate that their provisions must constitute no obstacle to any humanitarian initiative that the Committee might wish to undertake. In this way, the states adhering to the conventions would be obliged to facilitate – indeed, support – the ICRC's efforts on behalf of the victims protected by these treaties. It was to be hoped that these future Geneva Conventions would be acceptable to all the states from the four corners of the earth, thereby uniting a divided world around a single humanitarian ideal, symbolized by the Red Cross emblem. The ICRC's capacity for effectiveness would then be reinforced, and its role as neutral intermediary and guardian of Red Cross principles – the ICRC's raison d'être within the International Red Cross – would be preserved.

To attain these objectives, the ICRC gradually developed a strategy – with no Machiavellian overtones – which included its action in the Palestine-EY conflict. The ICRC's desire to act in Palestine, the way it approached the conflict raging in the territory of the Mandate, and the order it followed in developing its activities there, all actually reflected the stakes of the battle it was waging to defend its integrality and its functions.

From the moment when the attention of the USSR, the United States, and the United Nations began to converge on Mandatory Palestine, the ICRC – universally criticized, misunderstood in the role of neutral intermediary conferred on it by Article VII of the IRC Statutes, and with its prestige at a low ebb – naturally attached greater value to its operation on this territory, since its activities there would be publicly observed. Through its actions, it would be able to prove its usefulness as a neutral intermediary in the field, a role it would no longer be able to assume if it were internationalized or subordinated to an international body. It therefore was grateful for Britain's public appeal asking it to intervene in Mandatory Palestine to help the Arabs, since the latter would not accept the United Nations. The ICRC, in contrast to the UN, could gain access to both sides of the battlefront, Arab and Jewish, thanks to its Swiss composition and autonomous method of recruiting members – which, it will be recalled, were designed to guarantee its neutrality and independence.

Its publications therefore highlighted the appeal the Palestine government had made to it at the end of December, 1947.

Since Mandatory Palestine was attracting the attention of the entire international community, it was also the place of choice to conduct an operation with demonstration value. This was the reason that the ICRC undertook and conducted its activities in Palestine almost didactically. It began by emphasizing its independence regarding Britain's wishes, investigating the needs of all the parties, and proposing to them a plan of action of its own devising that would theoretically benefit each one. It also posed conditions: It would begin to act as neutral intermediary only when the parties to the conflict had undertaken to respect the essential principles of the 1929 Conventions – that is, when they had given the ICRC the legal grounds it needed to intervene. It would not begin supplying material aid until it had started its traditional activities as a neutral intermediary. With this methodical approach, the ICRC illustrated the arguments it had opposed to the idea that its effectiveness could be improved through the revision of the 1928 International Red Cross Statutes.

Not only did the Palestine conflict provide the ICRC with an opportunity to demonstrate its specific services, it was also, by virtue of its timing – coming as it did between the establishment of the old conventions and the adoption of the new and revised ones – an arena where the ICRC could hope to create precedents for the evolving international humanitarian law; the ICRC's practices there could in fact influence the development of that law.

From March, 1947, to May, 1948, the ICRC saw the conflict in Mandatory Palestine as a civil war. Wanting to promote an article that would make future conventions applicable to civil wars, which it perceived as both the conflicts of the near future and the leaven for more distant, generalized hostilities, the ICRC tried to interpose itself between the belligerents of several civil wars, notably those of Greece and Indochina. Of the authorities it approached, only the government of Mandatory Palestine was disposed to allow it to act unrestrictedly, according to its principles, on both sides of the battlefront. With the revision of the 1929 Conventions in mind, the ICRC naturally appreciated Britain's attitude. Moreover, a clear understanding of its operation in Palestine might increase the willingness of the authorities

CONCLUSION

of home or colonial territories where other conflicts of the same type were going on to accept the ICRC's offers of service.

The ICRC did not forget the development of humanitarian law when it created safety zones in Jerusalem for the protection of civilians, either. Although this project was not carried out in accordance with the drafts of the new legal provisions, that was due not to the Committee, but to the head of the ICRC delegation in Palestine, de Reynier, who for one thing was not a jurist, and for another, was not able to acquaint himself with the relevant drafts until late in the operation. This did not prevent the ICRC from capitalizing on the action; on the basis of the experiment de Reynier attempted in Jerusalem, in 1949 it successfully promoted the adoption of an article allowing belligerents to agree on the creation of neutralized zones in the new convention for the protection of civilians.

Mandatory Palestine was thus the site of a strategic game between the two sides of the Cold War, a place where the ICRC could demonstrate its usefulness, and a practice ground where new legal provisions could be tried out. It was also, for the ICRC, the place to make a gesture – the good Samaritan gesture that Britain had requested from it. Although to do so it had to adapt its code of conduct, which forbade it to collect and care for wounded combatants itself or to be anything other than an intermediary, the ICRC nevertheless found ways to compromise, as witness the services it provided to the government and private hospitals, as well as its actions in the battles of Nebi Daniel, Gush Etzion, Katamon, and Kfar Saba. By taking care of victims protected by the Geneva Convention and emphasizing the convention's role, the ICRC was able to remind the world implicitly that it itself was at the source of that convention, and of the entire Red Cross, having been the first to formulate its principles of action. Accordingly, its publications described at length its actions on behalf of the wounded in the hospitals and, as an extension of that idea, the establishment of safety zones in Jerusalem to protect noncombatant civilians against the effects of the war. They related anecdotes and counted up the ICRC delegates' acts on behalf of prisoners and the sick and wounded, categories it linked together while making a distinction between combatants and noncombatants – as the Geneva Convention had done since 1864. Its operations to help civilian populations and the wounded and sick were also of a nature to interest the USSR.

The Geneva Convention – the first version of which, dating from 1864, cannot be dissociated from the creation of the International Red Cross itself – had established the principle of the immunity of the wounded and sick, and had instituted, to designate the equipment and personnel assigned to assist them, a sign that served as a distinctive label: a red cross on a white background. In principle, military authorities were supposed to furnish hospitals with this sign so that the enemy could spare them. Since 1929, the Geneva Convention had also recognized the validity, for the same purpose, of two additional signs: the red crescent and the red lion and sun.

Substituting itself for the military authorities, the ICRC marked the hospitals and other fixed and mobile medical equipment with the emblem of the Red Cross, which it had used as its own since 1863, and which in its eyes symbolized the spirit of the movement it had founded and the principles it guarded. The Red Cross flag, which in Mandatory Palestine flew between the red crescent – a Moslem symbol – and the red star of David – a Jewish symbol not mentioned by the Geneva Convention – was to bear witness to the unity of the Red Cross and the uniqueness of its ideal. At the same time, the ICRC, which would have liked the signatories of the Geneva Convention to go back to using a single distinctive sign, the red cross, fought against the prospect of additional emblems in future conventions. It could not, however, take the risk of suggesting the elimination of the red crescent, as the Arab world was not prepared to make such a concession.

The struggle against the multiplication of distinctive emblems led President Paul Ruegger of the ICRC, whose Catholic sensibility supported his political will, to call on the states convened in 1949 for the purpose of adopting the Geneva Conventions to oppose the addition of the red star of David to the gallery of existing emblems. In doing this, he confused the protective function of the sign and its symbolic value. Succeeding in his appeal, he managed to keep the Arab states among the signatories of the conventions; if the red star of David had been accepted as a protective emblem in the new, 1949 Geneva Conventions, these states might have refused to accede to them. This would have been particularly unfortunate at a time when the ICRC had good reason to hope that two other antagonistic camps, the East and

CONCLUSION

the West, would find common ground in the new conventions and adhere to them.

I have shown that the ICRC's general concerns were acted out, in various ways, in the Palestine-EY conflict and influenced its action there; but did that action influence the ICRC's struggles to safeguard the spirit of the 1928 Statutes of the International Red Cross and to promote humanitarian law to come? We lack the documents for the detailed analysis necessary to answer this question. The Committee, controlled by a neutralist mentality that kept political intentions unvoiced, formulated no assessment in this respect. Nonetheless, certain effects of the Palestine-EY conflict on the ICRC's general orientations can be pinpointed:

- The agreement concluded between the League and the ICRC in August, 1948, dividing their tasks in the provision of relief to Palestinian refugees. This agreement, conceptually the work of the ICRC, was necessitated by the competition that had arisen, in the circumstances described in Chapter 6, between the League and the ICRC over aiding Palestinian refugees. It saved the ICRC from coming under the control of a higher international body for aid to Palestinian refugees, which would have opened the door to the attempts to reform the structure of the International Red Cross – attempts that aimed to place both the ICRC and the League under the direction of an international governing council of the Red Cross. With this agreement, which laid out the division of duties between itself and the League, the ICRC managed to save one of the elements of the International Red Cross's structural and democratic equilibrium: the possibility for the League and the ICRC to decide together, through discussion, on their respective spheres and competences, making the best use of their differences.
- The re-establishment of the ICRC's financial situation, thanks to the operation conducted on behalf of the indigent population of Jerusalem. This stabilization was all the more necessary because the ICRC's financial dependence on Switzerland fueled the criticism regarding its excessively Swiss character.
- The 1949 Diplomatic Conference's adoption of an article allowing the parties in a conflict to reach agreement on establishing neutral zones for the protection of civilian populations – a cate-

gory of victims that the ICRC saw, at the beginning of the Cold War, as likely to be the main sufferers in conflicts to come.
- The refusal – in conformity with the ICRC president's wishes – to recognize the red star of David as a protective emblem in the Geneva Convention of 1949. This, however, merits some comment. Since 1906, the ICRC had consistently lobbied for a return to the single emblem of the red cross. However, since in 1946 the Arabs had refused to accept the red cross, the ICRC decided in 1948 to give up promoting the single emblem. Insofar as it had consented to maintain a number of emblems, the ICRC was no longer in a strong position to argue against the 1949 Diplomatic Conference's adoption of additional ones, such as the red star of David. But if it had supported the Israeli request and the conference had voted in favor of adopting the Israeli symbol, the Arab states, which did not recognize Israel's legitimacy, would certainly have refused to accede to the 1949 Geneva Conventions – conventions which had been conceived precisely to unite a divided world.

Taking all these aspects into account, then, it can be said that the Palestine-EY conflict affected the ICRC's general strategy at the beginning of the Cold War.

The ICRC's operation in Mandatory Palestine, begun in January, 1948, allowed the ICRC to maintain an activity it could highlight as being representative of its traditional role as neutral intermediary up to August, 1951, during a time when its participation in international affairs was reduced and its operations in other strife-torn areas were either limited or non-traditional. The question arises, however, as to whether this operation, which the ICRC held up as an example, was also exemplary in terms of the principles the ICRC had chosen to embrace: humanity, impartiality, and neutrality.

The head of the ICRC delegation in Palestine navigated the conflict there with the Committee's general objectives as his only compass, objectives which he tried to translate first to the circumstances of the Mandate, then to those of the first Arab-Israeli war. He did not know how to attune himself either to the suffering of the victims or to the cultural and religious context in which he gave the ICRC's activities their general orientation, on the basis of his instructions from Geneva. This was unfortunate, since, similarly, he did not have the wisdom to associate the belligerents with the success of his plans, himself monopolizing the interpretation of the provisions and spirit of the Geneva Convention. A soldier with an authoritarian personality, de Reynier tried to compel rather than to convince. And what was even more serious, the head of the ICRC delegation in Palestine could not manage to exercise an apolitical charity impartially. Conditioned by his affinities for the Arab world, by his taste for strategy and prestige, and perhaps also by his anti-Jewish prejudices – of which the Committee did not appear to take any notice – he undoubtedly sought to serve, in varying degrees and under cover of humanitarian purposes, the transitory strategic and political interests of the British and the Arabs – sometimes the Palestinian Arabs, sometimes the king of Transjordan.

Of course, de Reynier himself had no sense of betraying the ICRC's general objectives, nor its ideal. He saw no inconsistency between the humanitarian operations and their political fruits, if they would save lives in any case. Thus, he was satisfied with the contribution he had tried to make to the demilitarization of Jerusalem by attempting to place it under the Red Cross flag, or, failing that, by increasing the number of safety zones, even if they sheltered no more than a few dozen refugees. In this sort of initiative he was aided by Ruegger, who himself was greatly attached to Switzerland's prestige and the interests of Great Britain – and who was undoubtedly nostalgic for the political role he had been able to play in his recent duties as minister of Switzerland in various important posts.

De Reynier and Ruegger formed a tandem, since as of May, 1948, the ICRC president had placed the activities of the ICRC delegation in the Arab-Israeli conflict under his own direct supervision. But neither de Reynier nor Ruegger differentiated sufficiently between their respective roles in the ICRC. The president, in charge of the organization's general orientations as defined by the Committee, was not in the best position to worry directly about the war victims every moment; whereas the sole purpose of the head of the ICRC delegation was supposed to be alleviating the plight of the victims for whom the organization had accepted responsibility, by exercising the role of neutral intermediary. In serving these victims, he was morally obliged to act as their advocate both vis-à-vis the belligerents and in contacts with the Committee, as Marti had done when he refused to abandon the refugees of the *Exodus 47* for a public relations mission in the Balkan countries. Marti was not, for all that, insensitive to such a mission's political utility for the ICRC. He had therefore begged for a compromise solution, for the good of the victims whom he had assumed the responsibility of assisting and to whom he had given a promise he could not break. Marti and de Reynier, however, did not have the same temperament, nor the same conception of their relation to the ICRC and its ideal. While on the *Exodus 47* Marti used the ICRC in order to implement a humanitarian ideal he had made his own, the credit for which could be attributed to the institution later, de Reynier took the opposite tack. He served the ICRC, sometimes at the expense of that for which the ICRC had been founded: the role of a neutral, independent intermediary between belligerents to see that they fulfilled their undertakings in respect to the victims of the war. By taking this approach, he did an injury to the dynamics of the ICRC's operation in the Palestine-EY conflict.

It was apparently the ICRC nurses – too rare, scattered among a few hospitals in Palestine – who were the closest to the most needy victims, and the most effective in helping them. They gave Arabs priority, because they were attached to former hospitals of the government of Palestine which were intended for Arabs. If the ICRC had called upon them to serve Jews as well, they would probably have tried to alleviate their sufferings with equal respect for the medical code of ethics. But it was the rank-and-file delegates who turned to best account the ICRC's role of neutral intermediary, its right to initiate humanitarian operations, and the spirit of the 1929 Conventions in their efforts to 'humanize' the war in Palestine. Whether they were more deeply committed to the cause of the Arabs in Palestine, like Courvoisier, or fascinated by the Arab Legion, like Munier, or more sympathetic to the Jews, like Gouy, and perhaps Lehner and Durand as well, it can be said, on the basis of the documents consulted, that they acted impartially, devotedly, and modestly, for the benefit of all the individuals, Jews and Arabs, whom they had to assist in that difficult and dangerous setting.

For those delegates as for Marti, working among the refugees of the *Exodus 47*, the ICRC seems to have been what it was supposed to be: a tool with which to serve their humanitarian ideal. Each of them, individually and to the best of his ability,

CONCLUSION

knew how to merge the institution and the man to help the people on the battlefield or in the camps and prisons. For a time in their lives, these delegates, with some exceptions, took for their own a 'red cross code,' a doctrine that forbade all discrimination except for that inherent in the categories of the 1929 Conventions. Because of their subordinate position, however, they did not have enough influence to propose to the Committee any major initiatives adapted to the daily problems they encountered. The idea did not occur to them, and it is not certain they would have been heeded merely on the basis of their humanitarian motivation.

My research in fact demonstrates that it was political interests more than humanitarian convictions that motivated the ICRC's great projects in the Palestine conflict, whether or not they had the result of improving the lot of the victims of that conflict; this was the case with the protection of hospitals, the establishment of safety zones, and the institution of large-scale aid for Arab Palestinian refugees and the indigent Arab population of Jerusalem. The victims were not the only beneficiaries of these actions. The way the ICRC conducted them often reflected the organization's efforts to preserve its own independence and maintain the unity, through the mode and spirit of its cooperation with the other bodies of the movement, of an International Red Cross threatened by structural reform and diverging interpretations of the nature of its vocation and its working principles.

CHRONOLOGY

1928 The XIIIth International Conference of the Red Cross at The Hague adopts the first Statutes of the International Red Cross.

1929:
July 27
Revision by a diplomatic conference in Geneva of the Geneva Convention for the Amelioration of the Condition of the Wounded and Sick in Armed Forces in the Field, and conclusion of the Convention Relative to the Treatment of Prisoners of War, also called Prisoners of War Convention.

1934:

The XVth International Conference of the Red Cross in Tokyo examines, for possible adoption by a future diplomatic conference, an international draft convention concerning the condition and protection of civilians of enemy nationality on territory governed or occupied by a belligerent.

1938:

A Commission of Government Experts examines the possibility of providing, by an agreement between the belligerents, for the establishment of hospital and safety localities and zones which would be respected by the belligerents. The experts assign the ICRC the task of studying the plan further.

1939:

May 17 — Great Britain publishes a White Paper limiting Jewish immigration to Palestine to 75,000 people in five years. After that period, immigration quotas will be subject to Arab consent. Palestine will become a state with an Arab majority by the end of ten years.

1941:

The ICRC accepts the League of Red Cross Societies as an associate in its actions by founding with it the Joint Relief Commission of the International Red Cross for assistance to civilian populations stricken by war.

1943:

USSR directs first criticisms against the ICRC.

1945:

February 10

The Hebrew Committee of National Liberation asks the ICRC to intervene on behalf of Jewish Palestinian deportees being held in the Anglo-Egyptian Sudan.

February 15

The ICRC issues a proposal to revise the old conventions and to look into drawing up new conventions for the protection of civilians (Tokyo Draft) and the protection of civilian populations (safety zones).

March 22 — The Arab League Pact is signed between Egypt, Syria, Lebanon, Transjordan, Iraq, and Saudi Arabia.

April 25–June 26

San Francisco Conference for the adoption of the United Nations Charter.

April 30 — Hitler commits suicide.

May 8 — Official announcement of the Allied victory in Europe.

CHRONOLOGY

May 11
: Carl Burckhardt, president of the ICRC, sends a telegram to Edward Stettinius, chairman of the United Nations Conference in San Francisco, explaining the ICRC's priorities during World War II.

May 29
: The ICRC decides to follow up the February 10 request of the Hebrew Committee of National Liberation. It asks its delegate in Cairo to take care of the matter.

June 26   Signature of the United Nations Charter.

July 17–August 2
: Potsdam Conference.

July 23
: The ICRC delegate in Cairo suggests to the ICRC that the delicate situation in Palestine makes it unwise to assist the deportees being held in the Anglo-Egyptian Sudan. The ICRC in Geneva agrees.

July 26   The Labour Party wins the elections in Great Britain. Churchill resigns.

July 27
: The Hebrew Committee of National Liberation insists: The situation of the Jewish Palestinians being held in a foreign land is very difficult. The ICRC does not react.

August 6   The first American atomic bomb is dropped on Hiroshima.

August 9   The second American atomic bomb is dropped on Nagasaki.

September 5
: The ICRC decides to remind the World War II victors of its desire to revise the 1929 Conventions, and, particularly, to extend their application to civilians of enemy

nationality who are on territory governed or occupied by a belligerent (Tokyo Draft).

September 7
The ICRC decides to help the Jewish Palestinian deportees, who are civilians of alien nationality being detained on territory occupied by Great Britain.

October 1   Ben-Gurion asks the Haganah to fight against the British presence in Palestine.

October 12   The Arab League announces that the creation of a Jewish state will lead to war.

November 1   Great Britain and the United States announce the formation of the Anglo-American Commission of Inquiry on Palestine.

1946:
March 5   Churchill's speech at Fulton: 'From Stettin on the Baltic to Trieste on the Adriatic, an iron curtain has descended across the Continent.' Churchill calls on the English-speaking people to fight against Soviet expansionist aims.

March 22
Independence of Transjordan.

March 26
The Colonial Office discourages the ICRC from continuing to intervene on behalf of the Jewish Palestinian deportees.

March 28
The Foreign Office expresses misgivings concerning discussion of a new convention for the protection of civilians of enemy nationality.

April 26
The ICRC decides to re-examine a pre-war issue, namely

the possibility of extending the applicability of future new or revised conventions to situations of civil war.

April 30   The Anglo-American Commission of Inquiry recommends the admission of 100,000 Jewish Holocaust survivors to Palestine.

June 12–1 July
The ICRC delegate in Cairo receives permission from British army headquarters to visit the Jewish Palestinian detainees at the Asmara camp in Eritrea. The ICRC delegate asks the Committee to intervene, but receives no response.

June 24   In Switzerland, Emil Anderegg, National Councilor for the Canton of St. Gall, proposes to turn entire countries into safety zones for war victims, under the Red Cross flag.
The Swiss government is opposed and prefers that the issue of safety zones be developed by the ICRC in a legislative framework, namely the revision of the 1929 Conventions.

June 29   The British arrest 2,000 leaders of the Jewish community in Palestine.

July 16
The Board of Governors of the League of Red Cross Societies meets in Oxford.

July 16
The American Red Cross and the Alliance of Red Cross and Red Crescent Societies of the USSR call for the liquidation of the Joint Relief Commission of the International Red Cross. The ICRC risks being excluded from relief actions to benefit civilian populations.

July 22   IZL attack on the King David Hotel in Jerusalem, the headquarters of the British administration.

July 26–August 3
Preliminary Conference of National Red Cross Societies for the Study of the Conventions and of Various Problems Relative to the Red Cross.

July 29 The Paris Peace Conference opens, charged with the task of drawing up peace treaties with the satellites of Nazi Germany.

July 30
Bernadotte is appointed chairman of the Standing Commission of the International Conference of the Red Cross.

July 30
Bernadotte proposes to internationalize the composition of the ICRC, in reaction to criticisms of the ICRC's weak efforts to aid the victims of Nazism and concern aroused by the fact that ICRC headquarters are in landlocked Switzerland, and that its members are of Swiss nationality.

September 1946–February 1947
The Yugoslav Red Cross expresses violent recriminations against the ICRC, accusing it of being an accomplice by omission in Hitler's crimes.

September 27
The ICRC decides to resume its activity on behalf of the Jewish Palestinian deportees in the Asmara camp in Eritrea. It requests that these detainees be tried by due process of law, if they are not to be released. It maintains that it lacks legal grounds for intervention, and that it is acting on the basis of the humanitarian principles that guided its actions on behalf of the Nazis' victims. It hopes that Britain will prove less intractable than Hitler.

October 1 The International Tribunal at Nuremberg gives its verdict.

October 4 Truman speaks out publicly in favor of the partition of Palestine into a Jewish state and an Arab state, and in favor of mass Jewish immigration to Palestine.

October 15　The Peace Conference completes its work.

November 1
The ICRC decides not to come to the assistance of the Jewish Palestinian detainees in Palestine, for they are nationals of their own state. Imposing on itself the same restrictions that it did during World War II vis-à-vis the Germans detained by Hitler, it considers that Britain could accuse it of interference in its internal affairs. Under the terms of the Tokyo Draft, the ICRC can only intervene on behalf of civilians of alien nationality.

November 23
　　The War of Indochina begins.

1947

January 1　Fusion of the American and British occupation zones in Germany.

February 10　Peace treaties are signed with Italy, Hungary, Bulgaria, and Finland.

February 18　Bevin announces to the House of Commons that London will refer the question of its mandate in Palestine to the UN.

March 2　Declaration of martial law in Palestine.

March 3
The HCNL asks the ICRC to send a permanent delegation to Mandatory Palestine. The ICRC hopes that this request will permit it to conduct an operation in a situation of civil war.

March 3　The Palestinian deportees in Eritrea are transferred to the Gil Gil camp in British Kenya.

March 12   Truman presents his 'containment' doctrine to Congress.

End of March
    The ICRC seeks to initiate contacts with the Jewish Agency in order to establish itself as a neutral intermediary between this organization, the representative of the Jewish community in Mandatory Palestine, and the British government. It learns that the Jewish Agency would be interested in operations benefiting victims of the White Paper policy – namely, illegal immigrants.

April 2
    The ICRC decides to take resolute action on behalf of the Jewish Palestinian deportees in Kenya, as well as the Jewish refugees interned in camps in Cyprus and Jewish Palestinians detained in Mandatory Palestine by the Palestine government. In this way it extends its field of operations to categories of victims who would be its responsibility if it carried out an operation in the 'civil war' raging in Mandatory Palestine.

April–July   Increasing tension between the Jewish extremists and the Mandatory power.

April 14–26
    Conference of Government Experts to revise previous conventions and draft new ones. The ICRC wants to introduce an article extending the applicability of the conventions to situations of civil war.

April 15–16
    The British hang members of the IZL in Acre.

April 28   In New York, an extraordinary United Nations session on Palestine opens. It decides to create UNSCOP.

May 14   In the United Nations, Andrei Gromyko indicates the USSR's interest in the Palestinian problem, and announces that the USSR will support UNSCOP's

CHRONOLOGY

　　　　　　conclusions, whether they favor the establishment of a Jewish-Arab state or the partition of Palestine into two states.

May 16
The ICRC decides to send a delegate to Palestine to make cautious overtures to the British high commissioner regarding the possibility of the ICRC acting as a neutral intermediary in Mandatory Palestine, now on the brink of civil war.

June 5　　　Inauguration of the Marshall Plan.

June–July
The ICRC, criticized for its excessively Swiss character, decides to free itself of its financial dependence on Switzerland and to seek lasting ways to universalize the sources of its funding.

June–July　　UNSCOP study mission in Palestine.

July 2　　　The USSR rejects the Marshall Plan. One week later, all the countries of Eastern Europe turn it down as well – even those that had already accepted.

July 12　　　The conference of countries accepting the Marshall Plan opens in Paris.

July 18　　　The *Exodus 47* is boarded by the British off the coast of Gaza.

July 24　　　France announces it will take in the Jewish refugees from the *Exodus 47*, subject to their consent.

July 24
At the request of the Hebrew Committee of National Liberation, the ICRC begins its action on behalf of the *Exodus 47* refugees at Port de Bouc.

July 29　　　The *Exodus 47* refugees arrive in Port de Bouc on British warships.

July 31   The IZL hangs two British sergeants.

July 31
> **The Jewish Agency asks the ICRC to act on behalf of the *Exodus 47* refugees. The ICRC agrees and immediately asks for advance financial assistance.**

August 1
> **After having consulted the British, the ICRC gives the Jewish Agency an affirmative response, emphasizing that the action is at the Jewish Agency's request.**

August 22–September 8
> The Jews of the *Exodus 47* are taken back to Hamburg by the British.
> **Three ICRC doctors accompany these victims of the White Paper policy.**

September 9   The Jewish refugees from the *Exodus 47* are transferred to displaced-person camps in the British zone of occupation in Germany.

September 22–27
> Creation of the Kominform.

September 24–October 1
> **Regional Conference of European Red Cross Societies in Belgrade.**

September 26
> Britain announces it will withdraw from Palestine.

October 7–15
> Meeting of the Arab League, which envisages a military intervention in Palestine.

October 9–29
> **An ICRC delegate visits the Jewish Palestinian detainees in Kenya.**

CHRONOLOGY

October–December
: Consultation between the ICRC and the Swiss government regarding the co-optation of the ICRC's new president, whose principal task will be to improve relations between the ICRC and the Communist world, and to rally the International Red Cross.

November
: Because of the accusations the Communists made in Belgrade against the Swedish Red Cross, Count Bernadotte considers giving up his plan to internationalize the composition of the ICRC. The Alliance of Red Cross and Red Crescent Societies of the USSR, however, as well as the National Societies of the USSR's allies, remains favorable to the idea. Bernadotte decides to support another plan, which involves placing the ICRC and the League of Red Cross Societies under the authority of a higher body, the Standing Commission of the International Conference of the Red Cross. The ICRC could, in either case, lose its essential powers: its role as neutral intermediary between belligerents and its role as guardian of the fundamental, uniform principles of the Red Cross. It proposes a different way of increasing its effectiveness: reinforcing its legal grounds for intervention when it comes time to revise the 1929 Conventions. The reforms anticipated imply the revision, as well, of the 1928 Statutes of the International Red Cross. This revision could lead to a schism in the International Red Cross, however. It can be done at the XVIIth International Conference of the Red Cross, which will meet in August, 1948, in Stockholm, under the chairmanship of Bernadotte. The future of both the ICRC and the International Red Cross will probably be at stake then.

November 29
: The United Nations pronounces itself in favor of partitioning Palestine into two states, one Jewish and one Arab, and placing Jerusalem under an international regime.

December 5
> The United States declares an embargo on arms to the Near East.

December 12
> Small-scale Arab attacks begin against Jews in Palestine and are answered with Jewish reprisals.

December 20–23
> Paul Ruegger, former minister of Switzerland in London, is offered the presidency of the ICRC. He confides in the Mountbattens, who encourage him to accept; according to them, the ICRC would be more acceptable than the UN in certain parts of the world.

December 31
> The government of Palestine issues an appeal to the ICRC through the press, asking it to send a delegation to Mandatory Palestine.

1948:
January 5
> The Colonial Office and the Foreign Office confirm the Palestine government's appeal to the ICRC.

January 5
> In London, a few members of the Special Commission to Study Ways and Means of Reinforcing the Efficacity of the Work of the International Red Cross Committee (including Bernadotte), all belonging to the Western camp, try to find ways of avoiding schism in the International Red Cross. Two ICRC members who are in London at the time are consulted on an informal basis. They find an ally in the British Red Cross, which opposes the internationalization of the ICRC and its subordination to a higher authority, and which believes the 1928 Statutes should not be revised, but merely amended.

January 12 National Councilor Emil Anderegg reaffirms his

CHRONOLOGY

idea of turning entire countries into safety zones under the Red Cross flag.

January 20–February 18
ICRC delegates carry out a mission to evaluate the needs of the population in Palestine. The head of the future permanent delegation in Mandatory Palestine, Jacques de Reynier, has received discreet instructions to institute safety zones.

February 15
The ICRC delegates perfect a plan of action which includes, notably, the creation of safety zones.

February 25 The 'Prague coup' succeeds.

End of February–March 10
The ICRC decides to ask the Special Commission to Study Ways and Means of Reinforcing the Efficacity of the Work of the International Red Cross Committee to seek its solutions in the reinforcement of the ICRC's legal grounds for intervention and in the improvement of the old conventions rather than in structural reforms affecting it or the International Red Cross.

March
The ICRC appoints a Russian-speaking delegate to the United Nations in New York, charged with following the debates concerning Palestine.

March–April
Two ICRC delegates make a fundraising tour through the countries of the Near East.

March 5 The Security Council asks its permanent members to brief it on the situation in Palestine and to make useful recommendations regarding the implementation of the partition plan. It calls on the peoples in Palestine and around it to do everything possible to reduce the disturbances.

March 12
: The ICRC calls on the parties to the conflict in Palestine to respect the essential principles of the Geneva Conventions. This appeal is transmitted all over the world.

March 19
: The United Nations, at the Americans' behest, decides to abandon the partition plan for the time being and to hand the administration of the Mandate over to the United Nations Trusteeship Council after the British leave.

March 20
: Last meeting in Paris of the Special Commission to Study Ways and Means of Reinforcing the Efficacity of the Work of the ICRC.

March 25
: The United Nations Commission on Palestine agrees to the operation of an ICRC delegation in Palestine after May 15.

March 28
: The ICRC intervenes in Nebi Daniel.

End of March
: The ICRC places the hospitals of the Mandatory power under its emblem.

April 1
: The United Nations Security Council asks the Jews and the Arabs to cease all violence immediately and to come before the Security Council to negotiate a truce. It requests the convocation of an extraordinary session of the General Assembly in Flushing Meadows to pursue the issue of the future government of Palestine.

April 1
: The Security Council asks the Jewish Agency and the Arab Higher Committee to conclude a truce.

April 3–7
: The parties to the conflict (Jewish Agency, Arab

CHRONOLOGY

Higher Committee) agree to apply the 1929 Conventions.

April 8–9 Massacre at Deir Yassin.

March–April
The ICRC delegate prepares to place under the ICRC's protection the hospitals of the Palestine government, to be transferred subsequently to the power that the United Nations will instate, after the British depart, either over the former Mandate territory or over Jerusalem. He does the same for Britain's administrative buildings in Jerusalem, which he turns into 'safety zones.'

April 14–29
The ICRC sets up its delegation in Mandatory Palestine.

April 16 The extraordinary session of the UN General Assembly opens in Flushing Meadows.

April 17 The Security Council declares that the Mandatory power is responsible for maintaining order in Palestine and promises to support it completely. It asks all the states to refrain from supplying arms to either the Arabs or the Jews.

April 19–22
The ICRC creates safety zones in Jerusalem.

April 23 The Security Council establishes a Truce Supervision Commission for Palestine.

April 26 The UN General Assembly decides that the maintenance of security and order in Jerusalem is an urgent issue, and asks the Trusteeship Council to determine the measures best suited to protect the city and its inhabitants.

May 1–6
The ICRC plans to turn all of Jerusalem into a safety zone under the Red Cross flag.

May 2 The Security Council invites all the warring parties to cease hostilities at midnight on May 22, and asks the Truce Supervision Commission to give absolute priority to a truce in Jerusalem.

May 3

The Trusteeship Council examines the British suggestion to appoint, before the end of the Mandate, a municipal commissioner for Jerusalem – who might be Jacques de Reynier.

May 3–4
ICRC intervention in Katamon.

May 6 The UN General Assembly recommends that the Mandatory power appoint a special municipal commissioner for Jerusalem before May 15, 1948.

May 12
At the United Nations, Gromyko considers that the ICRC is exceeding its humanitarian mission with its proposals to neutralize Jerusalem, and in this way is serving Anglo-Arab interests.

May 13
De Reynier sets up safety zones in Jerusalem, still hoping to turn the entire city into a neutral zone.

May 14 The British Mandate ends, Ben-Gurion proclaims the independence of the state of Israel, the United States grants de facto recognition to the new state, and the Arab armies begin to enter Palestine.

May 14 The UN General Assembly decides to appoint both a mediator and, before the end of the Mandate, a municipal commissioner for Palestine. One of the latter's duties will be to promote the well-being of the inhabitants of Palestine with the assistance of the appropriate agencies, such as the International Red Cross and the other apolitical govern-

	mental and non-governmental humanitarian organizations.
May 14–15	**ICRC intervention in Gush Etzion.**
May 16–28	Fighting between the Arab Legion and the Haganah around the Old City of Jerusalem. The Jewish Quarter of the Old City is surrounded by the Arab Legion.
May 17	The USSR recognizes Israel de jure.
May 19–21	**The ICRC calls on the belligerents in Palestine to respect the safety zones in Jerusalem; this appeal is widely publicized in the international press.**
May 21	Bernadotte accepts the post of United Nations mediator for Palestine, even though he believes his chances of success are only 1%.
May 24	**The ICRC issues an appeal to the two sides presenting its role as neutral intermediary and urging them to respect the 1929 Conventions.**
May 27	**The ICRC closes down the safety zone it had established around the Italian hospital, which has become a battle zone for the Arab and Israeli troops.**
May 28	**The president of the ICRC evacuates the residents of the Jewish Quarter, which is surrounded by Arab forces in the Old City of Jerusalem.**
May 29	The Security Council asks the parties to call a truce for four weeks, and to communicate their acceptance of this resolution on June 1. If the parties refuse, or violate the truce, the Security Council

will reconsider the matter in terms of Chapter VII of the United Nations Charter.

June 2
The ICRC begins its strictly traditional activities as a neutral intermediary (repatriation of wounded and visits to prisoners of both sides of the conflict, in particular) and its material relief operations for prisoners.

June 11   The first truce begins. The Israelis reinforce their military potential.

June 15
Bernadotte, the UN mediator, moves into the King David Hotel, in the middle of an ICRC safety zone.

June 15–July 15
An ICRC delegate carries out a study mission in Palestine to determine the material needs of the hospitals and prisoners.

June 17–30
Ruegger-Wolf-Pictet mission to the US.

June 28   The IZL is incorporated into the Israel Defense Force.

June 30
The ICRC president asks President Truman for his government's support for the ICRC's position at the Stockholm Conference, and sends a letter making the same appeal to Great Britain. In both cases, the ICRC's operation in Palestine is cited as an example of the organization's usefulness as a neutral intermediary.

July   The Arab League begins a campaign in favor of the Palestinian Arab refugees and makes political capital out of it.

July 7   Israel and Transjordan agree to the demilitarization of Mount Scopus under UN supervision.

July 8	The first truce ends.
July 9	Bernadotte leaves the King David precipitately. The Haganah takes up a position there.
July 9–17	Ten-day war. Egyptian attacks on establishments and equipment displaying the red star of David, and Israeli reprisals against buildings and ambulances bearing the red cross.
July 15	The Security Council deems the situation in Palestine to constitute a threat to peace in the meaning of Article 39 of the United Nations Charter. It orders a truce, the beginning date of which is to be decided by the mediator in consultation with the parties. It orders that priority be given to Jerusalem and that a 24-hour cease-fire be observed in the Holy City from the time this resolution is adopted. It asks the mediator to work towards the demilitarization of Jerusalem, without prejudice to its future status, and to insure that the holy places are protected and accessible to all.
July 17	The second truce begins.
July 22	**The King David-YMCA safety zone is terminated.**
August 2	Israel deposits its formal instrument of accession to the 1929 Conventions with the Swiss government. In accordance with official procedure, the accession will take effect six months later.
August 2	At Lake Success, Alexander Cadogan draws a parallel between the Jewish displaced persons in Europe and the Palestinian Arabs displaced as a result of the Palestine conflict.
August 15–17	**The USSR announces it will not go to the Stockholm**

Conference, primarily because of its grievances against the ICRC.

August 16
The first ICRC appeal that mentions relief for the Palestinian refugees.

August 18
Bernadotte calls on the UN and International Red Cross forces to aid the Palestinian refugees.

August 19 The Security Council declares that the parties are responsible for truce violations by both their regular and irregular forces, and that they should not gain any military advantage from them.

August 20–30
XVIIth International Conference of the Red Cross in Stockholm.

August 31
Agreement dividing responsibilities between the ICRC and the League of Red Cross Societies in the matter of aid to Palestinian refugees.

September 17
Bernadotte is assassinated in Jerusalem by the Lehi (Stern group).

October
The ICRC establishes a central delegation for Palestine in Beirut.

October 8
In the Government House safety zone in Jerusalem, the ICRC gives way to the United Nations. The zone is demilitarized under UN control.

October 19 The Security Council points out the difficulty of demarcating the truce lines and the problem of Jewish settlements isolated in the middle of largely

Arab-populated zones. In particular, it advocates that the armies retreat to the positions they held before the battle of the Negev. It encourages the parties to negotiate the issue of the Negev directly or through the UN.

October 22 End of fighting in the Negev.

November 4

The Security Council calls on the parties to negotiate permanent armistice lines and demilitarized neutral zones. Should agreement prove impossible, the UN mediator may impose an arrangement.

November 16

The Security Council invites the parties to facilitate the transition from the truce to armistice accords.

November 19

The UN establishes the United Nations Relief for Palestine Refugees (UNRPR).

December 4 Stanton Griffis, US ambassador to Egypt, is appointed director of the UNRPR.

December 10

The UN General Assembly issues the Universal Declaration of Human Rights.

December 11

The UN General Assembly votes for allowing those Palestinian Arab refugees who wish to return home to do so, and for the payment of indemnities to those who do not. It decides that Jerusalem, Bethlehem, and the surrounding region should be separated from the rest of Palestine and placed under the effective control of the United Nations. It asks the Security Council to do what is necessary to demilitarize the city, and advocates a maximum of local autonomy for the communities living in Jerusalem.

December 16
: **Agreement between the ICRC and the UN concerning the mechanics of their cooperation in assisting the Palestinian refugees. Following this accord, the ICRC opens a Commissariat to aid the Palestine refugees.**

December 17
: The UN refuses to admit Israel as a member.

December 29
: The Security Council requests a cease-fire in the Negev.

1949:

January 6 — Cease-fire agreement for the Negev between Egypt and Israel.

February–July
: **Mixed medical commissions examine the wounded and sick prisoners on both sides who are eligible for repatriation under the 1929 Prisoners of War Convention, and these prisoners are repatriated, most of them by the ICRC.**

February
: **The ICRC president plans to begin an operation to assist non-refugee indigent residents of Jerusalem.**

February 3 — Israel's accession to the 1929 Conventions goes into effect.

February 24 — Armistice agreement between Egypt and Israel.

March 23 — Armistice agreement between Lebanon and Israel.

March 30 — Coup d'état in Syria.

April 3 — Armistice agreement between Jordan and Israel.

April–August
: **Diplomatic conference in Geneva and adoption of the**

CHRONOLOGY

four Geneva Conventions of August 12, 1949, for the Protection of War Victims.

May 11 Israel becomes a member of the United Nations.

July 20 Armistice agreement between Syria and Israel.

1950:
April 30
> The ICRC Commissariat ends its activities in aid of Palestine refugees, which are taken over by the UNRWAPR. The ICRC also concludes its operation on behalf of the non-refugees of Jerusalem, turning it over to a number of organizations.

October 19
> The issue of revising the Statutes of the International Red Cross is taken up for re-examination: The ICRC and the League risk having their actions supervised by the Standing Commission of the International Conference of the Red Cross.

1951:
End of August
> End of ICRC activities in Israel and the Arab countries.

December 8
> The ICRC and the League of Red Cross Societies sign an accord aimed at preserving some of their respective functions.

1952:
July 26–August 7
> XVIIIth International Conference of the Red Cross in Toronto. Adoption of the revised Statutes of the International Red Cross, which are not substantially different from those of 1928.

1954: The USSR accedes to the four Geneva Conventions of 1949.

1955: The US accedes to the four Geneva Conventions of 1949.

LIST OF THE DELEGATES AND NURSES OF THE ICRC DELEGATION

Delegates:

Names	from ... to
De Reynier, Jacques	Jan. 48 ... July 49
Courvoisier, Jean	April 48 ... May 49**
Gaillard, Pierre	April 48 ... Oct. 49
Gouy, Robert	April 48 ... Nov. 48
de Meuron, Maximilian	April 48 ... June 48
Dr Pflimlin, Raoul	May 48 ... April 49
Dr Fasel, Pierre	May 48 ... Aug. 49
Dr Lehner, Otto	June 48 ...?
Moeri, Emile	July 48 ... March 49
Durand, André	July 48 ... June 49
Calpini, Pierre	July 48 ... June 49
Fillietaz, Emile	Sept. 48 ... Jan 49**
Iselin, Frederic	Oct. 48 ... March 49**
de Reynold, Franz	Jan. 49 ... June 49**
Gaberel, Gaston	Feb. 49 ...?
Horneffer, François	Dec. 48 ... April 49**

Collaborating closely with the ICRC delegation for Palestine:
Burnier, Georges, delegate in Beirut
de Cocatrix, Albert, delegate in Cairo

Nurses:

Bolomey, Nelly	April 48 ... April 49
Giauque, Marguerite	April 48 ... Oct. 48
Thorin, Gabrielle	April 48 ... May 49
Kalt, Rosa	May 48 ... April 49**
Rogivue, Violette	May 48 and April-June 49

Weber, Madeleine	May 48 ... March 49
Beauverd, Juliane	May 48 ... Jan. 49
Heer, Hulda	May 48 ... Jan. 49**
Cousin, Florence	May-June 48
Visher, Rosa	May 48 ... Jan 49**

** means that these employees were transferred to the ICRC's Commissariat for Refugees.

Source: Jacques de Reynier, *Rapport général d'activité de la délégation du CICR pour la Palestine – Janvier 1948 – Juillet 1949* (Lebanon: July 1949). IZG IV.28.3.3.

BIBLIOGRAPHY

I. Unpublished sources

I (a) Archives

Archives of the International Committee of the Red Cross:
– Classification system not designed for the use of the public.

Swiss Federal Archives, Bern, Switzerland:
– Handakten Petitpierre.
– Handakten De Haller.
– Swiss Legation in London.

Central Zionist Archives, Jerusalem, Israel:
– Political Department, Jewish Agency.

Israel State Archives, Jerusalem, Israel:
– Ministry of Foreign Affairs.
– International Organisations Section.

Public Record Office, Kew, Great Britain:
– Foreign Office: FO 371, FO 369.
– Colonial Office: CO 537.

Institut für Zeitgeschichte, Zurich, Switzerland:
– Fonds Paul Ruegger.

Middle East Library, St Antony's College, Oxford, Great Britain:
– Sir Alan Cunningham's Private Papers.

Michel Doret's Private Papers, Geneva, Switzerland.

I (b) Documents
(In chronological order)

XVIème Conférence internationale de la Croix-Rouge. *Résumé des débats de la Commission juridique.* London, June 1938. Mimeographed, non-consecutive page-numbering (ICRC Library).

LRCS. *Advisory Conference of Delegates of Red Cross National Societies. Proceedings.* Geneva, October 15–November 2, 1945. Stenographic transcript. 2 vols. (ICRC Library).

ICRC. *Preliminary Conference of National Red Cross Societies for the Study of the Conventions and of Various Problems Relative to the Red Cross,* Geneva, July 26 to August 3, 1946. *Documents Furnished by the International Committee of the Red Cross.* Vol. I. Contained in Conférence préliminaire des Sociétés nationales de la Croix-Rouge, Genève, 26 juillet au 3 août 1946. *Rapports et Documents.* Mimeographed, no date, non-consecutive page-numbering (ICRC Library).

CICR. *Procès-verbaux de la Conférence préliminaire des Sociétés de la Croix-Rouge pour l'étude des Conventions et de divers problèmes ayant trait à la Croix-Rouge. 26 juillet-3 août 1946.* Geneva, 1946. Mimeographed, non-consecutive page-numbering (ICRC Library).

ICRC. *Preliminary Documents Submitted by the International Committee of the Red Cross to the Commission of Government Experts for the Study of Conventions for the Protection of War Victims, Geneva, April 14 to 26, 1947.* Contained in Conférence des experts gouvernementaux, 14–26 avril 1947. *Documentation Présentée par le CICR.* Mimeographed, no date, non-consecutive page-numbering (ICRC Library).

CICR. *Procès-verbaux des séances plénières de la Conférence d'experts gouvernementaux pour l'étude des conventions protégeant les victimes de la guerre, Genève, 14–26 avril 1947.* Mimeographed, no date, non-consecutive page-numbering (ICRC Library).

ICRC. XVIIth International Conference of the Red Cross, Stockholm, August 1948. *Co-operation and Relations of the National Societies with One Another and with the International Committee of the Red Cross and the League in Time of Peace and in Time of War, Report by the International Committee of the Red Cross.* May 1948. Mimeographed. 13 pages (ICRC Library).

ICRC. XVIIth International Conference of the Red Cross, Stockholm, August 1948. *Relations of the International Committee of the Red Cross with the United Nations and Other International Organizations, Report of the International Committee of the Red Cross.* June 1948. Mimeographed. 6 pages (ICRC Library).

ICRC. XVIIth International Red Cross Conference, Stockholm, August 1948. *Financing of the I.C.R.C.* June 1948. Mimeographed. 4 pages (ICRC Library).

LRCS. XVIIth International Conference of the Red Cross, Stockholm, August 1948. *Co-operation and Relations between the National Societies and with the International Committee of the Red Cross and the League of Red Cross Societies in Peace-time and in War-time.* June 1948. Mimeographed. 7 pages (ICRC Library).

XVIIth International Conference of the Red Cross, Stockholm, August 1948. *Report of the Special Commission to Study Ways and Means of Reinforc-*

BIBLIOGRAPHY

ing the Efficacity of the Work of the International Red Cross Conference [sic – should be International Red Cross Committee]. June 1948. Mimeographed. 10 pages (ICRC Library).

XVIIème Conférence internationale de la Croix-Rouge, Stockholm, 20–30 août 1948. *Rapport complémentaire sur l'activité du Comité international de la Croix-Rouge (1er juillet 1947–30 juin 1948)*. Geneva, July 1948. Mimeographed. 87 pages (ICRC Library).

ICRC. XVIIth International Conference of the Red Cross, Stockholm, August 20–30, 1948. *Draft Revised or New Conventions for the Protection of War Victims, Addenda and Amendments, Report of the International Committee of the Red Cross (Under Item III of the Agenda of the Legal Commission)*. Geneva, August 1948. 16 pages (ICRC Library).

CICR. XVIIème Conférence internationale de la Croix-Rouge, Stockholm, août 1948.
– *Résumé des débats des sous-commissions de la Commission juridique*. No date, non-consecutive page-numbering (ICRC Library).
– *Sténogramme des séances de la Commission juridique*. No date, non-consecutive page-numbering (ICRC Library).

CICR. *Rapport général d'activité du Commissariat pour l'aide aux réfugiés de Palestine (Période du 1er janvier au 31 mai 1949)*. Beirut, 1950. Mimeographed. 23 pages and supplements (ICRC Library).

CICR. *Deuxième Rapport général d'activité du Commissariat pour l'aide aux réfugiés de Palestine (Période du 1er juin au 30 septembre 1949)*. Beirut, 1950. Mimeographed. 165 pages (ICRC Library).

CICR. *Troisième Rapport général d'activité du Commissariat pour l'aide aux réfugiés de Palestine (Période du 1er octobre au 31 décembre 1949)*. Beirut, 1950. Mimeographed. 162 pages (ICRC Library).

CICR. *Quatrième Rapport général d'activité du Commissariat pour l'aide aux réfugiés de Palestine (Période du 1er janvier au 30 avril 1950)*. Beirut, 1950. Mimeographed. 223 pages (ICRC Library).

Commissariat of the International Committee of the Red Cross for Relief to Palestine Refugees. *General Report on the Activities of the Medical Service*. 189 pages (ICRC Library).

CICR. *Collection des circulaires, (1945–1949)* (ICRC Library).

CICR. *Collection des communiqués de presse, (1945–1949)* (ICRC Library).

CICR. *Collection des appels publics, (1945–1949)* (ICRC Library).

II. Published sources

II (a) International Red Cross
(In chronological order)

IVème Conférence internationale des Sociétés de la Croix-Rouge. *Compte rendu*. Carlsruhe, 1887. 145 pages.

IXème Conférence internationale de la Croix-Rouge, Washington. *Compte rendu*. Washington, 1912. 362 pages.

Xème Conférence internationale de la Croix-Rouge, Genève. *Compte rendu*. Geneva, 1921. 266 pages.

Département politique fédéral. *Actes de la Conférence diplomatique convoquée par le Conseil fédéral suisse pour la révision de la Convention de Genève du 6 juillet 1906 pour l'amélioration du sort des blessés et des malades dans les armées en campagne et pour l'élaboration d'une Convention relative au traitement des prisonniers de guerre et réunie à Genève du 1er au 27 juillet 1929*. Geneva, 1930. 771 pages.

XVème Conférence internationale de la Croix-Rouge, Tokyo, 20–29 octobre 1934. *Compte rendu*. Geneva, Tokyo. 309 pages.

ICRC. Sixteenth International Red Cross Conference, London, 20–24 June 1938. *General Report of the International Red Cross Committee on Its Activities from August, 1934, to March, 1938*. Geneva: ICRC, 1938. 138 pages.

ICRC. Sixteenth International Red Cross Conference, London, 20–24 June 1938. *Supplementary Report by the International Committee on Its Activities in Spain*. Geneva: ICRC, 1938. 7 pages.

XVIème Conférence internationale de la Croix-Rouge tenue à Londres du 20 au 24 juin 1938. *Compte rendu*. Geneva, 1938. 140 pages.

CICR. *Projet de convention pour la création de localités et zones sanitaires en temps du guerre adopté par la commission d'experts réunie à Genève les 21 et 22 octobre 1938, Rapport du Comité international de la Croix-Rouge*. Geneva: ICRC, 1938. 33 pages.

CICR. *Rapport du Comité international de la Croix-Rouge sur le Projet de Convention pour la création de zones sanitaires en temps de guerre adopté par la Commission d'experts réunie à Genève les 21 et 22 octobre 1938*. Geneva, 1939. 41 pages.

CICR/LSCR. *Manuel de la Croix-Rouge internationale*. Eighth edition. Geneva, 1942. 561 pages.

ICRC. *Report Concerning Hospital and Safety Localities and Zones*. Geneva, May 1946. 16 pages.

ICRC. *Report on the Efforts Made by the International Committee in behalf of 'Partisans' Taken by the Enemy*. Geneva, Oct. 1946. 19 pages.

ICRC. *Summary Report of the Work of the Preliminary Conference of the National Red Cross Societies, Geneva, July 26–August 3, 1946*. Geneva, 1946. 37 pages.

ICRC. *Inter Arma Caritas. The Work of the International Committee of the Red Cross during the Second World War*. Geneva: ICRC, 1947. 135 pages.

ICRC. *Report on the Work of the Preliminary Conference of National Red*

Cross Societies for the Study of the Conventions and of Various Problems Relative to the Red Cross. Geneva, 1947. 143 pages.

ICRC. *The Work of the ICRC for Civilian Detainees in German Concentration Camps from 1939 to 1945*. Geneva: ICRC, 1975. 125 pages.

ICRC. *Summary Report of the Work of the Conference of Government Experts for the Study of the Conventions for the Protection of War Victims, Geneva, April 14–26, 1947*. Geneva, 1947. 156 pages.

ICRC. *Report on the Work of the Conference of Government Experts for the Study of the Conventions for the Protection of War Victims (April 14–26, 1947)*. Geneva, 1947. 332 pages.

Croix-Rouge yougoslave. Conférence régionale des Croix-Rouges européennes, Belgrade, 1er septembre-1er octobre 1947. *Compte rendu*. Belgrade, no date. 118 pages.

ICRC/LRCS. *Report of the Joint Relief Commission of the International Red Cross, 1941–1946*. Geneva, 1948. 462 pages.

ICRC. *The International Committee of the Red Cross in Palestine*. Geneva, July 1948. 23 pages.

ICRC. XVIIth International Conference of the Red Cross, Stockholm, August 1948. *Draft Revised or New Conventions for the Protection of War Victims, Established by the International Committee of the Red Cross with the Assistance of Government Experts, National Red Cross Societies and Other Humanitarian Associations*. Geneva, May 1948. 245 pages.

ICRC. XVIIth International Red Cross Conference, Stockholm, August 1948. *Report of the International Committee of the Red Cross on Its Activities during the Second World War (September 1, 1939–June 30, 1947)*. 3 volumes. Geneva: ICRC, May 1948.
– Vol. I. *General Activities*. 736 pages.
– Vol. II. *The Central Agency for Prisoners of War*. 320 pages.
– Vol. III. *Relief Activities*. 539 pages.

Seventeenth International Red Cross Conference, Stockholm, August 1948. *Report*. Stockholm, 1948. 113 pages.

ICRC. *Revised and New Draft Conventions for the Protection of War Victims. Texts Approved and Amended by the XVIIth International Red Cross Conference*. Revised translation. Geneva: ICRC, 1948. 171 pages.

ICRC. *Revised and New Draft Conventions for the Protection of War Victims. Remarks and Proposals Submitted by the International Committee of the Red Cross, Document for the Consideration of Governments Invited by the Swiss Federal Council to Attend the Diplomatic Conference at Geneva (April 21, 1949)*. Geneva: ICRC, Feb. 1949. 95 pages.

ICRC. *Report on General Activities (July 1, 1947–December 31, 1948)*. Geneva, 1949. 119 pages.

Federal Political Department. *Final Record of the Diplomatic Conference of Geneva of 1949*. Bern, 1950. 4 volumes.

ICRC. *Report on General Activities (January 1 to December 31, 1949)*. Geneva, 1950. 95 pages.

ICRC/LRCS. *Handbook of the International Red Cross*. Ninth edition (first English edition). Geneva, 1951. 592 pages.

ICRC. *Hospital Localities and Safety Zones*. Geneva: ICRC, 1952.

LRCS. *Report of the Relief Operation in behalf of the Palestine Refugees Conducted by the Middle East Commission of the League of the Red Cross Societies in Conjunction with the United Nations Relief for Palestine Refugees, 1949–1950*. Geneva: LRCS, 1951. 120 pages and appendixes.

ICRC. *Relief Scheme for the Poor of Jerusalem*. Geneva: ICRC, 1950. 14 pages.

ICRC. *Report on General Activities (January 1 to December 31, 1950)*. Geneva: ICRC, 1951. 99 pages.

ICRC. XVIII International Red Cross Conference, Toronto, July-August 1952. *Summary Report on the Work of the International Committee of the Red Cross (1st July 1947–31st December 1951)*. Geneva: ICRC, 1952. 112 pages.

ICRC. XVIIIth International Conference of the Red Cross, Toronto, 1952. *Report of the International Committee of the Red Cross Relative to Relief Distributed or Transmitted by the ICRC from January 1, 1947, to December 31, 1951*. Geneva: ICRC, 1952. 10 pages.

ICRC. XVIIIth International Red Cross Conference, Toronto, July-August 1952. *Proceedings*. Toronto, 1952. 194 pages.

ICRC. XVIIIth International Red Cross Conference (Toronto, July-August 1952). *Resolutions*. Geneva: ICRC. 24 pages.

ICRC. *Statutes of the International Red Cross and Rules of Procedure of the International Conference of the Red Cross* (Adopted by the XVIIIth International Red Cross Conference, Toronto, July-August 1952). Geneva: ICRC, 1952. 24 pages.

ICRC. *Report on the Work of the International Committee of the Red Cross (January 1 to December 31, 1951)*. Geneva: ICRC, 1952. 73 pages.

ICRC/LRCS. *Handbook of the International Red Cross*. Tenth edition. Geneva, 1953. 615 pages.

II (b) Other published sources

– *Documents diplomatiques suisses*, Vol. 12, 1937–1938. Bern, 1994.

– **United Nations Organization:**

UN. *Charter of the United Nations and Statutes of the International Court Of Justice*. New York. June 26, 1945.

BIBLIOGRAPHY

UN. *Plenary meetings of the General Assembly.* Vol I. *Summary Records of meetings. 16 April-14 May 1948.* Lake Success. New York, 1948.

UN. 'Progress Report of United Nations Mediator on Palestine submitted to the Secretary General for transmission to the Members of the United Nations in pursuance of par. 2. of resolution 186 (S-2) of the General Assembly of 14 May 1948'. *General Assembly Official Records.* Third session. Supplement 11 (A/648). Paris, 1948.

UN. Security Council. *Official Record.* Third Year. Lake Success, New York. 1948.

UN. Trusteeship Council. *Official Record,* Second Session, 1947–1948. Lake Success, New York. 1948.

Yearbook of the United Nations, 1947–1948 (New York: United Nations, 1948). 1,126 pages.

– **Anthologies and collections**

Laqueur, Walter, and Barry Rubin, ed. *The Israel-Arab Reader. A Documentary History of the Middle East Conflict.* Revised and updated edition (first edition 1969). Harmondsworth, Victoria, Markham, Auckland: Penguin Books, 1984. 704 pages.

Moore, John Norton, ed. *The Arab-Israeli Conflict.* Vol: III: *Documents.* Sponsored by the American Society of International Law. Princeton, N.J.: Princeton University Press, 1974.

III. Memoirs

Abdullah I, King of Jordan. *Memoirs.* New York: Philosophical Library, 1950. 278 pages.

Begin, Menahem. *The Revolt.* Tenth edition (first edition 1952). Tel Aviv: Steimatzky Ltd., 1983. 386 pages.

Ben Gurion, David. *Israel, Years of Challenge.* New York, Chicago, San Francisco: Holt, Reinhart & Winston, 1963. 240 pages.

Bernadotte, Comte Folke. *La fin, mes négociations humanitaires en Allemagne au printemps 1945 et leurs conséquences politiques.* Lausanne: Marguerat, 1945. 140 pages.

Bernadotte, Comte Folke. *Instead of Arms.* London: Hodder & Stoughton, January 1949. 200 pages.

Bernadotte, Comte Folke. *To Jerusalem.* Trans. Joan Bulman. London: Hodder & Stoughton, 1951. 208 pages.

De Azcarate y Flores, Pablo. *Mission in Palestine 1948–1952.* Washington: Middle East Institute, 1966. 211 pages.

De Reynier, Jacques. *A Jérusalem un drapeau flottait sur la ligne de feu.* Neuchâtel: La Baconnière, 1950. 244 pages.

Dov, Joseph. *The Faithful City. The Siege of Jerusalem 1948*. New York: Simon & Schuster, 1960. 356 pages.

Dunant, Henry. *Un Souvenir de Solférino*. Second edition (first edition 1862). Paris: Cherbullier; Torino: Bocca Frères; St. Petersburg: Jacques Isakoff; Leipsic: F.A. Brockhaus, 1862. 115 pages.

Dunant, Henry. *A Memory of Solferino*. English version by American Red Cross. Geneva: ICRC, 1986. 147 pages.

Glubb, Sir John Bagot (Pasha). *A Soldier with the Arabs*. London: Hodder & Stoughton, 1969. 460 pages.

Katz, Samuel. *Days of Fire*. New York: Doubleday, 1968. 317 pages.

McDonald, James. *My Mission to Israel, 1948–1951*. London: Victor Gollancz Ltd., 1951. 275 pages.

Troyon, Roland, (Major). *Révolte et Discipline*. Lyon: Jean Honoré, 1980. 226 pages.

Yalin Mor, Nathan. *Israël Israël. Histoire du groupe Stern, 1940–1948*. Paris: Presses de la Renaissance, 1978. 373 pages.

IV. Secondary sources

Antonius, Georges. *The Arab Awakening*. New York: Capricorne Books, 1965. 471 pages.

Attali, Jacques. *Un homme d'influence, Sir Siegmund G. Warburg, 1902–1982*. Paris: Fayard, 1985. 571 pages.

Bailey, Sidney, D. *Four Arab-Israeli Wars and the Peace Process*. Third ed. (first ed. 1982). London: Macmillan, 1990. 522 pages.

Ben Achour, Yadh. *Islam and International Humanitarian Law*. Geneva: ICRC, 1980. 11 pages.

Ben Tov, Arieh. *Facing the Holocaust in Budapest. The International Committee of the Red Cross and the Jews in Hungary, 1943–1945*. Geneva: Henry Dunant Institute; Dordrecht, Boston, London: Martinus Nijhoff Publishers, 1988. 492 pages.

Best, Geoffrey. *War and Law since 1945*. Oxford: Oxford University Press, 1995. 434 pages.

Bethell, Nicholas. *The Palestine Triangle, The Struggle between the British, The Jews and the Arabs, 1938–1948*. First ed. 1979. Tel Aviv: Steimatzky Ltd., in association with André Deutsch, London, no date. 384 pages.

Boisard, Marcel. *L'Humanisme de l'Islam*. Paris: Albin Michel, 1979. 436 pages.

Boissier, Pierre. *From Solferino to Tsushima, History of the International Committee of the Red Cross*. Geneva: Henry Dunant Institute, 1985 (original French ed. Paris: Librairie Plon, 1963). 512 pages.

BIBLIOGRAPHY

Bonjour, Edgar. *Histoire de la Neutralité Suisse, 4 siècles de politique extérieure fédérale*. Trans. from German. Neuchâtel: La Baconnière, 1949. 6 volumes.

Bugnion, François. *The Emblem of the Red Cross: A Brief History*. Geneva: ICRC, 1977. 81 pages.

Bugnion, François, *Le Comité international de la Croix-Rouge et la protection des victimes de la guerre*. Geneva: CICR, 1995. 1,438 pages.

Cohen, Michael, J. *Palestine and the Great Powers, 1945–1948*. Princeton: Princeton University Press, 1982. 417 pages.

Coursier, Henri. *The International Red Cross*. Trans. M.C.S. Phipps. Geneva: ICRC, 1961. 131 pages.

De la Pradelle, Paul. *La Conférence diplomatique et les Nouvelles Conventions de Genève du 12 août 1949*. Paris: Les éditions internationales, 1951. 423 pages.

Derogy, Jacques. *La loi du Retour: la secrète et véritable histoire de l'Exodus*. Paris: Fayard, 1970. 439 pages.

Des Gouttes, Paul. *La Convention de Genève pour l'amélioration du sort des blessés et des malades dans les armées en campagne du 27 juillet 1929. Commentaire*. Geneva: ICRC, 1930. 267 pages.

Djurovic, Gradimir. *The Central Tracing Agency of the International Committee of the Red Cross*. Geneva: Henry Dunant Institute, 1986. 259 pages.

Durand, André. *History of the International Committee of the Red Cross. From Sarajevo to Hiroshima*. Geneva: Henry Dunant Institute, 1984. 675 pages.

Duroselle, Jean-Baptiste. *Histoire diplomatique de 1919 à nos jours*. Ninth ed. Paris: Dalloz, 1985. 962 pages.

Favez, Jean-Claude. *Nouvelle Histoire de la Suisse et des Suisses*. Lausanne: Payot, 1982–1983. 3 vols. 996 pages.

Favez, Jean-Claude. *Une Mission impossible? Le CICR, les déportations et les camps de concentration nazis*. Lausanne: Payot, 1988. 429 pages.

Flapan, Simha. *The Birth of Israel, Myth and Realities*. New York: Pantheon Books, 1987. 277 pages.

Fontaine, André. *Histoire de la guerre froide*. Paris: Fayard, 1966–1967. 2 vols. 1,080 pages.

Forsythe, David. *Humanitarian Politics: The International Committee of the Red Cross*. Baltimore and London: Johns Hopkins University Press, 1977. 289 pages.

Freymond, Jacques. *Guerres, Révolutions, Croix-Rouge: réflexions sur le rôle du Comité international de la Croix-Rouge*. Geneva: Graduate Institute of International Studies, 1976. 222 pages.

Friedman, Wolfgang. *De l'efficacité des institutions internationales.* Paris: Armand Colin, 1970. 200 pages.

Gabbay, Rony, E. *A Political Study of the Arab-Jewish Conflict: The Arab Refugee Problem.* Dissertation for Graduate Institute of International Studies. Geneva: Droz, 1959. 611 pages.

Gilbert, Martin. *Jerusalem. Illustrated History Atlas.* First ed. New York, London: Macmillan, 1977; second revised ed. 1978. Tel Aviv, Haifa: Steimatzky, 1987. 128 pages.

Gilbert, Martin. *The Arab-Israeli Conflict. Its History in Maps.* Third ed.; first ed. 1974. London: Weidenfeld & Nicolson, 1979. 118 pages.

Gloor, Ernest. *Le Comité international de la Croix-Rouge et les Prisonniers de guerre soviétiques; Réponse à un étranger.* Renens: L'Avenir, Dec. 1943. 19 pages.

Golay, Jean-François. *Le financement de l'aide humanitaire, l'exemple du Comité international de la Croix-Rouge.* P.U.E. Bern, Frankfurt am Main, New York, Paris: Peter Lang, 1990. 313 pages.

Gresh, Alain, and Dominique Vidal, *Palestine 47, un partage avorté.* Brussels: Complexe, 1987. 256 pages.

Gutman, Israel, ed. *Encyclopedia of the Holocaust.* New York, London: Macmillan Publishing Company, 1990. 4 vols. 1,905 pages.

Haug, Hans. *Les relations de la Suisse avec les Nations Unies.* Bern and Stuttgart: Association suisse de politique étrangère, 1972. 208 pages.

Huber, Max. *Principles and Foundations of the Work of the International Committee of the Red Cross (1939–1946).* Geneva: ICRC, 1947. 40 pages.

Ilan, Amitzur. *Bernadotte in Palestine, 1948: A Study in Contemporary Humanitarian Knight-Errantry.* Oxford, London: Macmillan, in association with St. Antony's College, 1989. 308 pages.

Kimche, Jon and David. *Both Sides of the Hill, Britain and the Palestine War.* London: Secker & Warburg, 1960. 287 pages.

Kimche, Jon and David. *La première guerre d'Israël, 1948.* Paris: Arthaud. 316 pages.

Laqueur, Walter. *The Soviet Union and the Middle East.* London: Routledge & Kegan Paul, 1959. 366 pages.

La Morzellec, Joëlle, *La question de Jérusalem devant l'Organisation des Nations Unies.* Brussels: Bruylant, 1979. 565 pages.

Lorch, Netanel. *The Edge of the Sword: Israel's War of Independence, 1947–1949.* New York and London: Putnam, 1961. 579 pages.

Louis, Roger, and Robert W. Stookey, ed. *The End of the Palestine Mandate.* London: I.B. Tauris, 1986. 192 pages.

Ludwig, Carl. *La politique pratiquée par la Suisse à l'égard des réfugiés au* cours des années 1933 à 1935. Report addressed to the Federal Council for the use of legislative councils. Bern: 1955.

Mattar, Philippe. *The Mufti of Jerusalem, Muhamad Amin Al-Husayni and the Palestinian Question*. New York: Columbia University Press, 1988. 192 pages.

Moreillon, Jacques. *Le Comité international de la Croix-Rouge et la protection des détenus politiques; Les activités du CICR en faveur des personnes incarcérées dans leur propre pays à l'occasion de troubles ou de tensions internes.* Geneva: Institut Henry Dunant; Lausanne: Editions L'Age d'Homme, 1973. 303 pages.

Morris, Benny. *The Birth of the Palestinian Refugees Problem, 1947–1949.* Cambridge, New York, New Rochelle, Melbourne, Sidney: Cambridge University Press, 1987. 380 pages.

Pappe, Ian. *Britain and the Arab-Israeli Conflict, 1948–1951.* London: Macmillan, 1988. 304 pages.

Perruchoud, Richard. *Les Résolutions des Conférences internationales de la Croix-Rouge.* Geneva: Henry Dunant Institute, 1979. 469 pages.

Petitpierre, Max. *Seize ans de neutralité active; Aspects de la politique étrangère de la Suisse (1945–1961).* (Contributions, discours et notes d'entretiens publiés par Edouard Poulet avec la collaboration de Maryse Surdez et Roland Blätter). Neuchâtel: La Baconnière, 1980. 461 pages.

Pictet, Jean. *The Sign of the Red Cross.* Geneva: ICRC, 1949. 35 pages.

Pictet, Jean S., ed. *The Geneva Conventions of 12 August 1949: Commentary.* Geneva: ICRC, 1952, 1958, 1960. 4 vols.

Reverdin, Olivier. *La guerre du Sonderbund vue par le Général Dufour, juin 1847–avril 1848, d'après les lettres et des documents inédits.* First ed. 1948. Geneva: Editions du Journal de Genève, 1987. 134 pages.

Rosenne, Shabtai. *Israel's Armistice Agreements with the Arab States.* Tel Aviv: Blumenstein's Bookstores, 1951. 93 pages.

Roy, Michael. *La reconnaissance d'Israèl par la Suisse (1948–1949).* Typewritten degree dissertation, University of Geneva. 74 pages and annexes (Library of Faculté des Lettres, University of Geneva).

Seguev, Tom. *The First Israelis.* New York: Macmillan, 1986. 379 pages.

Shlaim, Avi. *The Politics of Partition, King Abdullah, the Zionists and Palestine, 1921–1951.* Revised ed. (First ed. 1988, under the title *Collusion across the Jordan*). Oxford: Oxford University Press, 1990. 465 pages.

Veuthey, Michel. *Guerilla et droit international humanitaire.* Geneva: ICRC, 1983. 451 pages.

Werner, Auguste-Raynald. *La Croix-Rouge et les Conventions de Genève, Analyse et synthèses juridiques.* Geneva: Georg, 1943. 447 pages.

Winkler, Stephan. *Die Schweiz und das geteilte Italien bilaterale Beziehungen in einer Umbruchphase. 1943–1945.* Basel, Frankfurt am Main: Helbling und Lichtenhahn, 1992. 647 pages.

Zanabili, Abdelmenim. *Les Etats arabes et les Nations Unies.* Doctoral thesis, Ecole de Sciences sociales et politiques, University of Lausanne. Aurillac, 1953. 216 pages.

Zasloff, Joseph J. *Great Britain and Palestine: A Study of the Problem before the United Nations.* Doctoral thesis, Institut de Hautes études internationales. Geneva: Droz, 1952. 187 pages.

Zorgbibe, Charles. *La guerre civile.* Paris: PUF, 1975. 208 pages.

V. Articles

Revue internationale de la Croix-Rouge, 1945–1952.

Best, Geoffrey. 'Making the Geneva Conventions of 1949: The View from Whitehall.' *Etudes et essais sur le droit international humanitaire et sur les principes de la Croix-Rouge en l'honneur de Jean Pictet.* Ed. Christophe Swinarski. Geneva: ICRC; The Hague: Martinus Nijhoff Publishers. pp. 5–15.

Bourgeois, Daniel. 'La porte se ferme. La Suisse et le problème de l'immigration juive en 1938.' *Relations internationales* 54 (Summer 1988): pp. 181–204.

Cunningham, Sir Alan. 'Palestine. The Last Days of the Mandate,' *International Affairs* (October 1948): pp. 481–490.

Durand, André. 'Origine et évolution des Statuts de la Croix-Rouge internationale.' *RICR* 742 (July-August 1983): pp. 179–213.

Graf, Christoph, and Maurer, Paul. 'Die Schweiz und der Kalte Krieg.' *Studien und Quellen* 11, Bern: Schweizerisches Bundesarchiv, 1985: pp. 5–82.

Hanna, Paul. 'The Middle East in the Post War World.' *Current History* (Jan. 1946). p. 49.

Huber, Max. 'The Principles of the Red Cross.' *Foreign Affairs. An American Quarterly Review* 26, No. 4 (July 1948): pp. 723–727.

el-Kauwkji, Fauwzi. 'Memoirs 1948.' *Journal of Palestine Studies* I, No. 4 (Summer 1972): pp. 27–58; and Vol. II, No. 1 (Autumn 1972): pp. 3–33.

Meron, Theodor. 'The Demilitarization of Mount Scopus: A Regime that Was.' *The Israel Law Review* III, No. 4 (1968).

Moreillon, Jacques. 'Le Comité international de la Croix-Rouge et la révision des Statuts de la Croix-Rouge internationale.' In Yvo Hangartner and Stefan Trechsel, *Völkerrecht im Dienste des Menschen, Festricht für Hans Haug.* Bern, Stuttgart: Verlag Paul Haupt, 1986: pp. 179–194.

Nasser, Gamal Abdul. 'Memoirs of the First Palestine War.' *Journal of Palestine Studies* II, No. 2 (Winter 1973): pp. 3–32.

Rosenne, Shabtaï. 'The Red Cross, Red Crescent, Red Lion, Red Sun and the Red Shield of David.' Pre-print, *Israel Yearbook of Human Rights* 5 (1975). 46 pages.

Sandoz, Yves. 'Le droit d'initiative du Comité international de la Croix-Rouge.' In Yvo Hangartner and Stefan Trechsel, *Völkerrecht im Dienste des Menschen, Festricht für Hans Haug*. Bern, Stuttgart: Verlag Paul Haupt, 1986: pp. 352–373.

Siordet, Frederic. 'Les Conventions de Genève et la guerre civile.' *RICR* 374 (Feb. 1950): pp. 104–122; and *RICR* 375 (March 1950): pp. 187–212.

Newspapers read at the ICRC in the years 1948–1949
(In alphabetical order)

Al Ahram
Basler Nachrichten
Das Bund
El Ba'ath Daily
La Bourse égyptienne
Courrier de Genève
Daily Mail
Egyptian Mail
Le Figaro
Gazette de Lausanne
l'Humanité
Journal de Genève
Journal suisse d'Egypte et du Proche-Orient
Manchester Guardian
Le Monde
Neue Zürcher Zeitung
New York Herald Tribune
New York Times
Palestine Post
Le Progrès Egyptien
La Suisse
The Times
Tribune de Genève
Tribune de Lausanne
Trud
Volksrecht
Voix Ouvrière

INDEX

Albania, 270
Abassieh camp, 218, 221–1, 229, 231
Abdullah (King, Hashemite dynasty) 102, 166, 185, 206, 211, 216, 289
Abdullah Tel, 181, 210, 217
Abyssinia, 20
Adler Rudel, S., 164, 178
Afula, 106, 193
Agreement between the Director of the UNRPR and the President of the ICRC (16.12.1948), 262–3
Agreement between the League and the ICRC (30.08.48), 260–1
Agreement between the League and the ICRC (8.12.1951), 277
Alliance of Red Cross and Red Crescent Societies of USSR, 16, 22, 24, 25, 27, 28, 140, 239, 246, 248, 249, 250, 280
American Colony, 145
American, 22, 177, 236, 245, 265; *see also* USA, American Red Cross, American Colony
American Joint Distribution Committee, 18, 78, 137, 162
American Red Cross, 21, 25, 27, 29, 244, 250, 255
Amman, 104, 182, 211, 232, 244, 254
Amman (ICRC delegation) 228, 230, 254, 269, 270

Anderegg, Emil, 157, 159, 247, 252
anti-Semitism (anti-Jewish, anti-Zionism), 48, 87, 120–2, 132, 168, 175–9, 182, 198, 221–2, 289; *see also* Aryan, Zionism
Anschluss, 40
Appeal of March 12, 1948, 117, 120, 122, 124, 239
Appeal of May 19, 1948 and Press communiqué of May 21, 1948, 173, 233
Appeal of May 24, 1948, 125, 126
Arab armies, 103, 125, 152, 195, 204, 215
Arab local authorities, 94, 106, 108, 123, 129, 151, 169, 170, 193, 198, 201, 205, 220
Arab countries, 89, 125, 127, 183, 218, 219, 232, 233, 240, 254, 258, 259, 260, 268, 270, 275
Arab non-refugees in Jerusalem (Poor of Jerusalem), 264, 266, 287
Arab governmental college, 159, 169, 184
Arab Higher Committee, 89, 103, 104, 105, 120, 121, 125, 128, 131, 166, 170, 181, 195, 201, 231, 258
Arab irregulars, 107, 183, 195, 199, 202, 203, 205, 207
Arab League, 110, 113, 123, 126, 166, 173, 183, 232, 254; *see also* Azzam Pasha
Arab Legion, 149, 173, 174, 176,

INDEX

181, 182, 184, 203, 206, 209, 210, 211, 212, 213, 215, 216, 217, 223; *see also* Glubb Pasha

Arab Liberation Army, 106, 107; *see also* el Kaukji

Arab Medical Association of Palestine, 104, 105, 142–3, 145, 153

Arab prisoners (POW and civilians), 97, 183, 193, 219, 220–1, 222, 226, 228, 231, 253; *see also* Atlit, Jalil, Sarafand, Tel Litvinsky, Um el Khaled

Arab refugees, 114, 176–7, 192, 226, 227, 234, 254–68, 287

Arab es Subeih, 192, 193

Arab world, 95, 98, 102, 104, 108, 127, 289

armistice agreements, 217, 218, 219

Aryan ('non-Aryans, aryanism'), 40–1, 121, 132

Asmara camp 119 (Eritrea), 50, 54, 55–6, 57–66, 68, 70, 96, 120

Assire Zion Committee, 61, 62

Assirenu, 69

Atlit, 220

atomic bomb, 157, 239; *see also* weapons of mass destruction

Augusta Victoria hospice, 149, 266; *see also* Mount Scopus

Australia, Australian, 275

Australian Red Cross, 137, 250

Austrian Jews, 40; *see also* Swiss border

Automobile Club, 248

Azcarate, Pablo, 115, 167, 206

Balkans, 21–2, 83–5, 289; *see also* European Red Cross Conference

Baltic countries, 27, 83

Bandak, Isa, 205

Beduin, 183

Beersheva, 141

Beirut, 254, 262; *see also* Sables Prison

Beirut (ICRC central delegation), 228, 229, 230

Belgian Red Cross, 25, 28, 52

Belgium, Belgians, 18, 30, 206

Belgrade, 27, 38, 83, 89; *see also* European Red Cross Conference

Ben Zvi, Itzhak, 101

Bergen-Belsen, 64

Bergson, Peter, 51, 52, 53, 66, 68; *see also* Hebrew Committee of National Liberation

Bernadotte, Count Folke, 3, 24–5, 27–9, 30, 60, 151, 179, 180–6, 208, 218, 227, 236–7, 246, 251, 255, 256–7, 258, 260; *see also* Swedish Red Cross, Standing Commission of the International Conference of the Red Cross, UN Mediator

Bethany, 145, 266

Bethlehem, 106, 194, 198, 205, 214, 217

Bethlehem French hospital, 204, 214, 215

Bethlehem mental hospital, 141, 142–3, 147, 154

Bethlehem prison, 62, 63, 66, 214–15

Bevin, Ernest, 56, 58, 66, 75, 244

Bey, Abdul Mahad, 107

Bichara, Dr, 153; *see also* Russian Compound

Biéri, Frédéric, 61, 71, 79–80, 87

Bishop, General, 87; *see also* Vlotho ICRC delegation

Bnei Brak, 141; *see also* Jewish hospitals

Bodmer, Martin, 37–8

'Bohemia Moravia', 133, 202

Bombay, 97

Brazilian Red Cross, 25

Britain, 1, 30, 39, 60, 66, 71, 72, 73, 75, 76, 77, 78, 80, 81, 86, 92–8, 100–1, 108, 111, 143, 154, 164, 225, 255

British authorities, 1, 22, 27, 29, 31, 50–2, 54–5, 58, 61–2, 68, 79, 94, 102, 107, 163, 199, 245

British administrative buildings,

INDEX

155–63, 172–5, 245; *see also* Safety zones

British army, 56, 59, 66, 103, 197, 233

British Mandate, 64, 69, 70, 73, 92, 103, 134, 143, 154, 155, 181, 197, 266; *see also* Mandatory Palestine

British Occupation zone, 81, 87; *see also* Vlotho ICRC delegation, N. Burckhardt, Poppendorf

British Red Cross, 25, 29, 39, 60

Bulgaria, 270

Bunche, Ralph, 186

Burckhardt, Carl, 18, 25, 37–8, 52, 54, 253

Burckhardt, Nicolas, 70, 87–8

Burma, 274

Burnier, Georges, 110

Cadogan, Alexander, 255

Cahen-Salvador, Georges, 241

Cairo, 66, 98, 107, 180, 232

Cairo (ICRC delegation), 55, 56, 59, 65, 90; *see also* Munier, de Cocatrix

Calpini, Pierre, 254; *see also* Arab refugees

calvinist, 47

Canaan, Tamous, Dr, 104; *see also* Arab Medical Association

cease fire, 199–202, 203, 209, 211; *see also* Gush Etzion, Jewish Quarter in the Old City of Jerusalem, Katamon, Kfar Saba, Nebi Daniel

Chamberlain's White Paper (1939), 51, 65, 75, 86; *see also* immigrants, *Exodus 47*, Cyprus

Chenevière, Jacques, 113, 269

Christian(s), 99, 100, 121, 122, 132, 146, 227, 274

China, 55

Chinese Red Cross, 25

Cilento, Raphael, 255

civil war, 9–10, 34, 35, 63, 66, 67, 68, 70, 188, 231, 239, 252, 271, 72, 80, 92, 94, 95, 96, 112, 124, 125, 188, 231, 239, 252, 271, 282, 284; *see also* Spanish civil war, non international conflict

civilian internees, 17–18, 23, 33, 36, 52, 53–4, 56, 58, 59, 60, 62, 63, 66, 70, 78, 124, 233, 282; *see also* Tokyo draft

civilians (individuals or populations), 21–4, 34, 66, 80, 83, 103, 109, 114, 119, 123, 156–9, 161, 187, 190, 192, 209, 210–11, 234, 238, 240, 246, 265, 266, 271, 272, 282, 285, 287; *see also* non-combatants

Clapp report, 268; *see also* Arab refugees

de Cocatrix, Albert, 123, 221; *see also* Cairo ICRC delegation, Abbassieh

Cold War, 2, 3, 14, 27, 28, 95, 137, 187, 270, 281, 288

Colonial Office, 57, 58, 61, 63, 64, 65, 68, 78, 80, 81, 88, 92, 93, 97, 111; *see also* Britain; British authorities

Commissariat of the ICRC for Refugees in the Near East, 263–4, 266–7, 268; *see also* Arab Refugees, Escher

common articles of the 1949 Geneva Conventions, 240, 271; *see also* non international conflict

Commonwealth, 39, 245

Communists, communist attacks against the ICRC, 14–16, 20–1, 24, 28, 37–8, 44, 59, 83, 85, 107, 112, 179, 238, 247, 249, 250; *see also* Poland, USSR, Yugoslavia

competent international body, 241

concentration camps, 18, 19, 25, 34, 61, 63, 64, 84, 221, 235; *see also* Hitler's crimes

Conference of Evian, 40

Conference of Government Experts for the Study of Conventions for the Protection of War Victims (1947), 35, 67, 72, 158, 239, 241

INDEX

Conference of San Francisco, 54
consular corps, 169
Conventions: 1929 'Geneva',
10–11, 45, 103, 106, 109, 112,
114, 116, 117, 121, 123, 125, 126,
127, 147, 150, 159, 190, 193, 195,
208, 220, 224, 238, 260, 282, 290;
development of the, 3, 33–7,
45–6, 54, 55–6, 58, 67, 83, 95,
110, 112, 113, 117, 118–20, 122,
124, 127, 138, 143, 193, 282–3,
284–5; *see also* Stockholm,
(drafts for), four Geneva
Conventions (1949) drafts
Courvoisier, Jean, 132, 188–91,
199–202, 206, 215–6, 227, 290
Cousin, Florence, 206, 208
Cunningham, Alan, 57, 66, 72, 90,
98, 106, 108, 115
Cyprus, 65, 71, 74, 85, 108, 230
Czechoslovakian Red Cross, 25,
28, 30

Damascus, 106, 107, 122, 166, 170,
222
Danzig, 37, 38; *see also* Burckhardt,
Carl
Dayan, Moshe, 217; *see also*
repatriation
Deïr Yassin massacre, 126, 128–30,
191, 220, 233, 258
Dejani, Mahmoud Taher, 104; *see
also* Bethlehem hospital
demilitarized 149, 165, 185, 190,
228, 289; *see also* Jerusalem,
neutralized
Depage, Pierre, 28–30, 81, 256; *see
also* subordination of the ICRC
deportations, deported,
deportees, 18, 50, 51, 52, 54, 57,
60, 64, 68, 69, 70, 258, 271
development of the international
humanitarian law, *see*
conventions (development of),
Stockholm (drafts for), Draft
revised . . .)
dogmatism, *see* ICRC doctrine,
Principles
Diplomatic Conference (1949),
36–7, 175, 237, 247, 250, 251,
253, 258, 264, 271, 272, 274, 287,
288
displaced persons, 27, 51, 86
Doret, Michel, 85–6, 88
Draft revised or New
Conventions for the Protection
of War Victims . . . adopted by
the XVII IRC Stockholm
Conference, 250
Drault, Paul, 6
Dubois, Georges, 79, 81, 83–5
Ducommun, Pierre, 79, 81, 83–5
Dunant, Henry, 7, 11, 32, 47, 80,
187, 194, 196, 209
Durand, André, 205–6, 208, 290

Effendi, Ibrahim Fahum, 191
Egypt, Egyptians, 98, 107, 125,
140, 150
Egyptian Red Crescent, 25
Ein Tzurim, 203–4
Emperor of Japan, 30, 265; *see also*
Japanese donation
Empire Rival, 75, 81, 82, 86
English mission hospital in
Jerusalem, 143
English-speaking countries, 275
Entr'aide française, 76, 82
Eritrea, *see* Asmara
Escher, Alfred, 263, 268; *see also*
Commissariat . . .
European Red Cross Conference,
Belgrade (1947), 27, 38, 83, 89
evacuations (transfers), 192–3,
204, 211, 213, 214, 216, 217, 219,
234, 244
exchanges, 212, 217–8, 223, 233
Exodus 47, 74–86, 93, 95, 121, 290
Eytan, Walter, 154, 178

Famagusta 74; *see also*
immigrants, Chamberlain
White Paper, Cyprus
Farran, Roy, 70
Fasel, Pierre, 133, 185, 202–4, 214
Fletcher Cooke, 165
Foreign Office, 56, 57, 58, 60, 78,
88

INDEX

France, French, 18, 31, 34, 52, 55, 71, 76, 77, 78, 79, 81, 86, 157, 241, 273
François Poncet, André, 278; see also Standing Commission, Statutes of the IRC (1952)
French Red Cross, 30

Gaillard, Pierre, 79, 132, 206, 269
Galilee, 188–94, 267
Gallopin, Roger, 25, 29, 44, 60, 73, 76, 78, 80–1, 269
Gaulan (Spiegel), Nahum, 215
Gaza, 75, 109, 141, 263; see also Egypt, repatriations
Geneva Convention (wounded and sick) (1864), 8, 10, 12, 13, 16, 33, 34, 46, 47, 238
Geneva Convention (wounded and sick) (1906), 10
Geneva Convention (wounded and sick) (1929), 10, 11, 35, 125, 134–8, 143, 148, 149, 153, 154, 174, 175, 187, 192, 193, 194, 197, 198, 199, 200, 204, 208, 213, 231, 285
'Geneva convention' (Prisoners of War) (1929), see Prisoners of War convention
Geneva Conventions, four (drafts) (1949), 3, 33, 36, 44, 47, 103, 117, 144–5, 156, 233, 237, 238, 239, 240, 247, 282, 286
Geneva Conventions (1949), 240, 270–6, 271, 273, 286, 288
'Germanisierung', 27
German assets, 30, 32
German Jews, 40
German prisoners, 20, 21, 52, 56, 76, 79, 94, 98
German Red Cross, 162
Germany, Germans, 16, 18, 21, 22, 27, 31, 37, 40, 51, 52, 66, 79, 81, 84, 86, 88, 99, 100, 111, 121, 132, 157, 177, 239
Gestapo, 40
Ghori, Emile, 104
Gil Gil camp, 68, 69, 73, 74, 78, 96, 120

Gloor, Ernest, 29, 38, 67, 83
Gouy, Robert, 132, 206, 216, 228–9, 230, 290
Government hospitals, 92–3, 151–4; see also hospitals, Bethehem hospital, Russian Compound
Government House, 156, 159, 161, 169, 183, 184, 185, 228, 251
Greater Berlin, 23
Greece, Greeks, 16, 67, 72, 92, 96, 243, 284
Gregson, Amiral, 77
Griffis, Stanton, 262
Gromyko, Andrei, 71, 167
Gruner, Dov, 72
Guerney, Sir Henry, 91, 101, 115, 116
Gush Etzion, 194–6, 202, 203–5, 207, 214, 215, 216, 233, 285

Hadassah hospital, 147–8
Haganah (Jewish and Israeli army), 79, 107, 128, 166, 172, 173, 181, 182, 183, 192, 199, 200, 206, 211, 212
Haïfa, 75, 106, 107, 109, 132, 141, 254, 258
de Haller, Edouard, 38, 263
health services, 134–5, 141, 203, 214
Hebrew Committee of National Liberation, 50, 51, 52, 53, 55, 56, 59, 60, 66, 67, 68, 69, 70, 71, 72, 73, 76, 78, 89; see also Bergson, Merlin
Hebrew University of Jerusalem, 147–8; see also Hadassah hospital, Mount Scopus, demilitarized
Hebron, 204, 254, 263
Helbling, Charles, 60, 66, 71–2, 74, 90
Himmler, Heinrich, 25
Hiroshima, 34, 157; see also atomic bomb, weapons of mass destruction
Hitler, Adolf, 19–20, 40, 95, 98
Hitler's (Nazi or 'Fascists')

INDEX

crimes, 2, 15, 19, 20, 60, 249, 258, 280
Hittim, 192
Holy See, 270, 275
hospital(s), 82, 84, 92, 93, 101, 134, 141–5, 152–5, 158, 165, 175, 234, 238, 245, 263, 254
hospitals and safety zones or localities, 34, 158–9, 168, 174, 209, 263, 274;
hostages, 206, 271
Huber, Max, 6, 37, 39, 125, 226, 245
Huber, Max-Henri, 76, 78
Hungary, 22
Husseini, Musa, 199, 214, 217
el Husseini, Abdul Kader, 106–7, 147
el Husseini, Hadj Amin, Grand Mufti, 98–100, 106, 123–4, 170, 190
el Husseini, Jamal, 163

ICRC, composition and tasks, 7–9, 13, 14, 19–20, 37
ICRC, doctrine and dogmatism, 36–7, 44, 48–9, 79, 86, 94, 97, 116, 131, 191, 193–4, 198, 208, 218, 226, 249, 291; *see also* Principles . . .
ICRC, finances, 23–4, 30, 32, 38, 44, 59, 73, 81, 93, 94, 97, 98, 100, 101, 104, 106, 111, 113, 114, 162, 243, 245, 252, 265, 287; *see also* Arab non refugees, German assets, Japanese donation
ICRC, propaganda, 15–19, 45, 54, 68, 69, 89, 92, 97, 114–15, 170, 200, 231–5, 244, 245, 284
ICRC, right of initiative, 12, 36, 242
immigrants, immigration, 71, 74–86, 102, 108
India, 275; *see also* New Dehli
Indian Red Cross, 250
Indochina, 67, 92, 243, 284
infiltrators, 269–70
International Center for Relief to Civilian Populations, 24

international conflict, 10, 95, 124, 125, 173, 233, 282
International Red Cross, 2–3, 6, 8, 13–14, 22, 27, 28, 29, 30, 38, 80, 92, 127, 137–9, 140, 150, 180, 187, 208, 235, 236–7, 239, 242, 244, 245, 255, 256, 259, 265, 281–2, 287
International Red Cross, reform of structure, *see* internationalization of the ICRC, subordination of the ICRC
internationalization of the ICRC, 24, 25, 26, 28, 30, 38, 60, 67, 92, 93, 237, 244, 280–1
Iran, 113, 181, 243
Iraq, Iraqi, 120, 125, 126, 128, 216, 228, 263
Iraqi Red Crescent, 122
Israel, Israeli, 1, 125, 127, 150, 152, 173, 176, 177, 178–9, 183, 184, 198, 214, 215, 218, 219, 220–3, 228, 229, 230, 231, 232, 258, 260, 267, 269, 273, 275, 288
Israeli Defence Forces, 215, 217
Italian school and hospital, 159, 176; *see also* safety zones
Italian Jews, 40–1
Italy, Italians, 16, 20, 38, 40, 41; *See* Swiss border
IZL, 51, 59, 71, 72, 74, 76, 128–30

Jabotinsky, Vladimir, 51
Jaffa, 106, 107, 109, 132, 141
Jalil, 220
Japan, Japanese, 20
Japanese donation, 30, 52, 244, 245, 265
Jenin, 124, 263
Jericho, 206
Jerusalem, 103, 104, 106, 107, 109, 111, 115, 121, 133, 141, 147, 151, 152, 154, 156, 159, 163–8, 170, 176–7, 178, 183, 184, 185, 190, 195, 207, 208, 209, 210, 211, 228, 229, 233, 234, 240, 248, 285, 287, 289; *see also* demilitarized
Jerusalem Old City, 103, 107, 133,

338

INDEX

152, 155, 156, 181, 182, 184, 206, 216, 219, 266
Jerusalem prison, 72
Jerusalem, west, 12, 133, 152, 166, 172, 178, 181, 182, 195, 199, 227
Jewish Agency, 73, 75, 78, 79, 80, 81, 85, 95, 101, 103, 104, 111, 117, 120, 123, 131, 134, 147, 149, 164, 166, 167, 170, 172, 174, 195, 199, 201, 202, 213, 229, 231
Jewish agricultural school for girls, 159, 169, 183; *see also* Government House
Jewish authorities, 94, 103, 106, 108, 123, 128, 151, 169, 193, 198, 201
Jewish extremists, 1, 66, 69, 72; *see also* IZL, Stern
Jewish hospitals, 149, 151, 206; *see also* hospitals, Hadassah hospital, Misgav Ladach, Russian Compound, Eytan
Jewish organizations, 53, 60–1
Jewish prisoners, 64, 66, 71, 97, 183, 184, 215, 221–4; *see also* Abassieh, Asmara, Bethlehem, Gil Gil, Latrun, Cyprus, Mafraq, Mazzé, Sables, Um el Djemal
Jewish Quarter in the Old City of Jerusalem, 103, 106, 107, 114, 172, 174, 176, 209–12, 224, 226, 228, 231, 233, 234, 244, 253
Jewish refugees at the Swiss border, *see* Ruegger, Aryan, Swiss border
Jewish refugees, 83–9, 93, 258, 270; *see also* Exodus 47, Swiss border
Jisr Mejama, 216
Joint Relief Commission of the International Red Cross, 21, 22–4, 226, 257, 265
Jordan, 269

Kadry, Ahmed, 258
Kahany, Menahem, 73–4, 80–1, 104, 122, 124, 146, 164, 178, 230, 269–70
Kaltenbrunner, Emil, 18, 25, 37, 52

Kaplan, Eliezer, 104
Karlsruhe (National Red Cross Societies Conference, 1887), 13
Katamon, 166, 167, 199–202, 207, 285
Katznelson, Abraham, 101, 154, 210, 214–5, 217, 232
el Kaukji, Fauwzi, 107, 124, 132, 166, 190, 191
Kenya, 70, 78, 85; *see also* Gil Gil
Kfar Saba, 192, 206, 207, 285
Kfar Yehuda, 206
Kfar Yona, 216
Khalidi, Hussein, 104, 121
Khan Yunis, 107
King David, 133, 141, 155, 156, 159, 161, 169, 170, 172–3, 180, 181, 182
Kohn, Leo, 101–3, 118, 147–51, 172–6, 299
Komintern, 56
Kook, Hillel, 51; *see* Bergson, Peter
Kristallnacht, 40, 239
Krikorian, Krikor, 100, 203
Kuhne, Paul, 44, 60, 73–4

Labis, Mahmoud, 107
Latrun camp, 74
League's Board of Governors: *see* Oxford, Stockholm
League of the Arab States, 89
League of Nations, 37
League of Red Cross Societies, 7, 13, 14, 21, 24, 29, 81, 140, 232, 233, 236, 250, 252, 256, 257, 258, 260, 261, 265, 266, 280, 287
Lebanon, 102, 104, 125, 126, 128, 228, 263
Lehner, Otto, 133, 202–4, 210, 213–14, 215, 221, 290
Lester, H.M.O., 100–1
Lie, Trygve, 262
Loker, Zvi, 275
London, 29, 38, 39, 93, 156
London (ICRC delegation), 57, 60, 61, 65, 78, 87
Lydda, 100, 206

Mafraq camp, 204, 215, 217, 223

Magen David Adom society (Israeli national society), 103, 127, 128, 143, 150, 151, 191, 260, 269
Maghar, 192
Mandatory Palestine, 1, 2, 39, 50, 51, 52, 54, 66, 71, 73, 74, 75, 78, 84, 85, 89, 94, 95, 96, 104, 105, 110, 152, 159, 169, 199, 211, 214, 228, 243, 253, 259, 260, 263, 283
Marseilles, 76, 90
Marshall plan, 83
Marti, Roland, 79, 81–5, 88–9, 95–6, 101–6, 111–14, 120–22, 166, 168–9, 178, 289–90
martial law, 66
material aid, 23, 69, 105, 114, 146–7, 211, 224, 225, 226, 227, 228, 244, 265, 266; *see also* reciprocity
Mazzé prison, 222–3
medical aid or services, 80–90, 101, 134, 224; *see also* material aid
Mendès France, Pierre, 71, 90
Metaxas, General, 67
de Meuron, Maximilian, 132
Merlin, Samuel, 71
Michel, William, 71, 76, 90–1
Misgav Ladach hospital, 174–5, 212
missing persons, 219, 229, 269, 270
Mitterand, François, 75
mixed medical commissions, 212, 213, 214, 218
Mizrahi, Eliahu, 200
Molotov, 16
moral authority, 116, 126, 131, 144, 187, 209
Moslem(s), 10, 39, 99, 107, 121, 140, 145–6, 148, 240, 286
Mossad leAliya Bet, 75, 77, 81
Mount of Olives, 103, 118, 266
Mount Scopus, 147–9; *see also* Augusta Victoria Hospice, Haddassah hospital, Hebrew University of Jerusalem, demilitarized
Mount Tabor, 192

Mountbatten, Lady, 39, 91, 141
Mountbatten, Lord, 39, 91, 141
Monod, Dr, 88
Mufti, *see* el-Husseini, Hadj Amin
Munier, Jean, 59, 61, 64–5, 90–1, 96, 98, 111–13, 120–2, 170, 217, 222–3, 228, 269, 290
Mussolini, Benito, 42

Najar, Emil, 273–5
Nazi(s), 38, 41, 59, 61, 64; *see also* Germany, Hitler's crimes
Nablus, 106, 132, 141, 188, 192, 216, 225, 244, 254, 267
Natanya, 216, 234
Nazareth, 106, 191, 192, 193, 267
Nebi Daniel, 194–8, 233, 285
neutralized zones, 251, 272; *see also* demilitarized, Jerusalem
New Dehli, 39, 91
Nobel Peace Prize, 2
non-combatants, 35–6, 285
non-international conflicts, 112, 117, 270; *see also* civil war

Ocean Vigour, 70, 75, 81, 82, 86, 87, 88
occupied territories, 36, 52, 54, 63, 239, 241, 271
O'Connor, Basil, 21, 29, 236, 257
Order of Malta, 248
Oxford, 21, 22, 24, 140, 263, 265, 266

Pacha, Azzam, 98–100, 122, 126, 166
Pacha, Glubb, 102
Pacha, Nukrachi, 98
Pakistan Red Cross, 275
Palestine Defence Emergency Regulations, 57–8
Palestinians Arabs, 69, 93, 98, 100, 101, 104, 105, 108, 128, 134, 146, 211, 216, 219, 227, 234, 254, 289
Palestinians Jews, 53–4, 58, 63, 69, 70, 71, 73, 74, 98, 100, 101, 102, 104, 108, 134, 146
Palestinian State, 166
Paris, 37, 71

INDEX

Paris (ICRC delegation), 71, 75, 89
partisans and resistance members, 2, 15, 16, 72
Parodi, Alexandre, 163
Pax Romana, 248
peace, 37
Petah Tikva, 206
Petitpierre, Max, 38–9, 157, 252–3, 270, 273, 275
Pflimlin, Raoul, 133, 178, 184
Pictet, Jean, 25, 244, 252
Poland, 20, 21, 113
Polish Red Cross, 27
Poppendorf, 88
Porchet, René, 76–7
Preliminary Conference of national Red Cross Societies for the Study of the Conventions and of Various Problems Relative to the Red Cross, Geneva (1946), 59, 139
Principles of the Red Cross and/or the Geneva Convention, 12, 14, 20, 26, 32, 46, 58; 59, 109–10, 112, 113, 117–20, 128; 187, 195, 198, 201, 205, 213, 226, 230–1, 239, 241, 245, 262, 271, 280, 284, 286, 288–9; *see also* ICRC doctrine and dogmatism
Prisoners of War Convention (1929), 10–12, 16–17, 19, 20, 112, 125, 218, 219, 220, 222, 224, 240, 242; *see also* Geneva conventions
protecting powers, 11, 19, 36, 162, 241, 242, 272; *see also* substitute of . . .

Quakers, 263
Qualkilya, 206, 233, 267

racial, 19
Rama, 192
Ramle, 206
reciprocity, 35, 112–13, 117, 123, 174, 190–1, 218; *see also* evacuations, material aid, medical aid

red crescent sign, 10, 100, 139, 140, 144–6, 149, 240, 273, 286
Red Crescent (societies), 151, 196; *see also* Red Cross or Red Crescent societies
red cross (sign, emblem and flag), 10, 13, 95, 110, 135–7, 139–40, 144–86, 196, 197, 199, 202, 207, 208, 209, 229, 240, 246, 286, 288
Red Cross (or Crescent) Societies, 7–8, 13, 22, 31, 32, 94, 136–7, 162, 179, 227, 252, 261, 265, 266
red lion and sun sign, 10, 139, 146, 240, 273
red neutral sign, 273
red star of David sign, 10, 103, 110, 140, 144, 146–7, 149, 152, 273–6, 286, 288
Red Star of David society, *see* Magen David Adom
removal of the wounded and dead, 199–202
repatriation, 153, 216, 219, 222, 223, 234
Resolution 181 (partition plan), 1, 39, 91, 92, 95, 101, 102, 108, 109, 134, 141, 152, 169
Revadim, 204
de Reynier, Jacques, 4, 95–6, 105, 111–12, 115–16, 120–2, 128–31, 133, 143, 146–51, 153, 155–6, 158–62, 164–6, 168–78, 183–5, 187–8, 201–2, 205–7, 209–10, 213–14, 221–2, 226–7, 229, 230, 232, 255, 274, 285, 289–90
Rhodes, 230
Romania, 22
Rome, 38
Roth, René, 76–8
de Rougé, Bonabès, 29
Ruegger, Paul, 4, 38–42, 91, 104, 141, 164, 180–4, 208–13, 222, 229–30, 233, 244–5, 247, 249–50, 252, 257, 265, 268–70, 273–5, 277, 286, 289
Runnymede Park, 75, 77, 81, 82, 88
Russian Compound hospital, 141, 143, 152–4

INDEX

Sables prison, Beirut, 104, 110
Safed, 106, 141, 192
safety zones, 110, 119, 155–63, 160–86, 191, 192, 195, 208, 209, 229, 231–2, 233, 238, 239, 244, 245, 246, 247, 248, 251, 272, 285
Sainte-Marie hospital, Hamburg, 88
Salameh, Hassan, 106–7, 206
Sandström, Emil, 278
Sarafand, 220
Sawfat, Ismaïl, 107
Scandinavians, 25
Scottish Mission in Nazareth, 191, 192
Scottish Mission in Tiberias, 191
Scout organization, 248
Sérot, André, 185
Sharett, Moshe, *see* Shertok
Shelley, William, 221
Shertok, Moshe, 126, 163, 173, 182, 229–30, 251, 267
Siordet, Frédéric, 83
Slavic people, 15, 20
Smith, Trafford, 63–4, 81
Soviet(s), 240, 252; *see also* USSR
Soviet Prisoners of War, 2, 15, 16, 112
Spanish Civil War, 35, 79, 84, 95, 217; *see also* civil war
Spain, Spanish, 35, 248, 249, 270
Special Commission to Study Way and Means of Reinforcing the Efficacity of the Work of the ICRC, 25, 26, 28–9, 30, 44, 78, 112, 119; *see also* internationalization of the ICRC, subordination of the ICRC
de St Aubin, Wilfred, 255; *see also* Arab Refugees, American Red Cross
St John of Acre prison, 72
Star of David, 146–7, 232; *see also* red star
Stalin, Joseph, 236
Standing Commission of the International Conference of the Red Cross, 26, 28, 29, 30, 38, 93, 179, 236, 248, 250, 252, 256, 257, 261; *see also* subordination of the ICRC
stateless, 18, 36, 41
Statutes of the ICRC, 7, 12, 14
Statutes of the IRC (1928), 6, 7, 9, 11–13, 14, 29, 30, 39, 44, 50, 70, 89, 92, 105, 115, 134, 176, 225, 243, 244, 248, 252, 253, 254, 256, 257, 260, 281, 281–4, 287
Statutes of the IRC (1952), 276
Steinberg, Arieh, 228
Stern group, 51, 71, 74, 107, 108
Stettinius, Edward, 54
Stockholm, 181, 184, 185, 250, 251, 256
Stockholm, draft conventions for, 33–6, 62, 112, 119, 137–8, 139, 140, 155, 158, 161, 166, 168, 169, 170, 172, 174–5, 176, 182, 212, 237–43, 247
Stockholm, XVII International Red Cross Conference, 26, 30, 31, 32, 36, 46, 112, 114, 117, 119, 140, 162, 166, 180, 181, 183, 184, 188, 207, 223–4, 231, 234, 236–7, 242, 243, 245, 247, 248–53, 257, 258, 261, 263, 266, 270
Straehler, Margarita, 163
subordination of the ICRC, 67, 80, 81, 237, 256, 259
substitute of protecting powers, *see* competent international body, ICRC finances
Sudan, Sudanese, 57, 64, 70, 86
Sweden, 34, 280
Swedish Red Cross, 20, 24, 25, 27, 30, 179, 185, 250, 256; *see also* Bernadotte
Swiss border, 38–42, 270
Switzerland, Swiss, 7, 10, 20, 24, 28, 30, 31, 32, 33, 37, 38, 39, 40, 45, 73, 78, 80, 81, 97, 100, 114, 127, 128, 136, 155, 157, 159, 161, 167, 202, 207, 241, 242, 243, 244, 247, 250, 251, 253, 263, 265, 270, 275, 280, 287
Syria, 102, 106, 107, 120, 125, 190, 222–3, 228, 236, 237, 258, 263

INDEX

Syrian Red Crescent, 121, 122, 258
Taibeh, 106
Tel Aviv, 103, 106, 109, 132, 141, 150, 151, 165, 166, 182, 230, 244, 269
Tel Aviv (ICRC delegation), 220, 228, 230, 232, 267, 270
Tel Litvinsky, 220
Templars, 111
Terra Sancta Franciscan school, 159, 169
Third World War, 23, 37, 44, 89, 244
Tiberias, 106, 109, 191, 192
Tobruk, 70
Tokyo Draft, 17–18, 33, 34, 36, 52, 53, 54, 56, 58, 62, 63, 66
Toronto XVIII International Red Cross Conference (1952), 253, 258, 265, 267
Transjordan (Transjordanians), 102, 106, 120, 183, 190, 211, 215, 219, 221, 223, 228, 263
Transjordanian Red Crescent, 203, 260
de Traz, David, 268–9
truce (first), 151, 152, 166, 227
truce (second), 183, 205, 253
Truman, Harry, 244
Tulkarm, 216, 234, 267
Turkey, 113

Um el Djemal, 223
Um el Khaled, 220
UN Mediator, *see* Bernadotte, Bunche
UN observers, 183, 184, 185
UN truce commission, 182, 206
UNESCO, 267
UNICEF, 264
UNO, 1, 34, 39, 54, 55, 71, 91, 92, 102, 111, 134, 143, 155, 156, 162, 163, 164–5, 167, 179, 180, 181, 185, 186, 209, 214, 218, 228, 244, 248, 251, 255, 256, 257, 261, 262, 263, 268, 283
UNRPR, 262, 263, 264

UNSCOP, 75, 102, 115, 116, 141, 142, 167
UNRWAPR, 268
USA (ICRC delegation), 57
USA, 22, 30, 31, 52, 55, 108, 127, 163, 239, 262, 265, 283
USSR (Soviet Union), 2, 14–16, 22, 23, 30, 39, 40, 55, 97, 108, 127, 163, 209, 236–7, 238, 239, 249, 250, 258, 259, 267, 270, 275, 280, 283, 285

Va'ad Le'umi, 69, 74, 141
Viet Minh, 67
violations, 19, 131, 191, 246, 249
visit of prisoners of war camp, 15–16, 219, 224, 229, 233
Vlotho, 87
Volksdeutsche, 20

war crimes, 241
Warburg, Anita, 44, 229
Warburg, Max, 44, 104
Weingarten family, 216
Weizmann, Chaïm, 44
Werth, Dr, 200, 201
weapons of mass destruction, 238
Western countries, 238
Wildi, Erwin, 85–8
Wolf, Max, 44, 104, 164, 178, 229–31, 265, 269
World Lutheran Organization, 268
World War I, 34, 156, 217
World War II, 2, 10, 15, 17, 18, 19, 20, 21, 24, 30, 33, 37, 42, 45, 52–3, 54, 56, 58, 61, 63, 68, 79, 98, 99, 112, 125, 128, 136–7, 156, 157, 190, 226, 234, 237, 238, 239, 240, 241, 248, 249, 270, 271, 280, 282

Yemin Moshe, 107, 172–3
YMCA, 133, 155, 159, 169, 172, 173, 177, 181, 182, 216
Yugoslav Red Cross, 20–1, 24, 27
Yugoslavia, Yugoslavs, 15, 16, 21, 60, 113

INDEX

el Zaim, Husni, 199, 214, 217
Zelnicher, Elimelech, 199
Zionism, Zionists (anti-Zionism, sionists), 44, 50, 90, 111, 126, 152, 220, 221, 258